T0092226

The Cooperative Neuron

The Cooperative Neuron

Cellular Foundations of Mental Life

William A. Phillips

Foreword by Matthew E. Larkum

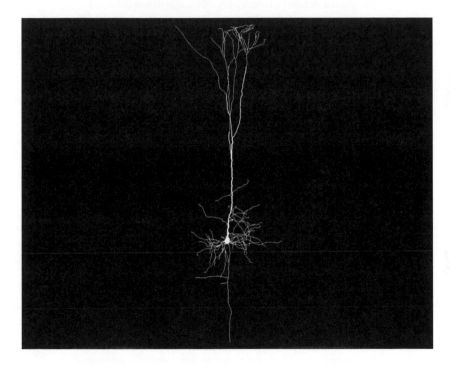

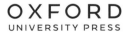

OXFORD
UNIVERSITY PRESS

OXFORD
UNIVERSITY PRESS

Great Clarendon Street, Oxford, OX2 6DP,
United Kingdom

Oxford University Press is a department of the University of Oxford.
It furthers the University's objective of excellence in research, scholarship,
and education by publishing worldwide. Oxford is a registered trade mark of
Oxford University Press in the UK and in certain other countries

Published in the United States of America by Oxford University Press
198 Madison Avenue, New York, NY 10016, United States of America

British Library Cataloguing in Publication Data

Data available

Library of Congress Control Number: 2022949982

ISBN 978–0–19–887698–4

DOI: 10.1093/oso/9780198876984.001.0001

Printed in the UK by
Bell & Bain Ltd., Glasgow

*To my wife, Rena
our children, Fred, Lowana, and Ned
our grandchildren, Charlie, Thomas, Andrey, and Daniel
and to all grandchildren, everywhere.*

Foreword

The history of science is replete with unexpected turning points that needed someone to put their finger on the right way to construe the emerging data. More often than not, it involves some insight, change in perspective or even a paradigm shift, that allows the known facts to be reorganized in a way that makes them appear to fall suddenly into place. It is usually difficult to identify turning points as they happen even though they frequently appear obvious with the benefit of hindsight. This is often because of the sheer amount, and often sheer disorganization, of the data. The Copernican Revolution required the marriage of hard-fought observations with a change in perspective. Similarly, Darwin's theory of Natural Selection made sense of a mountain disparate evidence with a fundamentally different starting assumption. In both these cases, and in numerous others throughout history, the critical insight itself is at first treated as improbable but eventually as obvious. I believe that *The Cooperative Neuron* has all the hallmarks of a perspective shift that will transform and endure in the best traditions of transformative science.

With this book, Bill Phillips attempts nothing less than to explain the relationship between the mind and brain, starting from bottom-up principles. Make no mistake, 'Here be dragons!'. There are many who would claim this is a foolhardy mission, both today and for the foreseeable future. Indeed, it is common to come across the opinion, including amongst neuroscientists, that, 'if the brain were so simple that we could understand it, we would be so simple that we couldn't'. So why should you expect this book to solve one of the last great mysteries of our time? And especially why should you invest the time and energy to embark on the trip Bill Phillips lays out from first neuroscience principles to psychophysics and information theory? Well, one reason is that it's fun all the way! Having spent time with Bill myself, I can attest to the fact that his enthusiasm is expressed in every bone and sinew. In this book, it pours out of the text. But the main reason is the multi-faceted intellect he throws at this problem. This is truly a book that only Bill Phillips could have written.

Also in the best traditions, the key insight of this book requires the reader to take on a perspective shift that runs against the current dominant dogma. It requires the reader to stop assuming that neurons of the brain are simple counting devices, but instead to take their complexities seriously. For a reader with no neuroscience experience, this might seem trivial. Why shouldn't neurons be complex? To be honest, I often find myself feeling a little bit like the little boy in the Emperor's New Clothes story. I mean, they do look complex, after all. And having recorded from thousands of real neurons, I can attest that their properties turn out to be more complex than their appearance already suggests. Nevertheless, the dominant description of a neuron in most models of the brain and artificial neural networks is not much more than a blob that counts how many signals arrive, and if and when enough do arrive, sends the signal on to the next unsuspecting blobs. In case you're tempted to say, 'that's absurd!', just remember that using only this description (embedded in a deep neural network) your phone can recognize your face, the best chess players of all time can be totally embarrassed, and everyday texts can be translated and even generated de novo in the style of different famous authors such as Shakespeare and Edgar Allen Poe. So, 'put that in your pipe and smoke it!', says the current and apparently unstoppable juggernaut of neuroscience and artificial intelligence research.

But have no fear! Professor Bill Phillips of Stirling University has done the heavy lifting for you in the form of this book. This book is really the distillation of the *important* complexities of the *important* neurons of the brain cast in the *important* abstraction of what their *important* function is. As you might guess from the title of the book, this involves the notion of the cooperative neuron. Having myself spent years interacting with Bill mulling over the morass of details one could focus on in describing real neurons and their function, I can say that this analogy works like all good insights in that it irresistibly instils in you that 'Aha!' feeling. However, as the author himself warns early on, you should not let yourself be satisfied with the first 'Aha!'. Rather, I would advise you to enjoy the various ways in which the cooperative neuron perspective solves one neuroscience problem after another as you progress through the book. Unless you're Bill Phillips or some other rare polymath, this is going to involve going to places you haven't yet thought about.

This book, therefore, introduces a kind of fiction in the best possible sense—the notion of the Cooperative Neuron. As Yuval Noah Harari points out in 21 Lessons for the twenty-first century, 'For better or worse, fiction is among the most effective tools in humanity's tool kit. By bringing people together, religious creeds make large-scale human cooperation possible. They inspire people to build hospitals, schools, and bridges in addition to armies and prisons. Adam and Eve never existed, but Chartres Cathedral is still beautiful'. He might have added that fiction is a great tool in the scientist's tool kit too. A simultaneously dangerous but powerful tool, so use the *The Cooperative Neuron* wisely!

Matthew Larkum
Berlin 2022

Preface

This book describes and contributes to a revolution that is occurring in brain and mind sciences. Twentieth-century psychology and systems neuroscience assumed that, in general, neurons sum all their synaptic inputs and signal the extent to which that exceeds a threshold. In contrast to that assumption, recent discoveries show that many neurons in the mammalian brain have two functionally distinct sets of inputs: one that provides the inputs about which the neuron usually transmits information, and one that amplifies that transmission when it is useful to do so in the context of information being transmitted by other neurons. This form of context-sensitive information processing is cooperative in that it seeks agreement between the active neurons, thus reducing mental conflict. This cooperative context-sensitivity provides cellular foundations for basic cognitive capabilities, so they have fundamental implications that are transforming our understanding of relations between mind and brain.

These discoveries use the Nobel-prize winning techniques of patch-clamping to explore processes of communication within individual neurons. They find that a special class of the pyramidal neurons that are widely distributed throughout the mammalian neocortex can do more than psychologists and systems neuroscientists have long assumed to be possible for any neuron. That is, they can use one subset of their inputs as a context within which to amplify transmission of information about their other inputs when that increases the coherence and usefulness of the system's overall activity.

The discovery of pyramidal neurons with context-sensitivity has fundamental implications for neuroscience. It casts new light on the systems level of organization, on intracellular communication, on the functions of ion channels in the cell's dendrites, and on the genes that either code for them or regulate their expression. Even more importantly, it has profound implications for psychology, neurology, psychiatry, and philosophy. This book shows that cellular context-sensitivity provides foundations for perceptual disambiguation, selective attention, working memory and imagery, emotional prioritization, cognitive control, and learning.

The book sketches evidence of evolutionary, developmental, and pathological variations in cellular context-sensitivity, and emphasizes the strong support this provides for the neuroconstructivist view of cognitive development. As these context-sensitive cellular mechanisms can malfunction in various ways, the book discusses these effect as they related to several pathologies, including epilepsy, psychosis, autism, and other neurodevelopmental disorders and helps explain what those disorders have in common and why there is such diversity both within and between them. As expected of findings with such widespread significance, these discoveries cast new light on enduring philosophical issues. They also provide cellular foundations for the theory of predictive processing within epistemology, for the selectivity of conscious experience, and for morality as cooperation.

This is the first book to argue for the fundamental importance of this new field of research. It is written for philosophers, psychologists, psychiatrists, and psychopathologists interested in the neural bases of mind, as well as for neuroscientists, neurologists, and anaesthetists interested in the philosophical and psychological significance of their work. It aims to make the neuroscience intelligible to psychologists, the psychology intelligible to neuroscientists and clinicians, and both fields intelligible to philosophers interested in relations between mind and brain. Finally, there are good grounds for supposing that it could also be of use to computer scientists who are developing machine learning algorithms inspired by neuroscience.

We are in the early days of this revolution in our understanding of the cellular foundations of mental life, however, so the discoveries on which this book is based will be unfamiliar to most people, including many neuroscientists, psychologists, and clinicians. Many of them are still committed to the assumption that neurons in general operate as simple integrate-and-fire point processors, and Chapters 3, 4, and 5 provide evidence for this newly emerging concept. Consequently, those chapters discuss complex esoteric issues, so each has a final summary of its contribution to the story overall. The first and last chapters summarize the essence of the perspective advocated.

The intellectual journey leading to this book was long and depended on essential contributions from a wide range of disciplines. It began in 1959 when I was an undergraduate student in the physics department of Manchester University where Ernest Rutherford had first split the atom in 1917. After just one year I switched to the study of psychology to pursue the answer to the central question that enthralled me as a young teenager (as it still does): how can minds be brains? I had, and still have, no doubt that the brains from which minds arise are composed of the matter whose properties have been revealed by physics and chemistry.

In switching from physics to psychology I took two key aspects of the physics mindset with me. First, I assume that what science seeks is a single coherent understanding of all we know. No part of that understanding can be a ghetto or island of knowledge entirely unto itself. Second, successes in that scientific search are likely to reveal realities that not only transcend what we knew already, but also, in some crucial ways, directly contradict what we thought we knew. Despite its many wonders, twentieth-century psychology is deeply unsatisfactory from that point of view. Few, if any, of its basic concepts are rooted in the cellular physiology and biophysics of the neurons that perform the information-processing operations inferred from psychological investigation. The conceptual framework outlined in this book aims to root basic psychological processes in their cellular foundations. It shows in partial, but considerable, detail how richly and deeply basic psychological processes are rooted in cellular processes, and especially in those of context-sensitive pyramidal cells.

A great deal of good fortune has been essential to making my intellectual journey possible. In addition to having had a long and healthy life with unwavering family support in a peaceful house and garden in the Scottish hills, I have had the great good fortune to meet and interact closely with many eminent world authorities in each of the disciplines on which our understanding of the cellular foundations of mental life depends. That good fortune began in 1966 when, as a PhD research student, I was part of a small seminar in the Australian National University in which eminent philosopher and member of the Vienna Circle Herbert Fiegl crossed swords with neurophysiologist and Nobel Prize-winner John Eccles. Their disagreement concerned free will, on which Eccles' views were largely formed by his Catholic faith. It seemed clear to me that, although Eccles knew far more about the brain, Fiegl was correct in insisting that the questions concerning free will were not only unresolved, but also not even adequately posed.

Now that we are developing a better understanding of the cellular foundations of mental life, we are more able to pose this issue in a form that can be explicitly related to brain function. I first became convinced that those foundations include cooperative context-sensitivity when I saw how that intuition can be made mathematically precise using the concept of three-way mutual information. That was about 30 years ago. Statistician Jim Kay, with his expert knowledge of information theory and neural networks, immediately saw the force of that intuition. Since then, he and I have worked closely together to improve and publicise it. Many eminent experts have now contributed to that goal by commenting on this book and suggesting corrections or improvements. In addition to Matthew Larkum, whose work is of central importance to this book, they include neuroscientists Javier DeFelipe, Albert Gidon, Peter König, Bjorn Merker, Danko Nikolić, David Nutt, Jan Schulz, Matthew Self, Gordon M. Shepherd, Gordon M. G. Shepherd, Stewart Shipp, Johan Storm, and Mototaka Suzuki; psychologists Jaan Aru, Victor Almeida, Talis Bachmann, Alan Baddeley, Peter Cahusac, Trevor Harley, David Heeger, Graham Hitch, Lotta Upanne, and Ivo Vlaev; cognitive neuroscientists Karl Friston, Lars Muckli, Lucy Petro, Viola Priesemann, Mac Shine, and Michael Wibral; neurologists and psychopathologists Kevin Bender, Chris Frith, Uta Frith, Alberto Granato, Avram Holmes, and Steve Silverstein; philosophers Andy Clark, Tomas Marvan, and Michal Polak; and computational neuroscientists Bruce Graham, Adam Linson, Tuomo Mäki-Marttunen, Verónica Mäki-Marttunen, Heiko Neumann, Leslie Smith, and Mike Spratling. Much support and encouragement has also been given by psychologists at the University of Stirling during my five decades there, and especially by Christine Caldwell, Ben Craven, Ben Dering, Martin Doherty, Peter Hancock, and Jan Kuipers.

An acid test of any conception of how brains work is whether it can be used to design algorithms that do useful things when applied to big real-world data. Ahsan Adeel has made a major contribution by showing that our conception of cooperative context-sensitive computation passes that acid test. From a long friendship with eminent logician and teacher of mindfulness Henk Barendregt, I have acquired a view of mental life that has shaped my attitude to many of the issues with which the book is concerned. Martin Baum and Jade Dixon at Oxford University Press, together with the copyeditor Michele Marietta, provided much needed encouragement and helped transform the raw draft into its final form.

Finally, this book, and the decades of work leading to it, would not have been possible without the unflagging support and patience of my wife, Rena. In addition to running daily life throughout our more than 60 years together, she has patiently listened to my perpetual musings about brain and mind. Her keen social insights have kept me, and the book, in touch with everyday reality.

Bill Phillips
University of Stirling
August 2022

Contents

Introduction to *The Cooperative Neuron*

A new era is dawning in the sciences of mind and brain. This book provides an overview of a conceptual revolution that is occurring in our understanding of the cellular foundations of mental life and its disorders. It relates conscious perception, thought, and action to recently discovered capabilities of pyramidal cells, a special class of neocortical neuron that has long been known to be widely distributed through the cerebral neocortex. The book describes in detail how many, though not all, of those cells are sensitive to context. Though this cellular context-sensitivity involves complex events that are unfamiliar to many neuroscientists and to most psychologists, the conceptual revolution to which these discoveries lead is, in essence, simple. It is now known that many pyramidal neurons in the neocortex have two functionally distinct sets of input: one provides the input about which the neuron usually transmits information, and the other can selectively amplify that transmission when it is useful to do so in the context of information being transmitted by other neurons. This form of context-sensitive information processing is cooperative in that it seeks agreement between the active neurons, thus reducing mental conflict. It provides cellular mechanisms that simplify the production of coherent percepts, thoughts, and actions that are usefully related to current goals and long-term needs. Selective amplification of the information that is currently relevant becomes both more difficult and more crucial as the information carrying capacity of a system's sensors, memory, needs, and effectors increases.

Discovery of this selective amplification is a fundamental advance in the field of neuroscience because it shows that some neurons can do more than was assumed possible for neurons in general. Twentieth-century systems neuroscience and psychology were largely based on the assumption that neurons operate as integrate-and-fire point processors. In other words, it was widely assumed that neurons in general sum all their many excitatory and inhibitory synaptic inputs to compute a net amount of excitation about which their outputs then transmit information. That summing of all synaptic inputs in a way that is the same across all dendrites has been memorably described as constituting a 'dendritic democracy'. That description has been shown to have

The Cooperative Neuron. William A. Phillips, Oxford University Press. © Oxford University Press 2023.
DOI: 10.1093/oso/9780198876984.003.0001

empirical validity in the case of neurons in hippocampal regions, which are a small (but much studied) part of the forebrain.

Pyramidal neurons in the neocortex are far more numerous and far more discerning than hippocampal neurons, however. Many of them can use one subset of their inputs to decide when the information that they transmit is currently relevant in the context of the system's overall activity. Neural systems containing that special class of neuron can operate with greater flexibility. When vital aspects of organism's environment change its chances of survival and success depend on the flexibility with which it can act in new ways when presented those new circumstances. Unfortunately, though often used in psychology and neuroscience, the notion of flexibility is rarely adequately defined. This book interprets it as implying activity that is adapted to the context within which it occurs. Cellular context-sensitivity increases the effectiveness and efficiency with which new actions can be generated in new situations, reduces the transmission of large amounts of information when it is currently irrelevant, facilitates discovery of the information that is relevant at higher levels of abstraction, and makes learning easier by helping to separate the information to be learned from a mass of background activity that would otherwise be a noisy nuisance. Thus, it increases the coherence, adaptability, and usefulness of the organism's overall activity.

The evidence for a special class of neurons that have two functionally distinct sites of integration, one of which can provide a context for responding to inputs to the other site, provides a new perspective from which to reinterpret many basic phenomena in psychology and cognitive neuroscience, and from which to discover new phenomena.

This broadly conceived field of research is growing rapidly, but is already substantial, as shown in later chapters. It can be called 'cellular psychology' where that phrase is used by analogy to the phrase 'molecular biology', the field of biological research that discovered how the aperiodic crystals DNA and RNA convey a vast amount of information from parent to child. That discovery showed that DNA and RNA molecules can do far more than was previously thought possible for molecules in general. Similarly, discovery of a large class of neocortical neurons that have exceptional capabilities for cooperating shows that those neurons can do far more than was previously thought possible for neurons in general. They are exceptionally good at cooperating, and that capability may be the root of the special magic of the mammalian neocortex, explaining why it has expanded and diversified so greatly during mammalian evolution, and how it set the scene for the evolution of the human intellect and the subsequent revolutions in human history.

This introduction summarizes the main topics discussed and inferences drawn in each of the book's ten chapters. It alerts the reader to some of the underlying assumptions on which those inferences are based. The evidence reviewed and arguments presented in this book are accompanied by a deep undercurrent of moral concern. It is sometimes claimed, or implied, that science shows nature to be pointless and life to be selfish. In contrast to that, I see progressive aspects of the history of nature as giving it direction and I see living things as marvels of cooperation. So, readers should not be surprised if they detect a bias toward that more positive view in the story that I tell.

Chapter 1 briefly outlines the discovery of neurons that are especially good at cooperating. It explains how these neurons are sensitive to the current context and can use that sensitivity to modify the strength of their output in ways that increase the coherence and usefulness of the system's overall activity. It also outlines further assumptions guiding the perspective presented in this book. Chapter 2 provides a brief description of the gross anatomy and functions of the mammalian thalamocortical system, which is the main stage upon which our mental lives are played.

Chapter 3 first outlines the standard conception of pyramidal cells as leaky integrate-and-fire point neurons. It then provides a more detailed overview of physiological experiments showing that many pyramidal cells in layer 5 of the neocortex have two distinct sites of integration. The front cover shows a single example of the hundreds of millions of such cells in the neocortex. The chapter provides detailed information about the anatomy of these types of cells, and outlines direct observations showing that excitatory activation of these apical dendrites can greatly amplify the cell's response to weak activation of its other dendrites. It explains how the anatomical distinction between the basal and apical dendrites is complemented by a mass of other anatomical and physiological data indicating that in the cooperative context-sensitive class of pyramidal neurons the basal dendrites convey the input about which the cell transmits information, whereas the apical dendrites specify the context within which that input is amplified when relevant. The chapter then summarizes the inhibitory and disinhibitory regulation of that apical amplification and emphasizes the diversity of pyramidal cell anatomy and function.

Chapter 4 first shows that there are quiet, active, and stressed states of wakefulness, and slow-wave or rapid eye movement states of sleep. An underlying assumption is that the overall level of arousal varies from being minimal during slow-wave sleep and increases upon waking, perhaps with critical transitions, to quiet, active, and highly stressed levels of maximal arousal. It is also assumed that, at any level of arousal, there are other fundamental ways in which mental states can vary. When asleep we can either be dreaming or not; when awake we can be engrossed in our own thoughts or in sensory or emotional experiences. These very different states of mind are distinguished by far more than the overall level of arousal. Transitions between mental states are regulated by modulatory neurotransmitters that can isolate the activation of apical dendrites from the soma during deep sleep. When awake they operate as a context that guides perception of the body and the external world, or as a way of sustaining perceptual experience in short-term memory, or as a way of generating them from long-term memory. Conscious experience consists mainly of perceptual experiences, memories, and thoughts, which led us to suspect that general anaesthetics might operate by blocking apical function. Chapter 4 validates that supposition. Nevertheless, it also argues that this new perspective on mental life raises doubts on current notions of 'consciousness' as something over and above the cognitive capabilities that operate when we are awake, but not when we are deeply asleep.

Chapter 5 is the book's main contribution to the conceptual perspective it advocates. It examines the psychological implications of the discovery of context-sensitive neurons with two points of integration. Though I have not been able to study all of the relevant evidence, the reader can be assured that the many papers that I have read and adequately understood are more than enough to justify the central claims. This chapter focuses primarily on cognitive functions including perceptual disambiguation, selective attention, working memory and imagery, emotional prioritization, and cognitive control. Learning is discussed last because, although of great importance, it is strongly dependent on the processes outlined earlier, which are all concerned with the moment-by-moment experiences in mental life. Thus, an understanding of their cellular foundations provides a new perspective on the nature and functions of conscious experience. Moment-by-moment decisions are therefore of great importance; that is why we are aware of them and why cooperative neurons have evolved to take as much of the currently relevant context into account as they can.

No great leaps of faith are required to relate the investigations discussed here to conscious experience. I have participated in all the psychophysical paradigms that I have used to study mental life, including those demonstrating subliminal perception. As I have direct phenomenological access to my own experiences in those paradigms, I can relate their findings to my own direct experience, which usually, though not always, seemed to be in harmony with what could be inferred about the conscious experience of others from their performance in those paradigms.

The first part of Chapter 6 sketches similarities and differences across species in the anatomy and physiology of neocortical cooperative context-sensitive neurons. The evidence reviewed indicates that they are common in six-layered mammalian neocortex, but not in the three-layered reptilian allocortex from which it evolved. It also indicates that this evolution includes increased differentiation in the inhibitory interneurons that prevent their overactivation, and that some aspects of cooperative neuronal function are distinctively human. It then briefly outlines similarities and differences across species in the cognitive capabilities that depend on cooperative context-sensitivity and explains that they are broadly as expected from the similarities and differences in the anatomy and physiology of cooperative context-sensitive neurons. Thus, those comparisons reveal cases where cognitive capabilities and neuronal mechanisms for them are known to be present in both species.

Such demonstrations in no way imply that there are no other mechanisms with those or similar capabilities. Walker (1983) reviews much evidence indicating that birds, but not fish or reptiles, have cognitive capabilities that are to a large extent comparable to those of mammals. Birds and mammals can both flexibly adapt their actions to novel circumstances. Both can learn the association between arbitrary stimuli or actions and activation of internal neural signals for rewards or punishments. Furthermore, dreaming has been observed in mammals and birds, but not in any other class of animal. This suggests that birds, like mammals, can generate perceptual experiences and/or motor commands from within, but cellular mechanisms for that in birds are unknown. They cannot be the same as those in mammals because the neocortex is specifically mammalian. There are clear signs of some form of intellect in the octopus, but exactly what their information processing capabilities are and how they are implemented remain unknown.

The second part of Chapter 6 sketches developmental changes in the anatomy and physiology of cooperative context-sensitive neocortical neurons and then relates them to psychological studies of cognitive development. It shows that this comparison resonates strongly with the neuroconstructivist perspective on cognitive development that has context dependence as a core principle, and neuroconstructivists were among the first to see the importance of physiological evidence for context-sensitive cells in the neocortex.

Chapter 7 shows that malfunctions of cellular context-sensitivity or its regulation have been convincingly, though incompletely, implicated in a surprisingly diverse range of mental health disorders, and it examines closely the way in which they have been implicated. It indicates that our notions of this mechanism—and of its information-processing functions—need to be upgraded. It discusses how, in some special cases, we can identify specific genes in the aetiology of the disorder, together with an explanation of how proteins for which they code are involved in the impaired aspects of mental life. Cognitive neuropsychology has focused on using the effects of localized brain damage to identify the role of different parts of the cerebral cortex in different domains of cognitive function. Chapter 7 explores how cellular psychopathology focuses more on malfunctions of cellular function that have widespread consequences across many different domains.

Chapter 7 also discusses five broad classes of pathology. Epileptic disorders that involve malfunctions of cellular context-sensitivity confirm its crucial role in conscious experience. Schizophrenic disorders confirm and cast further light on the role of cellular context-sensitivity in generating subjective aspects of conscious experience and in distinguishing them from objective aspects. It looks at the autoimmune disorder known as anti-NMDA encephalitis and its role in generating and distinguishing subjective experiences, and provides further evidence that NMDA receptors for glutamate have a key role in the mechanisms involved. Autistic disorders are highly diverse but most of them involve impairments of cognitive capabilities that implicate context-sensitive cells. Furthermore, as these malfunctions are acute from early in infancy, the chapter looks at their role in socialization and cognitive development in general. In special types of autistic disorder, such as fragile X, the predisposing genes, the proteins for which they code, the role of those proteins in ion channels, the role of those channels in cellular functions, and the role of those functions in the person's information processing capabilities can all be sketched with sufficient confidence to assure us that, although many details remain to be discovered, a firm understanding of the disorder is now within reach. Finally, it looks at foetal alcohol spectrum disorders (FASDs), which are far more common than widely realized and involve reduced growth of context-sensitive dendrites during prenatal development. These highly preventable cognitive consequences overlap with those of autistic disorders but are instead caused by exposure to alcohol during embryological development, rather than by any specific genetic predisposition. This shows that cognitive disabilities with lifelong consequences may have no heritable genetic bases. As prenatal exposure to alcohol is so harmful, it should be clearly and strongly discouraged, as it is in Canada for example.

Chapter 8 provides explicit mathematical definitions and quantification of cooperative context-sensitive information processing. Though many readers may not find explicit mathematical formalization illuminating, the history of science confirms it is needed. A minimal requirement of any explanation

of how the mind and brain work must be the ability to perform the information processing work that it purports to explain. The theory must specify
that work explicitly and show that the algorithms hypothesized to perform
it can (in principle) be implemented by systems composed of neurons. This
chapter outlines a long-standing theory that meets those requirements and
that is grounded in multivariate mutual information theory. It then shows
that when activities at both the cellular level and at the level of human observers in psychophysical experiments are quantified in that way, they do indeed operate as context-sensitive two-point processors. The chapter ends by
citing machine-learning algorithms inspired by advances in the neurobiology
of context-sensitive cooperative computing. As they are shown to be both effective and efficient we must be hypercautious in releasing them from their
biological constraints by implementing them in silicon.

Chapter 9 begins by noting some basic difficulties in the field of cellular
psychology, and then discusses the evidence for cooperative neurons as it
relates to predictive coding and the principle of free energy reduction—one
of the most influential of all current perspectives on relations between mind
and brain. The main aim of this chapter, however, is to emphasize some of the
main issues to be resolved by future research in cellular psychology. It makes
clear that many fascinating and well-formulated issues await exploration.

The final chapter speculates on possible implications of the findings reviewed in earlier chapters on three unresolvable but unavoidable issues implicit throughout our daily lives. The first concerns knowledge and doubt: how
can we determine the validity of the way things seem to us? The second concerns self-identity: what is it, and must it be defended? The third concerns
life's purposes: can they ever be anything other than those that we create for
ourselves?

The many empirical observations outlined in this book are interpreted
from a conceptual perspective that is sometimes presented via a precise mathematical statement, for example, in Körding and König (2000) and in Heeger
and Zemlianova (2020). The probabilistic theory of Coherent Infomax I developed with Jim Kay is outlined in Chapter 8, although the science of cellular
psychology is far too young to seek allegiance to any such theory. Premature
systematization and overgeneralization can do far more harm than good.
Information-processing algorithms based on cooperative context-sensitive
computation have not yet been shown to have capabilities comparable to that
of humans. Precisely quantified predictions based on those theories have not
yet been confirmed in a wide range of different tests. These theories have not
yet produced effective cures or management strategies for the pathologies to
which they are here related. These theories are therefore principally advocated

as a way of guiding explorers to territory in which there may be abundant riches. It is assumed that what is discovered there will often require those theories to be upgraded.

Although concerned with states of mind, this book does not discuss the cellular foundations of the act of mindfulness; this is a major omission. The practice of mindfulness, which increases peace of mind and reduces mental suffering, has been passed on, sometimes with improvement, for about two thousand years, so we can be confident that it contains much wisdom. I know of no publication in which its cellular foundations are adequately discussed. For interested readers who seek to understand more about both the nature and the logic of mindfulness, I recommend the papers by Barendregt and Raffone (2013, 2022). My hope, and expectation, is that cellular foundations for that logic will soon be identified.

The focus throughout is on cooperation which is shown to combine effectively with competition in Subsection 5.2.6. Though the focus is on cooperation between neurons, it assumes that cooperation is essential to life at all levels of organisation, including that of social interactions between people. Recent reviews providing strong support for that assumption are cited in Section 5.7.

Finally, although written mainly for those working within or studying the sciences of mind and brain, this book also aims to make its key messages comprehensible to readers in general. For those seeking an introduction to these sciences I recommend David Nutt's 2021 *Brain and Mind Made Simple*—Nutt is a leading authority on neuropsychopharmacology and its implications for social policies on drugs. For an outline of channels in the cell's membrane through which, when open, charged electrical ions can pass and of the resultant changes in electric potential across the cell's membrane, I recommend Ramaswamy and Markram (2015). Though one of many, their open access review is especially relevant here because it focuses on the specific class of neocortical neurons that epitomize those with cooperative context-sensitivity.

1

Life, Brain, and Mind

Marvels of Cooperation between Diverse Individuals

Many forms of organized complexity have arisen during nature's long journey from the uniformity of the Big Bang to the total disorganization that physicists predict to be its final fate. On earth, despite the ever-present forces of noise and disorder, evolutionary selection has created an endless diversity of living things that are complex but organized. Unicellular organisms are marvels of organized cooperation between the individual molecules of which they are composed. Multicellular organisms are marvels of organized cooperation between individual cells. At all levels of organization, from the genetic to the social, life depends upon cooperative interactions between diverse individuals. As their diversity increases, so does the need to coordinate their activities effectively and efficiently.

Cooperatively organized complexity is epitomized by mammalian brains and minds. The importance of cooperative organization in mental life is apparent in the human search for peace of mind. For more than two thousand years techniques for reducing mental conflict have been developed and passed from mind to mind by many meditative traditions. Psychologists have long studied the various strategies that have evolved for reducing dissonance and increasing harmony in mental life. Cellular neurophysiology is now providing evidence that this search for coherence is so important, and so difficult, that within the neocortex of mammalian brains it begins at the level of individual neurons.

The relations between minds and brains explored in this book are not easy to understand intuitively, and there is much to learn for readers who have no neuroscience background. For those who have some familiarity with neuroscience, other challenges may arise concerning the recent discoveries in cellular neuroscience, because they show that some basic assumptions taken for granted by twentieth-century neuroscience are misleading. Most prominent among these is the assumption that the function of neurons in general can be adequately conceived of as summing all their excitatory and

The Cooperative Neuron. William A. Phillips, Oxford University Press. © Oxford University Press 2023.
DOI: 10.1093/oso/9780198876984.003.0002

inhibitory synaptic inputs and informing other neurons of the extent to which that sum exceeds a threshold. In contrast to that assumption, recent discoveries show that a common class of neurons in the mammalian neo-cortex can use one part of their synaptic input to strengthen the information transmitted about the other part when doing so makes neuronal activity overall more coherent and adaptive. These discoveries have not yet reached the textbooks, so, although they are based on world-leading research (cited in the many notes that accompany the text), they will be unfamiliar to many readers. Nevertheless, these discoveries are of great importance and are beginning to provide cellular foundations regarding many aspects of our mental lives.

Although the evidence for cellular foundations of cooperative inter-actions emphasized throughout this book is not yet widely known, the func-tional importance of cooperative interactions is well-established. Notions of memories that arise from experience according to laws of association that specify which elementary ideas occur together, or in quick succession, are at least as ancient as Aristotle. Notions of cooperative interactions within the schema that store associative information have been common in studies of memory since Frederic Bartlett's (1886–1969) early work on memory, and Jean Piaget's (1896–1980) on cognitive development. Donald Hebb (1904–1985) provided a neural interpretation of such associative schema in the form of cell-assemblies in which recurrent facilitation between cells enables their activity to reverberate in the absence of the input that initiated their activity, for example, from the sensors; Hebb (1949) broadly defined them as providing cellular foundations for 'thought'.

Cooperative computation is central to Arbib and Érdi's (2000) schema theory, which shows how behaviour could arise from the concurrent coord-inated operation of cells in many different parts of the brain. Their extensive review mainly focused on the hippocampus and cerebellum, and outlined evidence from olfactory cortex, but they are not representative of neocortical regions. Others have questioned their relevance to the cognitive capabilities of the neocortex, and this remains unclear. An understanding of neocortical capabilities requires evidence of how the many components of a cell-assembly, associative memory, or schema within the neocortex can maintain their indi-vidual identity when they are active together with other components to form a mutually supportive whole. Later chapters in this book explore how coopera-tive neurons help accomplish this.

Although the primary aim of this book is to help us understand relations be-tween mind and brain, it also has a moral agenda. It suggests that cooperative context-sensitive computation in the thalamocortical system may have relevance to a common dilemma in our social lives: should the freedom of the individual or the organization of society be given priority when the freedom of the individual clashes with the needs of the whole of which it is a part. A central argument of this book is that individuality and cooperation are not (in essence) opposed. On the contrary—the more they cooperate, the greater the individual freedom, and the greater the individuality, the greater the benefits of cooperation.

I am able to view these issues from a broad multidisciplinary perspective because over the last five decades I have had the great good fortune to collaborate or communicate with eminent international authorities in each of the major disciplines involved. These include Wolf Singer, Matthew Larkum, Peter König, and Johan Storm in neuroscience; Talis Bachmann, Jaan Aru, Alan Baddeley, Graham Hitch, David Heeger, and many others in cognitive psychology; Lars Muckli and Lucy Petro in ultra-high-resolution neuroimaging; Steve Silverstein in experimental psychopathology; Alberto Granato in neurology; and with Andy Clark, Tomas Marvan, and Michal Polak in philosophy. Michael Wibral was the first to see that multivariate partial information decomposition can provide firm mathematical foundations for the viewpoint I advocate. In addition, I have learned much from being part of the ten-year, €1 billion Human Brain Project, which is a flagship of the European Commission's research on future and emerging technologies. A more recent and ongoing collaboration is with Ahsan Adeel, who is a leading expert on the use of cooperative context-sensitivity in artificial intelligence (AI) applications, and who has demonstrated, for the first time, a transformative computational potential of cooperative neurons that have the context-sensitivity I assumed long ago, thus showing how recent neurobiological breakthroughs could inspire advances in the design of more effective and efficient forms of machine learning. Last, but by no means least, the mathematical formulation of the theory of coherent infomax, as sketched in Chapter 8, arose from my long-lasting collaboration with Jim Kay, who has a deep understanding of the statistical foundations of information processing in neural networks. That chapter shows how mathematical foundations of cooperative context-sensitivity are provided by decomposition of the information transmitted by a local processor with two sets of inputs whose contribution to output are to be distinguished.

1.1 Enduring Philosophical and Psychological Issues Can Now be Explicitly Related to the Cellular Foundations of Mind

Attempts to understand the essence of truth, knowledge, and belief have long been central to the philosophy of mind. They are of particular importance during times in which deliberate deception is both rife and skilful. A perspective on these issues that is currently highly influential in philosophy, psychology, and neuroscience is focused on the use of predictive neuronal processing to deal with the omnipresent uncertainty in life. The empirical discoveries and conceptual advances outlined in the following chapters support much of that perspective, but they require it to be reinterpreted as being more concerned with enhancing the salience of coherent or relevant signals, rather than with fundamentally changing the information for which the signals code.[1]

The cognitive functions whose neuronal bases we seek are of far more than philosophical or academic interest. In addition to their close relations to pathology, they also have implications for crucial issues about which we must make judgements in everyday life, but about which we cannot be certain. Shakespeare's view of mental life, as dramatized in his plays, involves three recurring issues: knowledge and doubt, the notion of self, and conceptions of purpose in life.[2] Though he had no knowledge of neurons, Shakespeare understood that it is the brain that provides the stage on which mental life is played—as shown by his 147 references to brains! A central aim of this book is to relate these three enduring themes to the neurons of which that stage is composed.

Knowledge may seem to leave little room for doubt when making judgements about physical things—except for the endlessly many marginal cases: should I eat that wild mushroom? Will that branch hold my weight? Do I go right or left when lost in the hills? Is it safe to ski down that tempting off-piste run? The problem of knowledge most frequently raised in Shakespearian dramas, however, concerns knowledge of other minds. How could Othello know who to trust: Desdemona, his loving wife, or Iago, his faithful steward? Shakespearian dramas portray honesty as being the primary human virtue because it enables cooperation in the construction of things as ordinary as a conversation or as impressive as a well-organized society. As its foil, deliberate deception is portrayed as the primary human vice.

The notion of 'self' raises enduring philosophical issues. What is it? Is it fixed or can it change? If changeable, then by what? Do people express the same 'self' in whatever they do, or different 'selves' in different contexts? Are we, as Sartre declared, condemned to be free? Must we bear responsibility for our own actions?

The theme of 'purpose' as discussed here refers not only to our own personal goals, but also to the teleological notion intended when we speak of the 'purpose of life'. Does life itself have any plausible purpose, or are all our purposes no more than human inventions, whether shared or selfish? Is life 'but a walking shadow, a poor player, that struts and frets his hour upon the stage … a tale told by an idiot, full of sound and fury, signifying nothing' (5.5.25–29) as Macbeth memorably says when in despair; or do we agree with Hamlet, who declares 'What a piece of work is a man! How noble in reason, how infinite in faculty! In form and moving how express and admirable! In action how like an angel, in apprehension how like a god!' (2.2.303–307)?[3] As a way of exploring the potential relevance of the research outlined in this book to these fundamental questions about life's purpose, in Chapter 10 I reconsider them from the viewpoint to which that research leads.

Many aspects of mental life depend on the use of context to amplify and select relevant internal neuronal signals at each of the several levels of abstraction. These include: selection of the events that we notice; how we interpret them; our emotional reactions to them, and what we choose to think about, and thereby remember. Chapter 5 explains how this applies to perception in general—including what you are doing right now, that is, reading—and perhaps even to rationality, which is constrained by interpreting things in context. Our understanding of other minds is especially dependent on our ability to interpret things in context. Our understanding of social cognition may increase through a better understanding of how neocortical neurons cooperate by being sensitive to context. Although many of those neurons use context to cooperate in the creation of coherent percepts, thoughts, and actions, we are seldom aware of that context-sensitivity. It is mostly done automatically for us by processes within neocortical cooperative neurons and the multitude of local microcircuits of which they are the key components. Long-term goals of the cellular and psychological neuroscience that this book advocates include discovering the distinct contributions to mental life of basal dendrites, apical dendrites, and the inhibitory and disinhibitory interneurons that predominantly effect either basal or apical dendrites. Its central thesis is that the apical dendrites of many neocortical pyramidal cells provide those cells with cooperative, context-sensitive, information-processing capabilities that transcend the capabilities of the integrate-and-fire point neurons assumed by twentieth-century neuroscience.

1.2 Information-processing Operations Can be Distinguished from Information Content, and Both Can be Studied by Psychological and Neurobiological Methods

We now have a good idea of the meaning, or semantics, of the information processed by most parts of the brain. For example we know which parts are primarily visual and which are primarily auditory. However, we also need to find out what that 'processing' is when expressed explicitly in terms of the operations neurons can perform. Much of psychology has been concerned with basic cognitive functions, or 'theoretical constructs', for example, perceptual interpretation of sensory data, selective attention, working memory and thought, with properties that can be rigorously inferred from behaviour. We now seek to find out how those cognitive capabilities arise from operations performed by neurons.

My long-lasting collaboration with Wolf Singer, an internationally eminent neurophysiologist, convinced me that this can be done. Our first collaboration explored interactions between locally specific neural responses to the onset and offset of visual stimulation using both physiological and psychophysical methods. From many psychophysical experiments (performed initially on myself!) I inferred that somewhere at an early stage of the human visual system there is a form of reciprocal inhibition between signals of stimulus onset and signals of stimulus offset. That reciprocal inhibition prevents the transmission of contradicting messages, that is, that a specific visual stimulus appeared and disappeared simultaneously at a specific location in space. I assumed this was but one example of a general processing strategy that prevents early stages of sensory processing sending contradictory messages to higher perceptual levels. Singer's neurophysiological investigations showed that this reciprocal inhibition does indeed occur in the cat's visual system, and that it does so in the lateral geniculate nucleus, which is the first-order thalamic gateway through which data from the retina enters the neocortex. Knowing the functional consequences of those neuronal mechanisms, he and I together were then able to predict several phenomena that should be observable in the psychophysical paradigm, including some that are highly counter-intuitive. Further psychophysical studies then confirmed all those predictions, including the ability to recognize stimuli specified only by their disappearance![4] The psychophysical paradigm was then modified to explore other basic cognitive functions, such as visual short-term memory. Fundamental properties distinguishing sensory storage and visual short-term memory were predicted on the assumption that sensory storage occurs at an early level of the visual system that preserves precise spatial topography. In contrast, visual short-term memory occurs in higher cortical regions where the information extracted from the sensory data is far more abstract, less spatially precise, and more flexibly related to current sensory input. Again, the psychophysical results confirmed the neurophysiological predictions.[5]

I am therefore convinced that we are at a stage in the development of the psychological and neurosciences in which we should aim to explain how specific neuronal processes provide adequate mechanisms for the basic cognitive capabilities inferred from psychological studies of mind and behaviour.

To do this, we must clearly distinguish information-processing operations from information content. The information content of a neuronal signal is whatever it is used to transmit information about, which, in formal mathematical terms, implies some form of mutual information between a local processor's input and its output. These information-processing operations can be described in a general way that is independent of the information itself. To understand how these operations are related to the brain, they must be described in a way that is explicitly related to operations that neocortical neurons can perform. It is commonly assumed that neurons first integrate their many synaptic inputs to compute a net level of cellular activation, and that they then transmit information about that net activation from one place to another via the axons that connect them to other cells using connections called synapses. Long-term storage of information is thought to take place by modifying the strengths of those synaptic connections.

However, there is more to neocortical information processing than transmitting, storing, and retrieving information. The transmission, storage, and retrieval of video information are far from being equivalent to what happens when someone watches the video. Mental life, including watching a video, involves perceptual interpretation of sensory data, selectively attending to and thinking about things in that data, its interactions with the emotional state of the viewer, and using all the information to decide what to do—if anything. All this requires far more than transmission, storage, and retrieval. At the very least, it must include selecting the information relevant to current circumstances at each of several different levels of abstraction and within several distinct streams of processing, while interpreting and using that data in a way that is appropriate to the context within which it occurs.

1.3 Amplification of Pyramidal Cell Output if Relevant in the Current Context

Although there exist many complexities and subtleties about the perspective on brain and mind presented here, it is, in essence, rather simple. It argues that the selective transmission of information relevant in the context of concurrent activity elsewhere in the brain is crucial to mental life, and that distinguishing between relevant and irrelevant (incoherent, misleading, etc.) information is one of the most important and difficult tasks that brains have evolved to confront. Thus, the discovery that a large class of key pyramidal cells have already begun the task of amplifying what is relevant is of great importance. The following chapters provide grounds for supposing that it has deep implications for neurobiology, psychology, neurology, psychiatry, AI, and philosophy. On the face of it, so grand a supposition may seem to be either highly implausible or too vague to be useful. Nevertheless, the grounds outlined for it here are both strong and clear.

A key assumption of neuroscience and psychology throughout the twentieth century was that neurons integrate their excitatory and inhibitory synaptic inputs and tell other neurons whether and to what extent that net sum exceeds a threshold. The more it does exceed that threshold, up to a limit, the stronger the signal sent. Integration sometimes approximates simple linear summing, but often it does not: sometimes the net value computed is greater than a linear sum, sometimes less. Regardless, neurons are conceived of as transmitting information about a single value that is the net sum of all their synaptic inputs. As neurons combine all their inputs into a single integrated value, they can be described as point processors. This integrate-and-fire point neuron assumption offers explanations for a wide array of experimental findings. It has also inspired impressive advances in AI based on neural networks.[6]

On both theoretical and empirical grounds, this book argues that we must now advance beyond that simplifying assumption by building on evidence for neurons with two functionally distinct points of integration. In brief, such neurons can be described informally as those in which one subset of inputs is combined to produce a single integrated sum that can amplify transmission of information about the other inputs. This form of context-sensitivity amplifies the cell's output only when the net inputs to the two points of integration are both positive, and so it is a simple form of cooperation. Given that multiple cells interact via these contextual inputs, this becomes a form of intercellular cooperation that tends to increase the overall coherence and usefulness of the neural system's activity. It shows how the many highly specialized activities of the neocortex can be dynamically coordinated so that they work harmoniously together in the interest of the whole organism. It has long been supposed by many that holistic and localistic conceptions of mind and brain are opposed, but they are, instead, complementary. The greater the specialization of local functions, the greater the need to coordinate the whole (as in the theory of Gestalt psychology), and cooperative context-sensitive cells have evolved to meet that need.

Chapters 3 and 4 outlines for this class of neurons the anatomical and physiological evidence, which indicates that, in a key class of the pyramidal neurons that are plentiful in all regions of the neocortex, it is the input to their apical dendrites in layer 1 that provides the contextual input. Further, it is their basal dendrites and synapses near the cell body that provide the input about which information is transmitted.

The primary contribution of this book is to show how that class of cells have a central role in mechanisms for basic cognitive capabilities that psychologists have inferred from their studies of behaviour (Chapter 5). Chapter 6 provides a new viewpoint from which to consider fundamental issues concerning the evolution and development of mental life, and Chapter 7 demonstrates how these empirical and conceptual advances offer a new viewpoint from which to consider a surprisingly wide range of pathologies. Chapter 8 briefly outlines the way in which recent extensions to the foundations of information theory provide mathematical foundations for the notion of context-sensitive selectivity and for the development of radically new machine learning algorithms.

1.4 Clarification of Some Contentious and Ambiguous Terms

The notions of cooperation and selfishness are as contentious in science and philosophy as they are in politics and society generally. Is nature red in tooth and claw, or not? Are neurons and genes selfish, cooperative, both, or neither? Is the individual sovereign, or the community, or both, or neither? Interpretation of and responses to these questions depend in large part on the context within which they are raised. From an evolutionary viewpoint it may seem that the struggle for survival between organisms in competition for inadequate resources ensures that selfishness is paramount. Whether or not this is so is much debated, and the issue is unresolved because there is both cooperation and competition between organisms as well as between the cells of which they are composed. Resolution of such issues requires clearer notions of the terms involved.

This book is predominantly concerned with a field still at an early stage of development, and as such, its terminology is not yet settled. Therefore, we must clarify the way in which the terms 'context', 'modulation', 'coherence', and 'relevance' are used here. Zipser, Lamme, and Schiller (1996) introduced the phrase 'contextual modulation' to describe the effects of figure–ground organization on the responses of pyramidal cells in the primary visual cortex. Neuronal responses to elementary features of a figure were shown to be more salient than those to the background. Generalizing that notion, 'context-sensitivity' is used here to refer to modifications of the strength or salience of a signal without corrupting the information that the signal transmits. It can be either amplifying or attenuating, and is described as cooperative when it amplifies signals that are relevant to the context in which they occur. Some examples of amplification have previously been referred to as 'lateral facilitation' to contrast them with the long-known phenomena of 'lateral inhibition'. They are also often described as increases in 'excitability', which is vague unless adequately distinguished from 'excitation'.

'Context' is information that is used to modulate the strength or salience of a signal that transmits information about things *other than* the context. Thus, streams of processing in perceptual regions have two distinct functions: not only do they serve as a stage in a hierarchy of perceptual abstractions, but also they provide a context that guides interpretation of other parts of the sensory input. For example, symbols and words are often ambiguous, but are disambiguated by the context in which they occur, and Section 5.1 provides some simple examples. Thus, inputs are defined as being context because their effects are modulatory, and not because they convey information about a specific class of thing, for example, place or time. Modulatory interactions between regions typically involve both amplification and attenuation because by amplifying the outputs of a few selected cells they attenuate the outputs of cells with which they are in competition.

Coherence and relevance are concerned with the criteria by which signals are selected for amplification. Signals in separate cells or streams of processing are coherent if they are mutually supportive. They are relevant if they are coherently related to other perceptual signals, support ongoing tasks, or have high emotional significance. Chapter 3 provides examples at a cellular level of organization, and Chapter 5 does so at a cognitive level of organization. Chapter 5 also provides further discussion of the notion of relevance as used in several fields of research, including psycholinguistics.

Relevance and coherence must be clearly distinguished from the informativeness of a signal. Signals that are coherently related to the current task or stimulus context or have high emotional significance can be made more salient even if they are less informative than signals that are not. Various figures in Chapter 5 provide examples of how, by implicitly assuming coherence, context guides perception to inferences that correct misleading sensory data. They also provide examples showing that in the rare cases where the sensory data seems to be incoherent the perceptual system keeps searching for a coherent interpretation, and that coherence can increase the salience of coherent elements even though that makes them less informative.

1.5 Cellular Psychology Is Analogous to Molecular Biology

When I was young, the physical bases of heredity were unknown. The amount of genetic information to be transmitted between generations of a species is great, and complex processes must be involved in replicating that information with a small amount of random error and using it to guide an organism's development from conception to death. For these reasons, many biologists initially assumed that genetic information must be carried by a complex machinery composed of many molecules. It was not discovered until the 1950s that the DNA molecule is capable of carrying information in quantities far greater than previously thought possible. Within a few decades, the discovery of DNA changed human lives to such an extent that today's world is utterly different from that into which I was born.

Similarly, most of us, including most psychologists and systems neuroscientists, have until recently greatly underestimated the capabilities of brain cells. Now, virtuosic intracellular physiological investigations show that there is a class of neurons, referred to here as cooperative context-sensitive neurons, whose information-processing capacities are far greater than previously thought possible for neurons in general. This class of neurons uses their sensitivity to context to selectively amplify transmission of their messages when doing so increases the coherence and effectiveness of their activities overall.

The great divide between those who know about intracellular neurochemistry and those who know about mental processes became obvious to me when I offered final-year psychology undergraduates a course on neuropsychopharmacology (that was not its title, of course—if it had been, few would have taken it!). It was called 'Drugs and the Mind', which was highly popular, not least because in some ways the students knew far more about it than I did! To those taking the course it soon became obvious that, although there is a gulf between the disciplines of psychology and neuropsychopharmacology, there is no separation between minds and intracellular processes. The course was also of practical use to the students because it alerted them to the dangers of misusing psychoactive substances—legal and illegal. A better, and more widely known, understanding of the cellular foundations of mental processes is therefore a major goal for research and teaching in the sciences of brain and mind.

Though there are some excellent textbooks on neuropsychopharmacology, they are not well suited to a course on cellular psychology.[7] These textbooks usually have far more information on molecular structure than is needed, with more emphasis on behaviour than on mental life. The scarcity of psychology departments that teach the relevant parts of neuropsychopharmacology shows that psychology (as taught at present) is not grounded in its cellular bases. With this book, I hope to encourage the teaching of cellular psychology as a way of grounding psychology firmly in the cellular foundations of mind, thus bridging the current gap that separates what we know about neurons from what we know about minds. From that point of view, cellular psychology is concerned with cellular mechanisms of basic cognitive capabilities (see Chapter 5), that is, perceptual interpretation, conscious experience, selective attention, working memory, emotional prioritization, cognitive control, and learning. If evidence on relations between mental life and its cellular foundations continues to grow at its present rate, then psychology departments that do not teach cellular psychology will become as rare as biology departments that do not teach molecular biology. It will then become clear that the mental processes studied by psychologists have more complex cellular foundations than has been understood until now and that differences between psychiatric and neurological pathologies do not reflect an unbridgeable gap between mind and brain.

Cellular psychology, thus conceived, is related to neuropsychopharmacology but differs from it in two major ways. First, it is explicitly focused on relating basic hypothetical constructs that psychologists and cognitive neuroscientists have inferred from behaviour and macroscopic neuroimaging to their cellular foundations, and Chapter 5 reports some explorations of that vast territory. The second difference is that it is also concerned with relating both those mental processes and their cellular foundations to direct conscious experience, that is, phenomenology (discussed in several later chapters).

This book argues that, by being sensitive to context, neocortical pyramidal neurons can operate together in a way that increases the coherence and viability of the overall dynamic system of which they are a part. Thus, it implies that systemic coherence can arise from purely local interactions, if they are appropriately cooperative.[8]

Cooperative context-sensitivity in neural systems is analogous to epigenetics in molecular biology. Life depends on cooperation at the molecular as well as at the cellular and higher levels of organization:

> Whatever the mechanism by which the first replication was accomplished in the prebiotic world, it must surely have been a cooperative enterprise involving more than one type of molecule, accompanied by substantial flows of energy from one molecule to another. After all, this is the way the genetic material replicates itself at the present time, with DNA, RNA, and proteins all cooperating with each other.
>
> (Wills & Bada, 2000, p. 130)

Epigenetic processes modify gene activity without altering the DNA sequences that code for the proteins to be built. They have evolved to guide expression of the coding genes so that it occurs at the appropriate times and places, that is, in the appropriate contexts. Furthermore, they do so by activating some genes and silencing others. Similarly, context-sensitivity in the neocortex guides the expression of each cell's message, for example, the presence of a particular feature or object in the percept or thought. It does so in a way that increases the overall coherence of perception and thought. Another similarity between epigenetic and neuronal context-sensitivity is that each was discovered long after discovery of the processes of information transmission that they modulate. Therefore, it must be emphasized that cooperative context-sensitivity is only a part (though important!) of the broader field of dendritic computation (see, e.g., Poirazi & Papoutsi, 2020).

The analogy between epigenetics and neural context-sensitivity can even be given a mathematical formulation. Pica and colleagues (2017) show that the advanced form of information theoretic analysis used (Chapter 8) to quantify neuronal context-sensitivity can also be used to quantify the operation of gene regulatory networks.

1.6 Mental Life Is Not Behaviour

When specific neuroanatomical and neurophysiological findings are described as providing bases for behaviour, I interpret this to mean that they provide bases for internal processes upon which behaviour depends. However, note that those internal processes are *not* the behaviour itself. One reason for insisting on the distinction between mind and behaviour is that describing neurobiological observations as being directly related to observed behaviour deflects attention from the more fundamental task of relating neurobiological observations to theoretical constructs. For a hundred years or more, these inferred concepts have been laboriously and carefully deduced by psychologists via observed behaviours and their accompanying data. Many, but not all, of those inferences express deep insights into the essence of mental life. What is needed now are interdisciplinary interactions that guide psychology and neurobiology towards paradigms that clearly reveal the relations between internal mental processes and physical neural processes. The suggestion of eminent Yale neurobiologist Gordon Shepherd that this field of research be called Cellular and Psychological Neuroscience resonated strongly with me because it describes the overall aim of the research without any theoretical commitment other than to discover the ways in which fundamental psychological capabilities arise from their neuronal bases. Seen from a psychological perspective this field of research can be described even more succinctly as Cellular Psychology.

A second reason for insisting that relations between brain and mind be distinguished from relations between brain and behaviour is that much of mental life is internal and not directly expressed in behaviour in any reliable way. Many, though not all, of those internal mental processes are conscious and great Chilean neuroscientist Francisco Varela argued that our methodologies should include paradigms in which neurophysiological observations are related to direct experience, even though our beliefs about that experience are fallible.[9] I say this because many identify mental life with life that is consciously experienced. However, Freud argued that some mental processes are not conscious—a fact confirmed by many rigorous psychological experiments, one of which demonstrated the surprise that many people show when presented with their highly limited ability to keep information in mind for only a second or so.[10] Another false belief about our own conscious experience of particular relevance here is that we can focus our attention on individual elements of the sensory mosaic in a way that enables us to directly experience properties of those elements independently of the context in which they occur (see Chapter 5).

Notes

1. Clark (2015) presents a lucid and highly influential philosophical analysis of how minds deal with uncertainty by using predictive processing. The evidence and arguments presented here support a modified version of Clark's analysis in which, instead

of fundamentally changing what neural signals code for, predictions and other forms of contextual input to pyramidal cells modulate the salience of the signals that those cells transmit.

2. Philosopher Colin McGinn (2006) presents an extensive analysis of Shakespeare's philosophy as shown by basic issues on which characters in his plays reflect from their various viewpoints and in various states of mind. Relations between imagination and reality are one of the most basic. As I see it, McGinn makes the common error of endorsing the misleading supposition that a greater contribution of imagination leads to a greater deviation from reality. That is not necessarily so. See Figure 5.2, which demonstrates how internal knowledge is sometimes used to create percepts that are more objectively valid than the raw sensory data. Discovery of the laws of nature and technology's use of them to create new things that work depends on imagination and the use of abstract symbol systems within which old ideas can be combined in new ways. Furthermore, I am sceptical of McGinn's attribution of that misleading supposition to Shakespeare, who seems to me to focus more on raising enduring issues than on offering simple solutions to them. Nevertheless, I agree with McGinn in seeing the three underlying issues that he identifies as being basic themes that Shakespeare explored from many different perspectives.

3. *Kingsway Shakespeare*, 1927.

4. In studies of the reciprocal inhibition between responses to visual onsets and offsets Phillips and Singer (1974) and Singer and Phillips (1974) confirmed detailed predictions from psychophysics to neurophysiology, and vice versa. This includes the prediction that letters defined only by their disappearance can be recognized (confirmed by Wilson, 1981).

5. Phillips (1974) confirmed that sensory storage at early stages of the visual system and visual short-term memory differ in ways predicted by simple inferences from neurobiology.

6. Rolls (2016) reviews a vast amount of evidence for principles of neocortical operation that are understandable on the assumption that neurons operate as integrate-and-fire point processors.

7. Feldman, Meyer, and Quenzer (1997) is an excellent neuropsychopharmacology textbook but it is written for pharmacologists, not psychologists.

8. In political philosophy, anarchy is social organization that arises from purely local interactions. Its positive values have been effectively obscured by popular presentations of it as implying complete disorder, but when considered in more depth the term has no such implication. It literally means 'without a ruler or king' and emphasizes that a monarch (or single ruler of any kind) is unnecessary for social order. Supporters of anarchic modes of social organization tend to emphasize the benefits of local self-organization rather than any losses consequent upon the absence of a single ruler. As I see it, the presence of much essential order in societies with rulers who are incompetent or worse provides some support for that view, as does the preservation of many basic cognitive capabilities despite loss or impairments of the prefrontal cortex.

9. Varela and colleagues (2001) review arguments for neurophenomenology, that is, research paradigms in which consciously experienced phenomena are related to neurobiological observations.

10. Simons and Rensink (2005) review evidence showing that a common belief about conscious experience is shown to be false in the case of change blindness.

2
Cerebral Neocortex

Hierarchies of Abstraction in Physical Matter that Knows and Doubts, Thinks and Feels, Intends and Hopes

The cerebral cortex, together with the thalamus (to which it is tightly linked), is the structure that has increased most in both absolute and relative size during mammalian evolution. The cortico-thalamic system is the organ on which our mental lives most depend. After Francis Crick and James Watson discovered the DNA code, Crick spent the final few decades of his life working on theoretical neuroscience. In a popular book on consciousness, he described as an 'astonishing hypothesis' (Crick, 1994) the view that conscious mental life is due to neural activity in the cerebral cortex, but he was firmly committed to that view, nevertheless. People affected by dementia, a stroke, or other forms of cortical damage, or who care for someone so affected, know only too well that it is no mere hypothesis. Nevertheless, Crick is surely correct in describing it as astonishing. It could be seen as a 'miracle' in that, although minds arise from physical matter with properties as described by the laws of physics, we still do not know how minds arise from brains. When we finally do understand (as we are now beginning to) how minds arise from matter, then that will be even more miraculous!

2.1 Function Depends on Structure

In neuroscience, as in biology generally, structure provides strong clues to function—that is, if you know what to look for and how to interpret what you see. This applies at all levels of organization, from molecular biology to that of the whole organism. Later chapters in this book focus on the structure and capabilities of neocortical pyramidal neurons. This chapter focuses on the structure and function of the cerebral neocortex overall. At the level of its gross anatomy the human

The Cooperative Neuron. William A. Phillips, Oxford University Press. © Oxford University Press 2023.
DOI: 10.1093/oso/9780198876984.003.0003

neocortex is a crumpled sheet that is about 2–5 mm thick that is usually represented as being composed of six distinct layers. It is organized into regions that are both anatomically and functionally distinct, and which form hierarchies. The higher levels within these hierarchies are concerned with more abstract things.

The division of the neocortex into distinct regions is primarily concerned with what is processed where, and much is known about these processes. However, this book is concerned mainly with the operations performed at a cellular level of organization within the distinct regions of the neocortex. Although these intracellular processes will be unfamiliar to many, learning about them may be more worthwhile and less difficult than anticipated as there are only a few basic operational principles to be learned. These are common to the many distinct neocortical regions that are specialized to apply those operations to information about myriad different things. Thus, learning what information is processed by each part of the brain requires learning about the great variety of feedforward inputs about which the cells in each region transmit information. Although learning about the cellular information-processing capabilities outlined here may at first seem challenging, it requires the acquisition of far fewer specific facts: certain aspects of cellular anatomy and physiology are common to many different neocortical regions.

The necessity of knowing what to look for is exemplified by perception of the structure of the dendritic tree of the pyramidal cell shown on this book's front cover. Knowing about the context-sensitivity of these cells, as outlined in this book, I can see that it is the kind of cell that is likely to use inputs to its apical dendrites at the top of the tree as a context within which to strengthen the information that it transmits about its other inputs. That is because those dendrites are connected by a single long trunk to the cell body ('soma'), which is the darker spot at the base of the trunk. If there were no such single trunk, or if its branching occurred closer to the cell body, so that it looked more like a shrub than a tree, then I would see it as much less likely to use inputs to the upper dendrites in that way. Fletcher and Williams (2019) measured the length of the trunk needed for pyramidal cells to function in that flexible, context-sensitive, way. It is about half a millimetre (Chapter 3), which is a great distance relative to the size of the cell body, which is about 0.002 of a millimetre.

2.2 The Neocortex: A Vast Number of Neurons

Figure 2.1 is an old diagram drawn at a time when visible structure was skilfully portrayed and shows the human neocortex in relation to the whole brain. This image is useful here in that it shows the neocortex (the large, crumpled

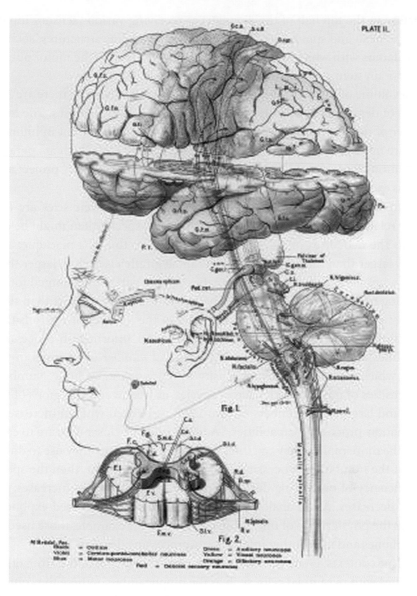

Figure 2.1 A schematic drawing of the cerebral neocortex in relation to the central nervous system overall. It shows the major sensory inputs to and motor outputs from the neocortex, which is depicted at the top of the diagram as a crumpled sheet surrounding various smaller structures, such as the thalamus, with the midbrain, brain stem, and cerebellum being shown separately lower in the diagram. There is no need to learn the anatomical names of all the various parts.

From DeFelipe, 2015, with approval from Javier DeFelipe. The original appears in a textbook published in 1899.

structure in the top half of the diagram) as receiving various sensory inputs from the head and spinal cord. It also shows surrounding structures, such as the thalamus with which it is closely intertwined, as well as the motor output via the brain stem, cerebellum, and spinal cord.

In a volume of the cortical sheet half a millimetre in diameter there are 270 metres of dendrites, about 30,000 neurons, and a billion synapses. The total number of neurons in the neocortex depends on the species, but in humans there are more than ten billion neurons in total, 70–80% of which are pyramidal neurons that release glutamate at the synapses to which they project and are thus excitatory.[1]

Figure 2.2 shows brains of several different species. Their sizes are less closely related to the cognitive capabilities of these species than might be expected. The neocortex of a deer is much larger than that of a macaque, and slightly larger than that of a chimpanzee, and a giraffe's is slightly larger than that of a human. These apparent anomalies can (in part) be accounted for by appealing to brain size relative to the body, but there is more to it than that. Gross brain size is not directly proportional to the number of neurons that it contains because neuronal packing density varies. Information-processing capabilities are more closely related to the *total number* of neurons in the cortex, which depends on packing density as well as on total volume. Numbers and densities of neurons varies across species, as well as across regions of the brain, and larger total numbers of neurons is associated with an increase in information-processing capabilities.[2] Additionally, the closer cells are to each other, the more rapidly they can interact and the less energy they use to do so. Thus, if the number of processing elements is kept constant, then the speed and efficiency of processing does not improve as physical size increases; rather, it decreases. As an analogy, computing power has increased exponentially as the physical size of microchips plummets, for example, those used in smartphones and many other information-processing devices.

In some contexts, I refer to 'neocortex' to explicitly distinguish it from other structures with pyramidal cells, such as the hippocampus. Where the context makes it unambiguous, I often refer simply to 'cortex'. The close interdependence between neocortex and thalamus is taken for granted.

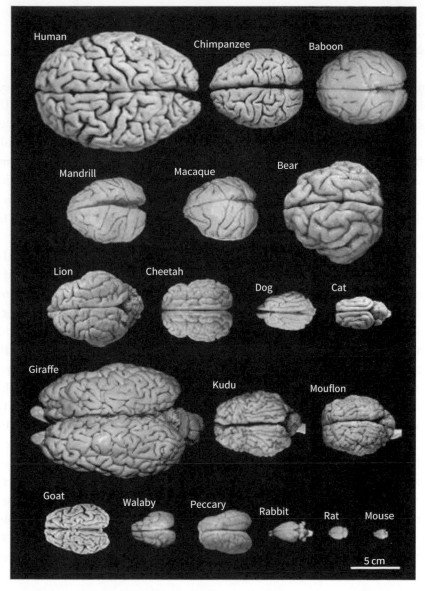

Figure 2.2 From top left to bottom right are the brains of a human, chimpanzee, baboon, mandril, macaque, deer, lion, cheetah, dog, cat, giraffe, kudu, mouflon, goat, wallaby, peccary, rabbit, rat, and mouse. They are all seen from above, with the head facing to the left, and all at the same spatial scale, as shown by the scale bar at the bottom right, which is 5 cm.

From DeFelipe, 2011, with approval from Javier DeFelipe.

2.3 The Neocortical Sheet: Six Layers, not Three

An internationally eminent neurophysiologist, for whom I have great respect, told me long ago that 'Hippocampus is perfectly good cortex'. It isn't. The assumption that it is has impeded our progress toward an adequate understanding of the neocortex, because evidence from hippocampal pyramidal cells has been taken as representative of pyramidal cells in general. It isn't. I have compiled a list of more than 20 functionally significant anatomical and biophysical differences between hippocampal and neocortical pyramidal cells. Although similarities do exist, these differences are surely relevant to the far greater evolutionary expansion of neocortex than of the hippocampus.

A simple and obvious anatomical property that distinguishes neocortex from more ancient structures (e.g. the hippocampus) is that it is composed of roughly six layers of cells, whereas the latter are composed of roughly three. I say 'roughly' because dividing the neocortex into six layers is (to some extent) conventional, rather than being a precise description of its anatomical structure. Nevertheless, Figure 2.3 shows that it is clearly a sheet-like structure organized into several different layers. It is also clear that there are about twice as many layers in the sheet of neocortex than in that of hippocampus. See Chapter 6 for an overview of the evolution of 'six' layered neocortex from the more ancient 'three' layered cortex of the hippocampus and reptilian cortex, for example, turtles.

Just as in gross brain size, the depths of the cortex in different species are less closely related to our initial ideas about the relative mental capabilities of those species than we might expect (Figure 2.3). The perspective advocated here argues that some key evolutionary modifications involve intracellular properties that are not visible at the spatial scale shown in Figure 2.3, microscopic though that is.

2.4 The Regions of the Neocortex

If the great sheet of the human neocortex were uncrumpled and laid out flat, it would occupy much of a square metre. Since the early twentieth century, the neocortex has been divided into many regions or areas based on their detailed internal cellular structure (Figure 2.4), most notably by the German anatomist Korbinian Brodmann (1868–1918), who distinguished 52 separate anatomical areas using different stains that reveal different aspects of their

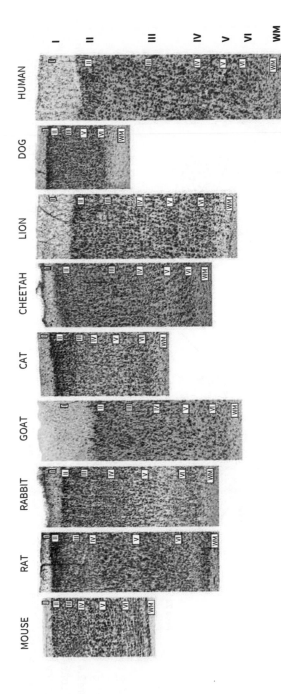

Figure 2.3 Photomicrographs of Nissl-stained sections down the depth of the neocortical sheet of nine mammals, all at the same spatial scale. Each is about 0.5 mm wide. The sections are 0.1 mm thick and from frontal regions. Maximal cortical depth is reached by human cortex, which, as here, can be up to about 4.5 mm deep. This kind of staining shows only cell bodies, which are the tiny dots. Many but not all of them are neurons. Most of the larger dots are the bodies, aka soma, of pyramidal cells. The different layers are labelled I to VI from top to bottom.

WM, white matter, or axons.

Adapted from DeFelipe, 2011, with approval from Javier DeFelipe.

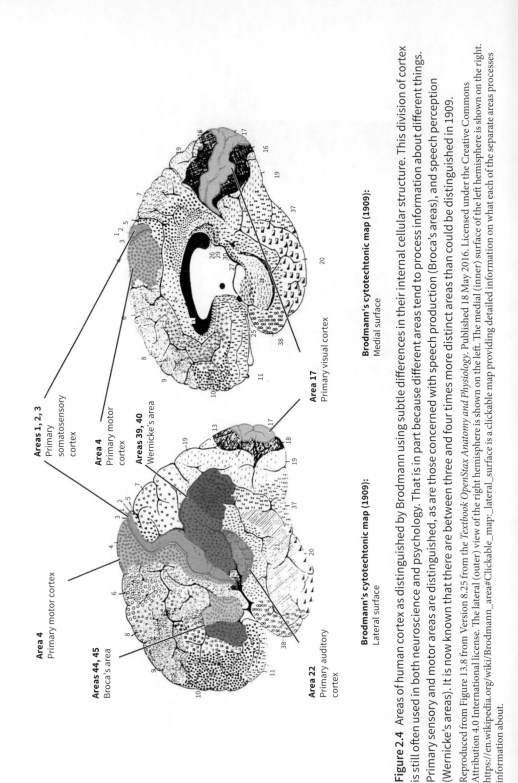

Figure 2.4 Areas of human cortex as distinguished by Brodmann using subtle differences in their internal cellular structure. This division of cortex is still often used in both neuroscience and psychology. That is in part because different areas tend to process information about different things. Primary sensory and motor areas are distinguished, as are those concerned with speech production (Broca's areas), and speech perception (Wernicke's areas). It is now known that there are between three and four times more distinct areas than could be distinguished in 1909.

Reproduced from Figure 13.8 from Version 8.25 from the *Textbook OpenStax Anatomy and Physiology*. Published 18 May 2016. Licensed under the Creative Commons Attribution 4.0 International license. The lateral (outer) view of the right hemisphere is shown on the left. The medial (inner) surface of the left hemisphere is shown on the right. https://en.wikipedia.org/wiki/Brodmann_area#Clickable_map:_lateral_surface is a clickable map providing detailed information on what each of the separate areas processes information about.

cellular composition. He numbered those regions in the order that he studied them, beginning with primary somatosensory cortex, and ending with an area near the border between the temporal lobe and the insula, which has a key role in emotion regulation. There is now detailed evidence for more than 40 regions in the neocortex of mice, and for about 180 in humans. The exact number may not be fixed but may vary across individuals and time depending on several things, perhaps even including the range of skills in which that individual brain has become proficient. The latest evidence shows that there are boundaries between regions that are too subtle to be visible to the techniques available to Brodmann. Furthermore, though boundaries between regions are sometimes sharp, they are also sometimes gradual.[3]

Much research in the sciences of brain, mind, and behaviour is concerned with relating the different contents of *what* we perceive, think, remember, and to different regional locations within the cortex. Learning about that therefore involves learning about the functions of about 180 regions with probabilistically defined boundaries, and which may not be fixed, particularly in regions concerned with higher levels of abstraction. Learning *how* we perceive, think, remember, and plan our actions may eventually turn out to be far easier and more useful than learning about *what* we perceive, think, remember, or do.

2.5 Organization of Neocortical Regions into Hierarchies of Abstraction

More than half of the neocortex consists of hierarchies of perceptual abstraction that are used for imagined percepts, as well as for objectively valid percepts. Therefore, it is no surprise that perception and imagination can sometimes become confused (as discussed elsewhere in this book).

The use of perceptual regions for thought may be an evolved modification of the more fundamental need to use internal knowledge to interpret sensory input. Bishop Berkeley (1685–1753), and other philosophers argue that internal ideas play a central role in perceptual experience. The great German physicist and neurobiologist Hermann von Helmholtz (1821–1894) argued that percepts are 'unconscious inferences' that use internal knowledge to interpret ambiguous sense data. The dependence of perceptual experience on information from internal sources is often directly demonstrated within psychology using ambiguous figures, such as the Necker cube, the Penrose triangle, and many other entertaining diagrams, which show that perceptual experience can change, although the stimulus does not. Ambiguity is far more ubiquitous than that, however. Later chapters in this book demonstrate how ambiguities are typically resolved using contextual information of various sorts, much of which involves interactions between different sensory modalities, as well as feedback from higher to lower levels of hierarchical abstraction. The depth of the abstraction hierarchy tends to be greater in more recently evolved species. Lower levels of abstraction and feedforward connections that flow up the hierarchy tend to arise earlier during ontogenetic development than higher levels, and thus also earlier than the feedback connections that flow down the hierarchy. This is as expected on the assumption that higher levels extract information that is in the input received from lower levels.

The number of cortical regions tends to increase with brain size. Figure 2.5 shows a map of 78 regions in the macaque neocortex. It preserves the relative positions and sizes of the different regions but excludes limbic regions, such as the hippocampus, which is not neocortex and has more ancient organizational principles.

The mean number of cells per cubic millimetre decreases from the lowest levels of abstraction in primary sensory regions to the highest levels in the prefrontal cortex, but the mean number of synapses per cell increases greatly. Thus, there are fewer, but far more complex, cells in frontal than in sensory regions. This difference between frontal and posterior regions increases greatly with brain size. Pyramidal cells in human frontal regions have far more synapses than in macaques, which, in turn, have far more than in marmosets. This reflects the depth of the abstraction hierarchy attained by those different species. Across the whole range of mammalian species, the organisation of their diverse primary sensory areas is much the same and privileged in several ways. They are the first to develop in the embryo and are modifiable by the input that they receive during post-natal development. Feedforward connections from lower to higher hierarchical layers develop before those in the reverse direction. Thus, the course of development tends to be from back to front, with cells in frontal regions developing over the longest time, and becoming less dense, but with more richly branched dendritic trees and far more synapses than cells at the sensorimotor base of the hierarchy. An evolutionary trend toward increasing depths of abstraction is clearly seen in the anatomy of neocortex across a wide range of species. The number of dendritic spines, and thus synapses, on pyramidal cell dendrites in temporal and frontal regions of humans is far greater than in mammals generally. As development proceeds, this difference increases greatly, which presumably reflects the large amount of information that humans acquire as they grow toward maturity and develop further through the life-course.[4]

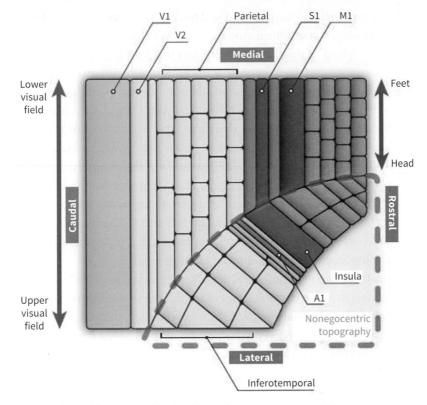

Figure 2.5 Hierarchically organized regions of one hemisphere of the macaque neocortex. Boundaries between each of the 78 regions are shown, with their relative sizes and positions being preserved. Primary visual cortex (V1), which is at the bottom of the hierarchy, is shown on the far left. This is at the back of the cortex, that is, it is caudal. Prefrontal regions, which are at the top of the hierarchy, are shown on the far right. They are at the front of the cortex, or rostral. The lateral to medial axis shows location relative to the outer and inner sides of the hemisphere. Most regions contain topographic maps of primary sensory inputs or motor outputs, though with far less spatial precision at higher levels. Here, such maps are described as egocentric. They include V1, V2, and the parietal regions that constitute the dorsal visual pathways that specify where things are and how to act on them. Regions in the wedge on the lower right corner do not map location relative to the organism, that is, their topographic layout is not egocentric. They include the inferotemporal visual pathway, that is, the ventral 'what' pathway that is concerned with identifying objects and events at various levels of abstraction.

Adapted from Finlay & Uchiyama, 2014. Use approved by Barbara Finlay, with permission from Elsevier.

Many key properties of feedforward and feedback connections have been discovered by in-depth anatomical studies (Markovkov et al., 2013, 2014) of the dorsal visual regions of macaques, which have much in common with those of humans. First, pyramidal cells transmit information in either the feedforward direction, or the feedback direction, but not both. Second, cells transmitting to higher levels are found in layer 5 as well as in layer 3, and cells transmitting to lower levels are found in layer 2 as well as in layer 5. Third, most feedforward and feedback interregional connections are to the nearest neighbour in the hierarchy, but a few skip a region or two. Those that skip regions in the feedforward direction come only from cells in layer 3. Those that skip in the feedback direction come only from cells in layer 5. Fourth, topographic mapping is more locally precise in layers 2 and 3 than in layers 5 and 6. Finally, cells providing feedforward output resonate at higher frequencies, that is, 40 Hz or more, than those providing feedback output, that is, 25 Hz or less.[5]

Findings from such studies are typically interpreted as showing that feedforward signals drive activity via inputs to dendrites in the central layers of the cortex, whereas contextual input, including feedback, amplifies selected activities via input to the outer layers, especially layer 1. If the contextual effects are to operate such that they preserve the validity of perceptual processing while increasing its usefulness, then they should not usually change the sensory data to fit the context. Instead, they should operate in a way that helps select the higher-level abstractions that best fit the sensory data. For the most part (although with some notable exceptions, e.g. imagination), the primary function of the feedforward flow of information from the senses through the many perceptual regions of the neocortex is to transmit information about the external world and the body that is both valid and useful. Selective amplification of sensory information that is relevant to current intentions and stimulus context can be referred to as 'purposeful objectivity'.

The evidence for hierarchical relations between cortical regions is clear and highly relevant to our understanding of context-sensitivity, and recent advances are discussed later in Section 9.8. However, this evidence can lead to some misleading assumptions, for example, it is often assumed that all contextual input to pyramidal cells is feedback from higher levels. Evidence for contextual input from other sources is cited in Chapters 3, 4, and 5. Another misleading assumption is that feedback is only from the next hierarchical level up, but studies of macaque visual regions show otherwise. A third misleading assumption is that there is only one hierarchy, but different modalities have distinct hierarchies in unimodal regions, and there can be distinct hierarchies within modalities, as in the distinct dorsal 'where' and ventral 'what' streams of processing in vision. An additional misleading assumption is that all feedforward transmission is driving, and all feedback is modulatory, but evidence indicates that, although uncommon, some feedforward transmission is modulatory and that some feedback is driving.[6] Thus, throughout this book, driving and modulatory inputs are distinguished by the effects that they have, and not by where they come from. A final misleading assumption is that the mode in which cells operate on their input is fixed. Again, evidence indicates otherwise, including some showing how the cells' mode of operation depends on their neuromodulatory state (outlined in Chapter 4 and emphasized in later chapters).

2.6 Neurobiological and Psychological Evidence for Common Neocortical Information Processing Operations

There is strong evidence from several methodologies for basic information processing operations common to all or most neocortical regions, including dynamic grouping by synchronized oscillations and the contextual guidance of learning and processing.[7] Although there is still no consensus on the extent to which cortical function depends on synchronized oscillations, that hypothesis has strong support and is being actively studied. It is highly compatible with the contextual guidance of learning and processing, as shown by Phillips and Singer (1997) and by Phillips, von der Malsburg, and Singer (2010).

There are five identified general themes on which variations are played across different cortical regions and species. First, there are three main classes of neocortical pyramidal cell that can be distinguished by the sites to which their axons directly project. One class of cells, located in layers 2, 3, and 5A, projects mainly to other higher cortical regions. They are referred to as intra-telencephalic (IT) cells. Another class is located in layer 5B and projects mainly to sub-cortical sites. They are referred to as pyramidal tract (PT) cells. The final class of cells is located in layer 6, and projects mainly to the thalamus. It is referred to as cortico-thalamic cells (CT). Misleadingly, 'pyramidal' in PT refers to the bundle of axons that convey information to subcortical locations via the pyramidal tract and brain stem, and the 'T' means different things in the three different acronyms. Nevertheless, despite these terminological ambiguities, these three classes of pyramidal cell clearly differ genetically, developmentally, anatomically, and physiologically.

The second general theme is that there is a flow of excitation from layer 4, where feedforward information is received, to cells in layers 2 and 3, and from there to cells beneath them in layer 5 and to cells in layer 4 of higher regions. As some feedforward input from lower regions also activates layer

5 cells directly, there is also some skipping of levels in this hierarchy of processing from one layer to the next.

The third general theme is that, in layer 1 of pyramidal cells whose cell body and basal dendrites lie in deeper layers, the apical dendrites receive input from diverse cortical and subcortical sources. This diverse input operates as a context that amplifies or attenuates the cell's responses to the feedforward input received by its basal dendrites (see Chapter 3).[8]

The fourth general theme is that the activation of apical dendrites is regulated by inhibitory and disinhibitory mechanisms that are distinct from those that regulate basal and perisomatic input. The final general theme is that the excitability of IT pyramidal cells in layers 2, 3, and 5A is regulated by input from both higher-order thalamus and sub-cortical arousal systems, with much of that regulatory input being to their apical dendrites, especially in humans.[9]

Notes

1. DeFelipe (2011, 2015) reviews quantitative information on brain size, numbers of cells, and synapses, etc., and discusses their relation to cognition.
2. Herculano-Houzel (2017).
3. Amunts and Zilles (2015) review much evidence showing that human neocortex can be divided into about 180 anatomically and functionally distinct regions.
4. For an in-depth review of anatomical differences between cortical regions, their hierarchical organization, and their differences across species, see Finlay and Uchiyama (2014).
5. Markov and colleagues (2014) report extensive studies of the feedforward and feedback connections between macaque visual regions.
6. Markov and Kennedy (2013).
7. Phillips and Singer (1997).
8. There have long been arguments and evidence for the existence of a common theme, on which different neocortical regions play different variations. Harris and Shepherd (2015) review ample evidence for a recent version of that view. Schuman and colleagues (2021) clearly establish the central role of layer 1 in various forms of context-sensitivity. Although they emphasize top-down sources of input to layer 1, they also cite ample evidence for lateral, intraregional, thalamic, and other sub-cortical sources.
9. Shapson-Coe and colleagues (2021) from Jeff Lichtman's Harvard lab report electron microscopic studies of human temporal cortex, which, among many other things, confirms that the anatomical distinctions between apical and basal dendritic trees are particularly clear in humans.

3

Neocortical Pyramidal Cells that Cooperate by Sensitivity to Context

Pyramidal cells are the workhorses of neocortex. About three quarters of the several thousand million neurons in human neocortex are pyramidal cells. Most of the others are there to support and regulate pyramidal cell function. As pyramidal cells are excitatory and transmit most of the excitatory signals in mammalian neocortex, including that of humans, we can safely assume that they have a central role in mental life.

In contrast to many other classes of neuron, neocortical pyramidal cells are not adapted to a particular prespecified purpose, but rather they are multipurpose, as shown by their ability to adapt to whatever input they receive as well as by their wide distribution throughout all cortical regions, including those concerned with visual, auditory, somatosensory, motor commands, thoughts, and executive functions, such as those referred to as 'cognitive control'.

Recent discoveries in the labs of Larkum and Schulz in Europe, Stuart, Williams, and Palmer in Australia, Magee, Svoboda, and Harnett in the USA, show that many neocortical pyramidal cells can cooperate by adapting the salience of their output to the context of activity elsewhere in the brain. They can do so because, in addition to the input from which they abstract the information that they transmit, they also receive information from many other sources, and use that as a context within which to increase the strength, or salience, with which they transmit their own message. These discoveries support the notion of 'psychic cells' that the great Spanish neurobiologist Ramon y Cajal (1852–1934) inferred from his anatomical observations (reviewed in depth by DeFelipe, 2010).

Perception and attention, thought and action, learning and memory—these all require the ability to select signals that are relevant in the current context. Thus, a better understanding of cellular mechanisms for amplifying selected signals is likely to have major implications for psychology and neuroscience. First, before discussing those mechanisms in detail Section 3.1 asks you to temporarily suspend doubts that you may have concerning all attempts to relate mind to cellular processes, and Section 3.2 summarizes a widely held

The Cooperative Neuron. William A. Phillips, Oxford University Press. © Oxford University Press 2023.
DOI: 10.1093/oso/9780198876984.003.0004

assumption about neuronal function that is a useful starting point beyond which we must now advance.

3.1 Common but Misleading Assumptions about the Cellular Bases of Mind

It is often assumed that any attempt to relate mind to cellular processes is necessarily ruthlessly reductionist. Indeed, Tomas Marvan, a philosopher with whom I collaborate, told me that my perspective is likely to be seen by many as 'reductionism on steroids' because it relates psychological processes to detailed aspects of intracellular physiology. I disagree. Rather, it puts cellular physiology in the context of cortical activity overall and then places that in the context of our place in nature. I see the long-term goal of this research as seamlessly situating psychology within a broad scientific view of nature. That implies a multilevel view of life as mechanisms-within-mechanisms, with no level of organization being assumed to be more 'real' than the others. That is in stark contrast to reductionism, ruthless or otherwise, which privileges lower levels.

Water, which can be fluid, solid as in ice, or gaseous as in water vapour, provides us with an opportunity to observe the great difference between the macroscopic properties of a system and the microscopic properties of the elements of which it is composed. However, a single molecule of H_2O cannot be in any of those states, because they apply only to large collections of molecules. Nevertheless, the properties of large collections of molecules depends on the properties of the molecules of which they are formed. The properties of molecules of H_2O are very special: few, if any, other molecules combine with each other to produce a solid state that floats on its liquid state. It is the same with context-sensitive cooperative neurons—they are also highly distinctive. When combined with each other, and with other classes of neuron (as in the neocortex), they generate very special macroscopic system properties, as outlined in this book.

It is also often assumed that, apart from synaptic strength, processes within individual neurons are fixed and are (at least in principle) predictably deterministic, but this is not so. Activity-dependent intracellular processes, such as trafficking, can insert or retract molecules known as ion channels into the cell's membrane within a few seconds or so, and this action applies to both synapses and non-synaptic parts of the cell. As outlined in this chapter, these ion channels have major effects on the cell's activities, so those activities are far less fixed and predictable than is often assumed. We are slaves neither to our neocortical neurons nor to our genes. Both have evolved ways of taking a broad context into account, with consequences that are, in practice, far from being wholly predictable. That is especially so in the case of the pyramidal cells described here because their activities are sensitive to a context that is exceptionally wide, diverse, and constantly changing. The intracellular processes on which we focus put local processing in the context of activity elsewhere in the neural system, thus making moment-by-moment neuronal dynamics more holistic than reductionist.

It is common to think that learning about intracellular processing is more difficult than learning about what is processed where in the brain: this is only partly valid. On the one hand, it is more difficult because intracellular processes are usually described in a way that is comprehensible to physicists, electronic engineers, and cellular neurophysiologists, but not to neuroscientists, psychologists, or philosophers. On the other hand, processes within individual pyramidal cells, and the local microcircuits in which they are embedded, offer a way of looking at mind in terms of a common underlying theme on which many variations can played. Thus, a few core insights about cellular and microcircuit functions may cast light on endlessly many psychological, physiological, and pathological phenomena. An understanding of those insights does not require learning exactly what is dealt with where in neocortex, which is complex, varies across species, and can even vary greatly within species (e.g. during development and across individuals).

It is often assumed that, apart from being either excitatory or inhibitory, neurons are essentially all the same. In contrast to that, neuroscience has long known that there are functionally distinct kinds of neuron. Even within the broad group classified as 'pyramidal', there are differences with important implications for function, for example, between those in different layers of the neocortex and between those in prefrontal and in sensorimotor regions. Later in the book, Section 9.8 highlights recent reviews that indicate that the higher a region is in the cortical hierarchy, the greater its dependence on cooperative context-sensitivity.

It may be thought that intracellular processes have little more than academic interest but nothing could be further from the truth. Many psychoactive drugs operate by affecting these processes, with major consequences for perception, consciousness, cognition, mood and emotion. This applies both to legal substances (e.g. alcohol, nicotine, caffeine, and to prescribed psychoactive medications) as well as to illegal substances. By learning about the intracellular processes that can be affected by psychoactive substances, people will better understand their effects and thus make better-informed judgements about whether and how to use them.

There is also a widely held assumption that it is only at the network level that brains evolve, and that the neurons remain unchanged; this is also untrue. There have been several major evolutionary advances in the complexity and intracellular capabilities of neurons, with many of those advances being at the sites where they receive inputs from other cells.[1] A major part of the evolutionary history of which we are a product involves changes at the cellular level that make possible new advances at the macroscopic network level.

Finally, the view of intracellular processes explored here is most radical in that it builds on grounds for supposing that we must now advance beyond the simple integrate-and-fire conception of neurons on which most of twentieth-century neuroscience is based.[2] Before discussing those grounds, however, Section 3.2 because much has been explained using that concept, and because familiarity with it provides a foundation upon which we can advance our understanding of cells with two functionally distinct points of integration.

3.2 Pyramidal Cells as Leaky Integrate-and-Fire Point Neurons

Although the advances in neuroscience that are emphasized throughout this book constitute a revolution, that revolution is peaceful. Cooperative neurons are mainly, or even wholly, neocortical, so can easily be combined with conceptions of other brain regions, even if all neurons in those other regions function only as point processors. Furthermore, it is only a subset of neocortical pyramidal cells that are able to operate as two-point processors, and those may (in some circumstances) be able to revert to operating as point processors. Thus, the evidence for cooperative neurons does not imply that we must completely reject the point neuron hypothesis. It has been, and remains a useful simplification, although it can be seriously misleading if we assume that it applies to neurons in general.

Pyramidal cells are neurons with a 'pyramidal' shaped cell body, or soma, and two distinct sets of dendrites. Figure 3.1 shows the typical anatomy of a pyramidal cell's dendrites, synapses, and axon. The basal dendrites feed directly into the soma (cell body) that houses its nucleus and DNA, etc., which is shown as a small black shape at the bottom of the apical trunk, into which feed the apical dendritic branches, aka 'tuft', which are much further away from the soma

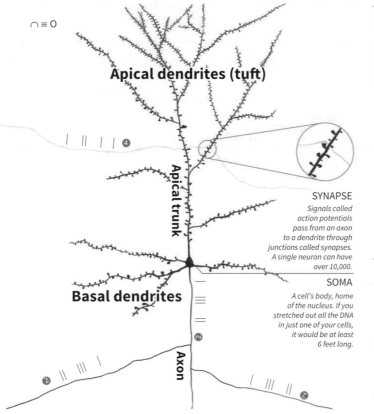

∩ ≡ 0

Apical dendrites (tuft)

Apical trunk

Basal dendrites

Axon

NEURON
ANATOMY

SYNAPSE
*Signals called
action potentials
pass from an axon
to a dendrite through
junctions called synapses.
A single neuron can have
over 10,000.*

DENDRITES
*Signals come in through
dendrites. These vast,
tree-like branches grow
up and out from the soma.
Dendrites are thicker than
axons and covered
in synapses*

SOMA
*A cell's body, home
of the nucleus. If you
stretched out all the DNA
in just one of your cells,
it would be at least
6 feet long.*

AXON
*Signals go out through
axons, which branch
many times and stretch
vast distances. Neurons
send action potentials
down their axons and
through synapses they've
formed to communicate
with other cells. The
longest axons in your
body reach from your
toes to your spine.*

Figure 3.1 The anatomy of a neocortical pyramidal cell, and examples of its single branching axonal output and one of its several thousand inputs (the wavy thin line), which are the axons bringing the all-or-nothing action potentials, or spikes, from many other neurons.

Adapted from image licensed under the Creative Commons Attribution-Share Alike 4.0 International license. Original available at: https://commons.wikimedia.org/wiki/File:Anatomy_of_a_Neuron_with_Synapse.png

The soma is only a tiny proportion of the cell, most of which consists of the dendrites that receive thousands of distinct inputs and the axon that transmits the cell's message to thousands of other cells, both nearby and far away. The dendrites receive inputs from other cells via synaptic junctions, which are narrow clefts about 0.1 micron wide. Within less than a millisecond, the neurotransmitters released by the incoming axon flow across the gap to affect the receptors on the receiving side, referred to as 'post-synaptic'.

Figure 3.1 shows the many tiny, mushroom-shaped, protrusions with which dendrites are covered. They are referred to as 'spines', and their exact shape changes in ways that depend on both the stage of development and learning.

Most spines have excitatory synapses, so the number of spines, which ranges up to several thousand per cell, depending on age, region, and species, is a lower limit on the number of excitatory inputs per cell. Chapter 7 discusses spine abnormalities that are involved in several neurological and psychiatric disorders.

Imagine gross pyramidal cell anatomy as being like a tree with roots, trunk, and branches. The soma is at the base of the trunk, the basal dendrites are shaped like roots that surround the soma, and the apical dendrites are like the upper branches and twigs of the tree. These are connected to the soma via the apical trunk, which is also sometimes referred to as the apical shaft. The cell's output is conveyed by its axon, which extends for long distances and divides into many branches that transmit all-or-nothing action potentials, that is, spikes, to many other cells.

There is no consensus on the terms used to refer to the apical dendritic tree. By implication 'the apical dendrite' describes what is here referred to as the apical trunk because there is only one per cell. Because there are several per cell, the branches of the apical tree are referred to here as the 'apical dendrites'— also often called the 'tuft'.

Figures 3.2 and 3.3 show the immensely dense packing of cell bodies, dendrites, and axons in neocortex. Size matters, and varies across a huge range, even at this microscopic scale. For example, the width of human cerebral cortex is about 3 millimetres (i.e. 3×10^{-3} metres). The width of a pyramidal cell body, or soma, is between $20–120$ μm (1 μm $= 10^{-6}$ m). The apical trunk is a few microns in diameter and the tips of their apical dendrites are about 0.1 μm in diameter.

A synapse is about 1 μm wide and the gap between axon and dendrite at the synapse is about 0.1 μm, which is too small to be visible by light microscopy, though it can be seen by electron microscopy. The cell's membrane is about 0.005 μm thick, and the diameter of the channels in the membrane through which charged particles called ions pass is about 0.0005 μm. Thus, relative to the size of the soma, the tips of the apical dendrites are far away. The soma of cells in layer 5 are about 20 μm in diameter, but their apical dendrites in layer 1 are more than 400 μm away, as indicated in Figure 3.3.

An emphasis upon the complexity of structures and events at and below the scale of microns may help to correct a tendency to equate size with computing power. Neanderthal brains were a little larger than ours, but that does not imply that they had superior information-processing capabilities. Indeed, there are good grounds for assuming that miniaturization does not reduce computational capability; rather, it can even enhance it. The Elliot computer that I used to run psychophysical experiments in the 1960s filled a large room,

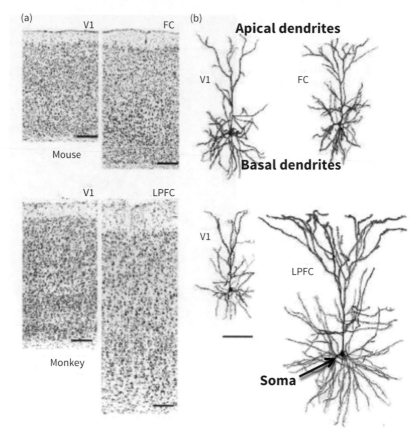

Figure 3.2 Layer 2/3 pyramidal cells in primary visual cortex (V1) and frontal cortex (FC) of mouse and monkey. In panel A only the cell bodies, or soma, are stained, and are visible as many small dots. Although most are the soma of pyramidal cells, some are those of inhibitory interneurons, including all those sparsely distributed throughout the top white band (i.e. layer 1 of the six layers). Although the differences between the other five layers are not clear in this figure, they are reliable and much clearer with other forms of staining (scale bar is 0.2 mm). Each of the four cells in panel B shows the soma and dendrites of one of the many pyramidal cells in layer 3 on a magnified spatial scale (scale bar is 0.1 mm). The two at the top are from a mouse. The two at the bottom are from a monkey. Although monkeys are highly visual animals, the cells in their primary visual cortex (V1) are slightly smaller than those of mice. In contrast to that, pyramidal cells in monkey lateral prefrontal cortex (LPFC) are much larger than the closest equivalent in mice (FC), with a much clearer distinction between apical and basal dendrites. That distinction is even clearer for pyramidal cells in layer 5, whose apical trunks are much longer.

V1, primary visual cortex; FC, frontal cortex; LPFC, lateral prefrontal cortex. All are shown at the same spatial scales.

This figure is adapted from Luebke, 2017, with her approval.

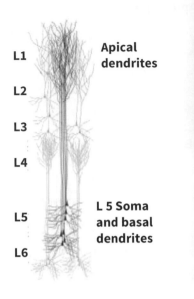
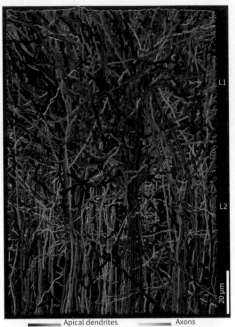

Figure 3.3 Left Panel: A diagram of pyramidal cells in layers 2, 3, 5 and 6. The apical trunks of those whose soma are in layer 5 (shown in red), are substantially longer than those of layer 2 and 3 cells (shown in green) and of layer 6 cells (shown in orange). Right Panel: An electron microscopic image of the dense canopy of the neocortical forest showing the apical dendritic branches (in shades of blue and green) and inhibitory axons (in shades of yellow and orange) in layers 1 and 2 of mouse neocortex. Excitatory axons, of which there are many in L1, are not visible in this image. The scale bar in the bottom right-hand corner shows 20 µm. The apical branches of pyramidal cells in layer 5 are more than 400 µm away from their soma, so, on this scale, they are far away from the site in the soma from which the cell's outputs are generated.

Left panel: adapted from DeFelipe, 2015, with approval from Javier DeFelipe. Right panel: adapted from Karimi et al., 2020, as approved by Moritz Helmstaedter.

but its capabilities were far less than those of my smartphone. It is no accident that computing power has improved as size has decreased. Miniaturization saves energy and time, which are far more crucial to the processing of large amounts of information rapidly than is sheer bulk. Thus, what happens at tiny scales of space and time has major functional consequences. Furthermore, the greater the capabilities of the elements of which an information processing system is composed, the greater the capabilities of the system overall.

Figure 3.1 shows the inputs to a pyramidal cell as a sequence of short red lines, which represent the all-or-nothing 'action potentials', or 'spikes', by which neurons typically communicate. Pyramidal neurons receive inputs via a few tens of thousands of excitatory synapses and a few thousand inhibitory synapses. Most of the excitatory inputs use glutamate as the transmitter. Inhibitory inputs typically use the transmitter gamma amino butyric acid (GABA). In addition, as outlined in the next chapter, they also receive input from subcortical centres, such as those that regulate arousal. When the cell is in a neutral state with little synaptic input, that is, 'at rest', the balance of osmotic and electrostatic forces produces more negative than positive ions inside the cell such that the voltage difference across the somatic membrane is around −70 millivolts. Put simply, the standard view of the effects of synaptic inputs to a neuron is that excitatory inputs make the membrane potential less negative, whereas inhibitory inputs make it more negative.

That integrate-and-fire point neuron assumption has been developed and improved in various ways.[3] Technically, the integration is usually referred to as 'leaky' because it is not literally a simple linear sum of the positive and negative inputs, which can leak through the cell's membrane before reaching the soma. Nevertheless, whether linear or not, the assumption is that the output is determined by first combining all inputs into a single net sum. This standard view of a pyramidal cell has been neatly described as being a 'dendritic democracy' because all synaptic inputs are assumed to be equivalent in that they have the same chance of affecting the cell's output, no matter how far they are from the site that generates output.[4]

Figure 3.3 shows how pyramidal cells operate together with other cells in a narrow column of neocortex about 50 μm wide. They form what are known as population codes in which much the same message is conveyed by each of a population of cells within a neocortical minicolumn. As all pyramidal cells are excitatory, so are most of the long-range connections within and between neocortical regions. However, about 15% of cells in the neocortex are inhibitory, so by activating them, pyramidal cells can have inhibitory effects. The inhibitory cells typically affect only cells within their own local neighbourhood (Section 3.5) so they are referred to as interneurons. Thus, pyramidal cells can transmit excitatory signals via direct connections, and inhibitory signals via inhibitory interneurons; they usually do both.

Changes in the strength of the synaptic connections between neurons are referred to as 'synaptic plasticity'. These changes depend on cellular activity and are the intracellular basis for learning. They depend on the endless interactions between our genetic inheritance, what happens to us, and what we choose to think and do.[5] Though neocortical synapses become less changeable with age, the neocortex is a perpetual construction site where change is always being possible. Much has been discovered about the processes underlying synaptic plasticity and learning, and there are many published introductions to that aspect of cortical function. The selection of *what* to learn—a central aspect of learning—is now viewed differently due to evidence for two-point neurons. Throughout the waking day in the neocortex, vast and constantly changing patterns of neuronal activity occur, most of which have no more than passing significance, if any. A key problem, therefore, is how to distinguish between aspects of the ongoing activity that are worth learning from, and those that are not. Essentially the same problem also concerns decisions about what is and what is not relevant to current information processing, and it is the latter with which we are primarily concerned here, as learning is a consequence of the ongoing processing that depends upon what signals are amplified.

The endurance and pervasiveness of the point neuron assumption are easy to understand. First, for many cortical neurons, including some pyramidal cells and many (if not all) inhibitory interneurons, it may be an adequate approximation. Second, in 1943, McCulloch and Pitts proved that neural nets composed entirely of such neurons can, *in principle*, compute anything computable. Third, only a few labs worldwide have the high level of technical skill required to observe interactions between different parts of the same cell when they are far apart, microscopic, and densely packed alongside other cells. As most neuroscientists are experimentalists, it is difficult for them to be enthusiastic about observations that they cannot make for themselves. Finally, the definitions of information provided by Claude Shannon, who invented information theory, are restricted to quantifying the capacity of a channel with a single input and a single output. They do not provide definitions that are adequate to quantify the different contributions to an output that are provided by different components of the input. That requires definitions of multivariate mutual information that have only been available since the study of 'partial information decomposition' began in 2010. Though still young, that field of research has already developed definitions that are adequate for our purposes (Chapter 8).

3.3 Context-sensitive Two-point Neurons

Although the conception of neurons as simple point processors has been (and remains) dominant within neuroscience, some neuroscientists have long argued that neurons are more than simple summing nodes. Much of the case for that view was foreseen by Wilfred Rall, the founder of dendritic studies (see Segev et al., 1995). Recent empirical and computational studies now clearly show dendritic computation to be a major subfield within neuroscience (Poirazi & Papoutsi, 2020).

The distinction between basal and apical dendrites is clear in the visible anatomy of pyramidal cells. It is also clear in what is known about the very different sources of input to those two sets of dendrites. The functional significance of these structural differences is less obvious, however. It was not until the final years of the twentieth century that direct physiological evidence showed that some neocortical pyramidal cells can function as context-sensitive neurons with not one, but two, points of integration.[6] Furthermore, in some pyramidal cells, inputs to their apical dendrites have effects on the cell's output that differ fundamentally from those to its basal dendrites. Basal and apical dendrites receive information from different sources, and that information is used for different purposes within the cell. These pyramidal cells increase the strength with which they transmit information about their basal input when the depolarization that it causes coincides with depolarization of the apical dendrites. Depolarization of the local post-synaptic potential at the soma makes it less negative and therefore more likely to generate an action potential that is transmitted to other cells via its axon. As the apical input arises from diverse cortical and subcortical sources it provides a broad context within which the cell can increase the salience of its message when that is likely to increase the coherence and effectiveness of neocortical activity overall.

3.3.1 Anatomy Suggests Distinct Functions of Apical and Basal Inputs

Apical and basal dendrites receive inputs from very different sources and basal dendrites are much closer to the soma. That raises the possibility that these two sets of dendrites have different functions. Basal dendrites of pyramidal neurons in perceptual regions receive inputs that usually convey information about current sensory stimulation. Basal dendrites in the same column of a few hundred cells in primary sensory regions receive inputs from similar sets of sensory receptors, but those in distant columns of the same cortical region typically receive their basal inputs from nonoverlapping parts of the sensory surface. Basal dendrites in regions that are higher in the hierarchy of perceptual abstraction convey information that arises from larger areas of the sensory surface, but neurons in specific columns in those higher regions respond only to highly specific things, such as the presence of a face, or even a particular face.

In contrast to the narrowly specified inputs to basal dendrites, inputs to apical dendrites come from a wide diversity of sources, including input from the prefrontal cortex (PFC), which is broadly concerned with making strategic decisions. Thus, apical dendrites convey information from diverse sources, rather than from the more narrowly specified sources to which that specific cell is selectively sensitive.[7] In addition to receiving input from different sources, apical and basal dendrites also differ in the distribution of the nonsynaptic neuromodulatory ion channels that regulate their activity.

3.3.2 Regulation of Synaptic Input to Apical Dendrites by Nonsynaptic Voltage-dependent Ion Channels

Ion channels are molecules in the cell's membrane that undergo changes in their shape such that they switch between open or closed states. When they are open, charged ions of specific kinds pass in or out of the cell at a rate of up to 100,000 ions per millisecond. Ion channels are selectively permeable to sodium, potassium, calcium, or chloride ions, or to specific subsets of them, and they open or close in response to a neurotransmitter released at the synapse, or in response to the electrical potential across the cell's membrane at that location if they are 'voltage -dependent', or to both. Some kinds of ion channel underlie synaptic transmission. When a specific neurotransmitter is released into the narrow synaptic gap and attaches to an ion channel in the membrane of the receiving cell, the channel opens briefly before closing again. Another kind of ion channel underlies transmission of signals by the axonal action potential, or 'spike'; these types are not opened by synaptic input. There are no synapses in the axon. Instead, their opening depends on the voltage difference across the membrane at that location, so they are referred to as being 'voltage-dependent'.

There are other voltage-dependent ion channels, however, with functions that are less widely known, and these are crucial to communication between parts of the same cell that are far apart, as are the apical branches and the soma. The effects of synaptic input can spread passively over short distances, but passive spread along a dendrite dissipates or leaks away as its distance from the soma increases. As a result, there can be up to a fortyfold attenuation of the effects of apical stimulation before it reaches the soma.[8] This attenuation can be overcome, however, by specific classes of voltage-dependent ion channel in the apical trunk that actively transport the effects of apical input to the soma. The operation of these ion channels varies with the state of arousal, as well as with several other things. The effects of apical input on the cell's output are therefore far more dynamically variable than is often assumed.

Several classes of voltage-dependent ion channel are particularly relevant to the effects of apical dendrites because that is where they are most dense. These include hyperpolarization-activated cyclic nucleotide-gated (HCN) channels. They are partly open when there is no synaptic input, and they move the resting level at the soma slightly closer to the threshold above which action potentials are generated by allowing positively charged ions to enter the cell. This current flow through HCN channels is referred to as I_h, and it is far more important to mental life than most psychologists and neuroscientists realize. In addition to opposing too much inhibition, these channels also oppose too much activation. Current flow through HCN channels has excitatory effects at sites near the soma but reduces the effects of input to the apical dendrites by decreasing the extent of spatiotemporal integration.[9] Therefore, current flow through these channels tends to minimize the effects of apical input on action potential output. The operation of HCN channels is strongly regulated by the adrenergic and cholinergic arousal systems, so they have a central role in variations of apical function that depend upon arousal (see Chapter 4).

3.3.3 Apical Activation Can Amplify Response to Basal Activation: Direct Physiological Evidence

The discoveries summarized in this section depend upon an exceptional level of technological expertise. Figure 3.3) shows a 50-μm wide minicolumn of pyramidal cells diagrammatically on the left. In the cortex, it would contain a few hundred densely packed pyramidal cells. Their apical dendrites are near the top of neocortex in layers 1 and 2, where they meet with a host of incoming axons from diverse sources. The right side of the figure shows a real image of the canopy of this dense neocortical forest, which shows the great difficulty of studying intracellular processes that convey information from a specific apical dendrite to a specific cell body which may be far away in layers 5 or 6 and thus not visible in this image.

However, studies exist that describe communication between the apical dendrites and the soma using a technique known as 'patch-clamping', which involves gently pushing the tip of an ultra-fine glass micropipette against a tiny part, or patch, of the cell to control and measure the local electrical currents or voltages at that location on the membrane. The patch thus formed can cover a single ion channel. It can be used to measure the local post-synaptic potential that results when current is injected at that specific site on the cell. Bert Sakmann in Heidelberg, together with Erwin Neher, was awarded the Nobel Prize in 1991 for developing the patch-clamping technique that made this possible. They showed that a tiny electrode within the micropipette could record the opening and closing of a single ion channel in the cell's membrane, and this enabled them to measure the resulting electrical potential inside that tiny patch of dendrite. By forming patches at different parts of the same cell, and measuring the effects of injecting current, both at that local patch and at distant parts of the same cell, multi-site patch clamping has revealed processes of integration and communication within individual pyramidal cells that transcend those assumed by previous theories of neuronal function. Research on dendritic computation using these and other recently invented techniques is a rapidly growing field of neuroscience sometimes referred to as 'dendritic computation'. The distinctive functions of apical dendrites play a leading role in that young field of research.[10]

Patch clamping individual pyramidal cells at two or three well-separated locations on the apical trunk of pyramidal cells in layer 5 of rat somatosensory cortex has revealed a zone near its top that integrates input to their apical branches. This is referred to here as the apical integration zone, but it is also known as the apical spike initiation zone, or nexus. When activation of the apical integration zone exceeds a threshold, it triggers a calcium spike that conveys activation to the soma via the apical trunk. The key discovery is that apical activation that has little or no effect on the soma by itself can greatly increase the cell's response when there is also some basal activation. Figure 3.4 shows how apical activation that has no effect by itself on the cell's output can transform the response to weak basal activation from one action potential into three action potentials that occur in rapid succession. Such effects are often referred to as supra-additive because three is greater than one plus zero. These effects of apical input are more than that, however, because they produce a brief but rapid burst of spikes, similar to signalling urgency by knocking on a door two or three times in rapid succession with pauses in between each burst of action potentials.

Describing the effects of apical activation as supra-additive can be misleading because addition is symmetric, whereas the effects of basal and apical inputs are highly asymmetric. The asymmetry between basal and apical dendrites is obvious in the anatomy of pyramidal cells, and especially so for cells in layer 5 (Figure 3.3). The asymmetry is also clearly shown by physiological observations in the case of context-sensitive pyramidal neurons. Activation of the soma is necessary to generate axonal spikes, and direct activation of the soma via basal dendrites is sufficient to specify its selective sensitivity.

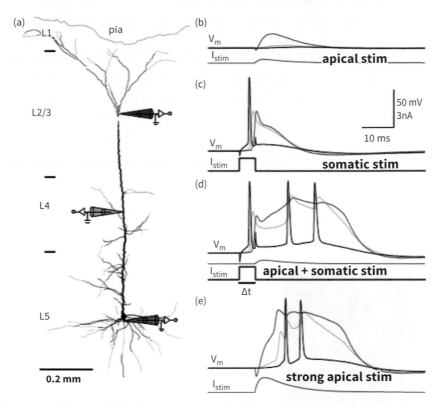

Figure 3.4 Apical amplification: stimulation that has no effect on output by itself has a large effect if combined with brief stimulation of the soma. a) Micropipettes in the soma (black), mid-apical trunk (blue), and trunk top (red) were used to insert current and measure the resulting potential difference (V_m) in layer 5 pyramidal cells in slices of rat somatosensory cortex. b) Apical stimulation (I_{stim}) alone activates the membrane locally Vm (red curve) but has little or no effect on the soma (black line). c) A 5-ms current pulse to the soma produces a single action potential (black spike). d) When the apical stimulation immediately follows the somatic stimulation, it transforms the response of a single spike into three spikes occurring in rapid succession. e) If the current injected into the top of the apical dendrite is strong enough it can generate two or three output spikes in rapid succession.

Adapted from Larkum, Zhu, & Sakmann, 1999, as approved by Matthew Larkum, with permission from Springer.

Activation of the apical integration zone is not necessary, and it is not usually sufficient. Amplifying effects of apical input that rapidly add a few extra axonal action potentials to one triggered by basal input are of central importance to the cooperative context-sensitivity with which this book is concerned. Those effects are referred to as 'apical amplification'.

Figure 3.5 gives examples of the contrasting sources of input that basal and apical dendrites receive from the thalamus. The division of pyramidal cell dendrites into basal and apical subsets is echoed by the division of the thalamus into two distinct groups of nuclei. First order (specific) thalamic nuclei convey specific unimodal sensory information to the cortex connect to the basal dendrites and perisomatic synapses. Higher-order (nonspecific) thalamic nuclei that receive input from various intracortical sources and project back to cortex connect to apical dendrites. In primary sensory regions basal dendrites receive input from current sensory stimulation via a specific nucleus in the thalamus both directly and via cells in layer 4 not shown in Figure 3.5. Information abstracted from that is then relayed up the perceptual

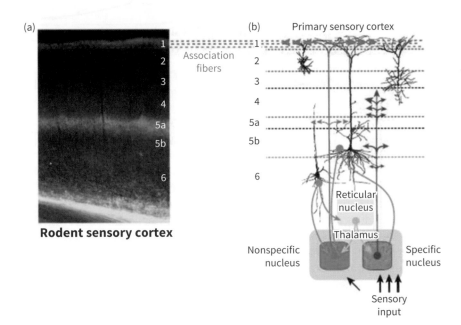

Figure 3.5 Basal dendrites in layers 2, 3, 4, 5b, and 6 receive ascending sensory information via specific thalamic nuclei (red). Apical dendrites in layer 1 and dendrites in layer 5a receive information from nonspecific nuclei and from various other sources (green). a) Axons from a specific thalamic nucleus (red) and a nonspecific thalamic nucleus (green), made visible by injecting red and green fluorescent proteins into the respective thalamic regions, from where they were transported by axons to the cortex. b) Schematic representation of the long-range input to the primary sensory cortex in rats. The colour scheme follows the fluorescent protein colours in a) for easy comparison. Association fibre axons carrying information from other cortical regions are shown overlapping with the nonspecific thalamic input in layer 1. Connections from cells in layer 6 to the reticular nucleus contribute to the regulation of arousal.

Adapted from Larkum, 2013, with approval from Matthew Larkum, and permission from Elsevier.

hierarchies via the basal dendrites in higher regions. In contrast to that, apical dendrites receive input from higher-order nuclei in the thalamus and from various other cortical and subcortical regions via the dense 'association fibres' in layer 1 that convey information about activity elsewhere in the brain.

Figure 3.5 shows how a recurrent feedback loop connects neocortical pyramidal cells with thalamic cells. A simple, but key aspect of this anatomy is that the feedback from the nonspecific, higher-order, thalamic nuclei to neocortex is to the apical dendrites in layer 1. Halassa and Sherman (2019) provide ample evidence that this recurrent cortico-thalamic loop has a central role in several basic cognitive functions (discussed in later chapters).

In contrast to the specificity of basal inputs, apical inputs are highly diverse. Excitatory inputs to apical dendrites arise from distant parts of the same neocortical region or other regions at similar levels of the abstraction hierarchy, from higher cortical regions (both directly and via the nonspecific thalamus), and from subcortical centres, including the amygdala, which deals with threat and anxiety.[11] They also receive inhibitory input from specific types of local inhibitory interneuron (see Section 5.5). Last, but not least, they receive input from subcortical systems that regulate waking, sleeping, and dreaming (see Chapter 4).

The long-range inputs to apical dendrites are not those about which the cell is adapted to transmit information, for example, tactile input in the case of the cell in Figure 3.4. Nevertheless, if the net input to the apical integration zone is excitatory it can amplify response to excitatory basal inputs with which they coincide. Therefore, it has been suggested that apical dendrites provide a cellular mechanism for wakefulness (Chapter 4) and for basic cognitive functions, such as perceptual disambiguation and the contextual guidance of selective attention (Chapter 5). Inputs to layer 1 are therefore collectively labelled 'context' in Figure 3.6. From that perspective, apical input is defined as operating as an amplifier when it increases the strength or salience with which information is transmitted about the feedforward input to basal dendrites.

Figure 3.6 shows interactions between apical and somatic integration zones that involve backpropagation-activated calcium-spike firing (referred to as BAC firing). 'Backpropagation' here refers to the propagation of action potentials toward the apical integration zone via the apical trunk, as well as to other neurons via the axon. Depending on the strengths of these activations, calcium spikes may then be triggered at the apical integration zone and propagated to the soma. In the limit, activation of either integration zone alone can trigger an apical calcium spike and action potential output if sufficiently strong. Activation of the apical branches that is not strong enough to trigger a

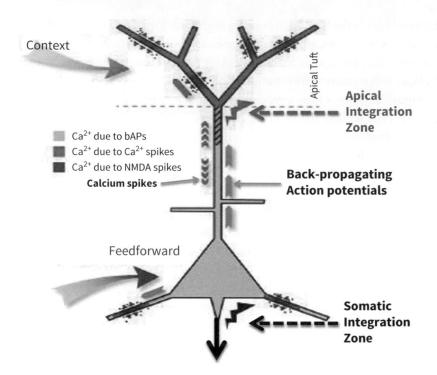

Figure 3.6 This diagram shows how contextual input to the apical dendrites of some neocortical pyramidal cells can amplify the strength of their response to feedforward input. In sensory and perceptual systems feedforward inputs from the external world are fed directly into the somatic integration zone via the basal dendrites. Diverse inputs from various sources feed into the apical integration zone. When an axonal output spike is triggered by feedforward input, shown by the black lightning strike, that spike also propagates to the apical integration zone where it combines with input from the apical dendrites to increase the probability that a calcium (Ca^{2+}) spike, shown by a red lightning strike, will be initiated and actively propagated to the soma where additional action potentials are then generated. Integration in both basal and apical dendritic trees is dependent upon NMDA spikes, shown as blue dots. Grey arrows going upwards from the soma to the AIZ are called back-propagated action potentials (bAPs).
Adapted from Larkum & Phillips, 2016, with permission from Cambridge University Press.

calcium spike by itself can amplify the cell's output when it occurs at about the same time as a BAC, or action potential, from the soma. Figure 3.4d shows a case where the apical calcium spike then generates another two output spikes in rapid succession following the first, which is called a 'burst'.

As these effects of apical input occur if the two integration zones are activated at around the same time their function has been described as coincidence detection. The exact nature of those timing requirements depends upon several factors. For pyramidal cells in layer 5 the effects require apical activation within about 15 ms either before or after direct somatic activation, but in some other pyramidal cells it occurs only if apical activation occurs within about 15 ms after somatic activation. In the rodent PFC, the class of pyramidal cells that provides the main output from the neocortex requires the coincidence to be much more precise than do those that project to other cortical regions.[12]

The phrase 'coincidence detection' is also used to refer to the nonlinear interactions that occur between near simultaneous inputs to small dendritic segments or spines. As the operation of N-methyl-D-aspartate (NMDA) receptors for glutamate is voltage-dependent, it can produce a supralinear summation that is common to both apical and basal dendrites. It must be distinguished from the coincidence between apical and basal activations for which BAC firing is a mechanism.

BAC firing is not the only mechanism for apical amplification. In rodents, BAC firing has been most convincingly demonstrated in layer 5b cells, but, for humans (at least), apical amplification may also occur in layer 2 and 3 cells by other mechanisms. One important difference between cells in the upper and lower layers is that the apical trunks of pyramidal cells in higher layers are substantially shorter and thinner. Another is that NMDA spikes may be adequate to enable apical input enhanced response to feedforward input in pyramidal cells that are in layers 2 and 3.[13] NMDA spikes involve the activation of a particular class of synaptic receptor for the excitatory neurotransmitter glutamate. Chapter 7 discusses psychotic and neurological disorders involving reduced ion flow through NMDA receptors.

Although it is difficult to study apical function directly in individual pyramidal cells in the whole living brain, it has been done in the motor cortex of anesthetized mice. It is especially difficult when animals are not anesthetized but awake, but studies have been done in rodents, for example, in the somatosensory cortex, in the PFC, in the somatosensory cortex, and in the whisker cortex while the animals performed an object-localization task.[14]

So far, I have focused on evidence for amplification of the response to basal activation by apical activation. Figure 3.4e shows that, if strong enough, direct activation of the apical integration zone can drive a brief burst of output spikes by itself in the absence of direct somatic stimulation. Similar effects of strong apical activation have also been observed in other labs. Here they are referred to as apical drive. If this occurs in perceptual systems outputs generated solely by will need to be distinguished from amplification, because the former could be misperceived as arising from events in the external world, rather than from internal sources. However, apical drive has most often been observed in physiological experiments where the apical integration zone is directly activated. That avoids the various dendritic and inhibitory mechanisms that constrain the level to which it is usually activated, so those findings may not be representative of the cell's usual mode of operation. Indeed, direct recordings of pyramidal cell responses to physiologically realistic somatic and apical inputs found that very few were generated by apical activation alone.[15] Nevertheless, there are also good reasons to suppose that apical drive does sometimes occur naturally, with fundamental implications for dreaming (Chapter 4) and for our understanding of relations between perception, memory, and imagination (Chapter 5). I assume that other complexities and subtleties of intracellular operations with implications for cellular and psychology will be discovered as evidence continues to accumulate about the cellular foundations of mental life.

3.4 On the Diversity of Pyramidal Cells

It is always tempting to treat individual members of a large population of similar things as being essentially equivalent. That works well for simple things such as atoms, and is the basis of thermodynamics, which is one of the most validated theories in physics. However, it is far from adequate to ignore differences between more complex things, such as neurons or people. Assuming that, from a functional point of view, all pyramidal cells can be treated as though they are all simple point neurons greatly underestimates their capabilities and diversity, and thus those of the systems that they together create.

Pyramidal cells vary depending on species, age, neocortical region, cortical layer, apical trunk length, apical branch size, projection sites, intrinsic electrophysiological properties, gene expression, and other molecular differences.[16] Furthermore, given the complexity of their dendritic trees and axonal projections, it is unlikely that any two pyramidal cells have identical inputs or outputs. The potential merits of diversity are easy to see by analogy to the specialization of human labour, which creates ways of life that would be impossible without it. By making distinctive contributions that are well suited to the whole of which they are a part, they greatly increase the chances that both they and it survive and flourish.

There is an important distinction between pyramidal cells in the neocortex and those in the primary olfactory regions or hippocampus. The six-layered neocortex has expanded greatly on an evolutionary timescale, but the more ancient three-layered cortex of olfactory regions and hippocampus have not.

That difference in evolutionary potential may be due to the enhanced ability of neocortical pyramidal cells to operate as context-sensitive two-point processors. There is some evidence that hippocampal pyramidal cells may have two functionally distinct sites of integration, and that has inspired an algorithm that can rapidly learn different maps for different places and use them in the appropriate contexts[17]. Nevertheless, it is probable that neocortical pyramidal cells have evolved more effective and efficient context-sensitive cooperative computational capabilities (Chapter 6).

Within the neocortex, pyramidal cells are also differentiated by the sources of their inputs, by the cortical layer in which their soma is located, by the anatomy of their dendrites, and by the targets of their outputs. Much of the excitatory input to neocortical pyramidal cells comes from nearby pyramidal neurons of the same class, with only a minority of feedforward input from distant sources. Pyramidal cells in layers 2 and 3 receive up to about 70% of their excitatory input from nearby cells in the same layer. They receive some of their feedforward input directly and some via cells in layer 4. Cells in layer 5 receive much less of their excitatory input from nearby cells, but it is still only a small proportion of their excitatory input that comes from distant feedforward sources. Nevertheless, despite their long-range feedforward inputs being in a minority, pyramidal cells in these local cortical microcircuits can reliably extract information from their inter-regional feedforward inputs and transmit it onwards for further processing.[18]

Pyramidal cells in layer 5 differ from those in layers 2 and 3 in that their apical trunks are longer. The lengths of apical trunks can vary even within a cortical region, with major functional consequences. The part of the rat primary visual cortex that is sensitive to things moving above them, such as predators, is thinner than other parts of their primary visual cortex, so the apical trunks of layer 5 cells there are shorter. Consequently, those neurons are more electrically compact. Figure 3.7 shows how excitatory input to these apical dendrites spreads to the soma, where it is integrated with other inputs to generate action potentials. In other parts of visual cortex where the apical trunks are longer, apical inputs are integrated separately from those of the basal inputs to the soma and contribute to output in a way that is fundamentally different from that of basal inputs.[19] Thus, differences in the length of apical trunks due to differences in cortical thickness are closely associated with differences in apical function. In most mammals, most of neocortex is at least as thick as that associated with the presence of pyramidal cells that have a functionally distinct site of apical integration. The extent to which the length of the apical trunk predicts apical function across regions and species is not yet clear, but

NEOCORTICAL THICKNESS GRADIENT

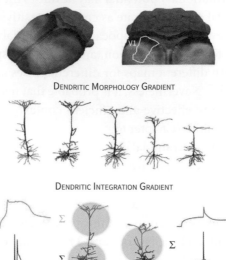

DENDRITIC MORPHOLOGY GRADIENT

DENDRITIC INTEGRATION GRADIENT

Figure 3.7   Rat neocortex is thickest (red) in frontal regions, and thinnest in posterior regions (blue). It can vary even within a single region (e.g. primary visual cortex, V1). The layer 5 cells shown are from progressively thinner parts of V1. Those with apical trunks longer than about 480 μm function as two-point neurons with a functionally distinct apical site of integration, as depicted by the blue summation sign. Those with shorter trunks function as point neurons.

Adapted from Fletcher & Williams, 2019, as approved by Stephen Williams, with permission from Elsevier.

it is likely that many parts, though not all, of the neocortex contain context-sensitive cooperative neurons.

Pyramidal cells can also be differentiated by their projection sites. All project to other cells in or near their own cortical column, but their long-range projections differ. Section 2.6 discusses how pyramidal neurons that project to distant sites within the neocortex are referred to as intra-telencephalic (IT) cells. Those that provide output from the neocortex to subcortical sites (including the pons, striatum, brainstem, and thalamus) are referred to as pyramidal tract (PT) cells. Finally, those that project to primary sensory specific thalamus, or to nonspecific thalamus, or to both are referred to as cortico-thalamic (CT) cells.

The subtype of pyramidal cell that provides the paradigmatic example of context-sensitive cooperative neurons are the PT cells that provide output from all regions of cortex, including primary sensory regions. The cell bodies of these cells are in the lower parts of layer 5 and have more extensive apical branches in layer 1 than other classes of pyramidal neuron. These thick-tufted layer-5 neurons have a pivotal role in neocortical information processing and are the principal output pathway from the neocortex to other sites. Within the neocortex, they have strong recurrent connections with other pyramidal cells in the same cortical column and have modulatory effects on neocortical pyramidal cells in other columns via their effects on the higher-order thalamus. They are sensitive to input to all cortical layers, either directly or via pyramidal cells in other layers. They have long apical dendrites, and the highest density of HCN channels. Nevertheless, the mean activity level of these layer 5 cells is high. As they have the most extensive dendrites in layer 1, they are among the most context-sensitive of all neurons. Those that receive feedforward input from the senses provide the most direct and fastest route into and out of the cerebral cortex. They also operate on a coarser spatial scale than cells in levels 2 and 3, so they may contribute to a processing style that operates at a coarse spatial scale initially, but which rapidly becomes more spatially refined. Finally, synaptic plasticity in these cells is highly dependent on the calcium currents in their apical dendrite, so the contribution of these cells to learning is highly context-sensitive.[20]

As thick-tufted cells in layer 5 have the widest local dendritic and axonal trees, they can be seen as specifying the extent of a local neocortical microcircuit. Francis Crick used his final three decades of life to explore potential relations between brain and mind and concluded that these layer 5 pyramidal cells have a key role in conscious experience.[21] As noted in later chapters, that view is supported by evidence that their apical dendrites are a key link in corticothalamic reverberatory loops. Nevertheless, as suggested above in 3.3.4, those may not be the only pyramidal cells that can function as context-sensitive cooperative neurons. Even if it is only that class of layer 5 pyramidal cells that are context-sensitive in mice, other classes may also be able to operate in that way in humans (see Chapter 6). Furthermore, even if layer 5 PT cells were the only subtype of pyramidal cell to be sensitive to context, that sensitivity would be conveyed to all the other neocortical pyramidal cells to which they project, either directly or indirectly via higher-order thalamic nuclei.

3.5 Inhibition and Disinhibition of Apical Function

Dynamic constraints on apical function are necessary because positive feedback via apical dendrites would produce overactivation if not appropriately restrained. Chapter 4 discusses ways in which apical function is both engaged and restrained by subcortical arousal systems. Here, the focus is on the local neocortical microcircuit where inhibitory interneurons regulate the balance between the effects of basal and apical inputs by inhibiting or disinhibiting apical dendrites with great local specificity. One subtype of inhibitory interneuron directly inhibits the soma, and another inhibits apical function and disinhibits the soma. A third produces disinhibition by inhibiting the other two, but it disinhibits apical function more than it disinhibits the soma, thus enhancing the extent to which the cell's output is sensitive to context.

Let us embrace the complexities of the wide array of inhibitory interneurons. In perceptual systems, information about the external world reaches the soma via the basal dendrites, whereas information from the stimulus context and internal sources is conveyed to the cell via its apical dendrites. So, when the effects of context are suppressed by inhibitory interneurons that specifically target apical dendrites, the cell's output becomes less context-sensitive, and more dependent simply on feedforward input. When interneurons that inhibit apical dendrites are themselves inhibited by another class of interneuron, however, then a window of opportunity is opened for apical input to amplify the cell's response to coincident basal input. This highly selective disinhibition of apical dendrites has radical implications for mental life (see Chapter 5).

3.5.1 The Three Main Classes of Inhibitory Interneuron

Figure 3.8 shows the inhibitory interneurons that densely surround pyramidal cells in the neocortex. They are activated by long-range input and inhibit nearby pyramidal cells and other interneurons, producing complex effects that are sometimes counterintuitive. All inhibitory interneurons are to some extent activated by the pyramidal cells that they inhibit. It is now clear that inhibitory interneurons can be classified into subtypes depending upon whether they predominantly affect basal and perisomatic locations or the more distant apical locations. Parvalbumin positive (PV) interneurons inhibit the basal dendrites and perisomatic regions of nearby pyramidal cells. Somatostatin positive (SST, aka SOM) and neurogliaform (NGF) interneurons inhibit their apical integration zone and apical branches. Vasoactive intestinal peptide positive (VIP) interneurons inhibit the other classes of inhibitory cell but inhibit SST cells most strongly. These subtypes of inhibitory interneuron have been shown to differ in several ways: in their shape, in their inputs and outputs, in the layers in which they are found, and in their distinctive molecular

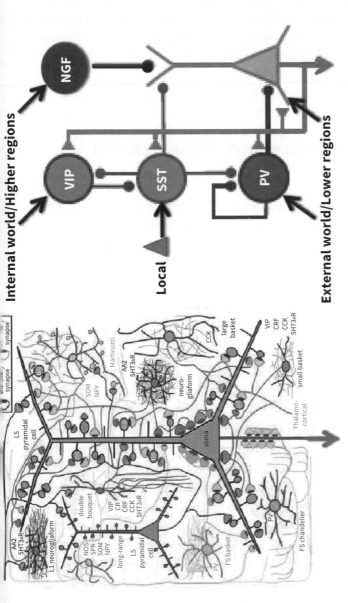

Internal world/Higher regions

Local

External world/Lower regions

Figure 3.8 Pyramidal cells are surrounded by inhibitory interneurons. The left panel shows nine kinds of inhibitory interneuron. Many inhibit themselves or other inhibitory cells in addition to the effects that they have on pyramidal cells. The right panel simplifies these complexities by putting inhibitory interneurons into sub-groups shown as circles. Only the strongest connections are shown. Somatostatin positive cells (SST cells, aka SOM cells) predominantly inhibit apical dendrites, whereas parvalbumin positive (PV) cells inhibit the basal dendrites and soma. Vasoactive intestinal peptide positive (VIP) cells inhibit several other classes of interneuron, but they inhibit SST cells more strongly than they inhibit PV cells. Pyramidal cells activate PV, SST, and VIP cells, thus tending to generate inhibitory feedback to themselves. Neurogliaform cells (NGF) also inhibit distal apical dendrites. Although several complexities remain to be discovered, there is now adequate evidence for distinguishing inhibitory regulation of apical input from that of basal/perisomatic input.

The panel on the left is from Kubota et al., 2016, as approved by Yoshiyuki Kubota. The panel on the right is modified from Wang & Yang, 2018, as approved by Xiao-Jing Wang, with permission from Elsevier.

contents (from which the labels PV, SST, and VIP are derived). The molecular differences play a leading role in guiding the embryological and developmental processes that construct the underlying skeleton of neocortical microcircuitry. This empirically based classification of inhibitory interneurons has been inferred from diverse methodologies that are logically independent of the evidence for the conception of cooperative two-point neurons. Therefore, it further strengthens and develops that conception.[22] The molecular contents also distinguish primate from rodent cortex, and the evolutionary variations on these inhibitory and disinhibitory themes are discussed in Chapter 6.

3.5.2   Two Classes of Interneuron Selectively Inhibit Apical Dendrites

SST and NGF interneurons both inhibit apical dendrites, but not the basal dendrites or soma. SST interneurons differ from other inhibitory interneurons in that their synaptic inputs are facilitating, which means that they respond to the second of two input pulses more strongly than to the first. The consequence of this is that activating SST cells tends to restrict pyramidal cell bursting to one or only a few bursts. Activating SST cells also inhibits interneurons that inhibit the soma, so, in addition to inhibiting apical function, they also disinhibit the soma. Thus, SST cell activation weakens the effects of input to the apical dendrites while strengthening the effects of more direct inputs to the soma. Thus, it weakens the effects of context relative to the effects of feedforward inputs, which, in neocortical perceptual systems, comes from external sources.

Inhibition restricted specifically to apical function was directly demonstrated by combining paired apical and somatic stimulation with stimulation of a nearby inhibitory interneuron located in the upper layers of neocortex. Figure 3.9 shows the clear results. Inhibition from that specific kind of interneuron blocked the burst of spikes that was dependent on apical input, but not the initial output spike that was dependent on direct somatic input.[23] This apical inhibition lasted up to 400 ms, which is long lasting on the physiological timescale of cognitive operations in the neocortex. It is also long lasting on the timescale of interactions between the effects of stimuli presented at slightly different times as studied in psychophysical experiments.[24]

Studies of interactions between the two cerebral hemispheres have cast further light on the effects of inhibition of apical function and its relation to basic cognitive phenomena. Psychologists and neurologists have long known

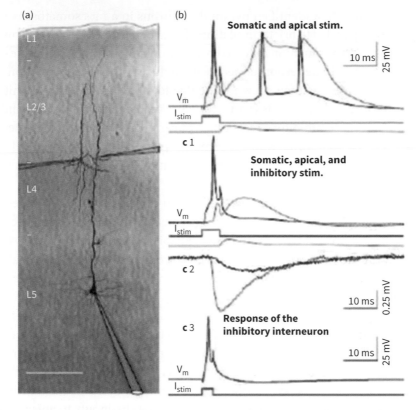

Figure 3.9 Activation of an inhibitory interneuron (blue in panel a) blocks effects of apical depolarization but does not affect the initial output spike caused by somatic depolarization. Microelectrodes for stimulating and recording responses are shown in black at the soma, in red at the top of the apical dendrite, and in blue at the inhibitory interneuron. Three output spikes (black in panel b) are produced when the apical integration site is activated soon after the somatic site. If the inhibitory interneuron is also stimulated (blue in the bottom traces), then the initial output spike produced in response to somatic stimulation is unaffected, but the two additional spikes due to coincident apical input do not occur.

Modified from Larkum, Zhu, & Sakmann, 1999, with the approval of Matthew Larkum and permission from Springer.

that sensitivity to stimulation on one side of the body is reduced by coincident stimulation of the matching site on the opposite side of the body. They also know that several disorders of attention, such as unilateral spatial neglect, arise from impaired interaction between the hemispheres. These interactions have much to tell us about apical function because the cross-hemisphere connections target apical dendrites and their inhibitory interneurons, and also because selective attention involves apical dendrites. Experiments capitalizing on that potential first identified pyramidal neurons in a rat's somatosensory cortex that responded to brief stimulation of a particular site on one of its hind paws. When that stimulation followed brief stimulation of a matching site on the other hind paw the response was greatly reduced. This large reduction in the cell's response was then shown to be due to a particular class of inhibitory receptors that have effects lasting for more than a hundred milliseconds. Activation of these inhibitory receptors by nearby interneurons disconnects the apical integration zone from the soma by activating potassium ion channels and by blocking calcium ion channels, both of which are plentiful in apical dendrites.[25]

The effects of apical inhibition have also been clarified by studying slices of rat somatosensory cortex. In the absence of apical inhibition, bursting occurs if the soma is activated when both basal and apical dendrites receive physiologically realistic excitatory inputs. The apical contribution to output, that is, the burst, is suppressed if inhibitory receptors on the apical dendrites are activated together with the excitatory inputs.[26]

Consequences of inhibition that should be more widely known, are its effects on the leakage current flow through the HCN ion channels outlined in Section 3.3. These highly idiosyncratic ion channels are mainly located on the apical dendrites and are open when pyramidal cells are at or below the action potential threshold. When open, these channels decrease the extent of spatiotemporal integration, thus reducing effects of the inputs to apical synapses that are distant from the apical integration zone. As the pyramidal cell becomes activated, however, leakage through the HCN channels is reduced, allowing apical inputs to affect the cell's output.[27] Thus, inhibition of apical dendrites tends to reduce the effect of apical inputs on the soma by opening HCN channels. Apical disinhibition has the opposite effect: it increases the pyramidal cell's sensitivity to its contextual input. Consequently, the selective disinhibition of apical function, to which we now turn, has rich functional implications.

3.5.3 Some Interneurons Selectively Disinhibit Apical Dendrites

Though much remains to be discovered about disinhibition, there is an emerging consensus that VIP interneurons predominantly disinhibit apical function. They do so by suppressing activity of the inhibitory interneurons that project to the apical dendrites, that is, SST interneurons. SST interneurons project to the apical dendrites of most pyramidal cells in their neighbour-hood, thus casting a wide blanket of inhibition over apical function. The disinhibitory effects of VIP interneurons have a more limited spatial extent, however, so they make temporary holes at a few selected places in that blanket of sustained apical inhibition.[28]

Disinhibitory effects on apical function have long been thought likely. The little evidence available in 1999 suggested that, under normal circumstances and with background inhibition, the activity of pyramidal cells depends mostly on somatic integrative properties alone until the inhibition of apical input is released for long enough for it to contribute to the cell's output.[29] Thus, disinhibition of the apical inputs to selected pyramidal cells increases their context-sensitivity. It disinhibits the effects of excitatory apical input and reduces the disinhibition of basal/perisomatic excitatory input. So, activation of the disinhibitory VIP interneurons increases the extent to which pyramidal cell activity is affected by internal mental state, current goals, and stimulus context.[30]

We now know that VIP interneurons mediate effects of stimulus and task context and receive inputs from sources that have information about that con-text. Their inputs are diverse, including excitatory inputs from higher cor-tical areas and the higher-order thalamus. Furthermore, a large part of the input to VIP inhibitory interneurons from higher cortical regions is from the layer 5 cells whose activity is so sensitive to apical inputs. During auditory discrimination, VIP neurons in the auditory and prefrontal areas are acti-vated by reinforcing signals. Excitatory inputs to VIP interneurons from the motor cortex disinhibit the relevant pyramidal cells in sensory cortex when rodents are actively using their whiskers to explore the environment. Input to VIP interneurons from the cingulate region of the PFC to layer 1 of the pri-mary visual cortex (V1) enhances its response to visual input and improves visual discrimination. Local activation of axons in V1 from the cingulate re-gion of neocortex amplifies responses to feedforward input at that location and attenuates responses to input at nearby locations as in centre-surround suppression. Thus, SST interneurons may contribute to surround suppres-sion, whereas VIP interneurons are crucial for centre facilitation. Together with much other anatomical and physiological evidence, this all suggests that a common feature of long-distance communication in the cortex involves dis-inhibition of apical contributions to the outputs of pyramidal cells in a few highly selected cortical columns.[31]

Though this inhibitory–disinhibitory theme applies to all neocortical re-gions, there are variations. In sensory and motor regions, interneurons that inhibit apical dendrites are less abundant than interneurons that inhibit the soma. In cortical regions that are more distant from the sensorimotor surface, however, there are three to five times more interneurons that inhibit apical dendrites than those that inhibit the soma. Therefore, context-dependent selective disinhibition may be more differentiated in higher than in lower cortical regions.[32]

Implications for cognitive function and malfunction of apical inhibition and disinhibition are discussed in later chapters. Here, we note just two simple implications. First, as these inhibitory effects are often silent (in the sense that they are not observable at the soma unless it is active), they cannot be due to any simple summing of excitatory and inhibitory inputs. Thus, this provides direct evidence against the widespread assumption that all pyramidal cells function simply as leaky integrate-and-fire point neurons.[33] Second, there are also implications for the popular hypothesis that descending feedback signals suppress transmission of matching feedforward signals to compute what are referred to as 'prediction errors'. On the contrary, the evidence for coincidence detection reviewed here indicates that feedback amplifies the transmission of information about the feedforward signals when that coincides with activation of the apical dendrites in layer 1 by information from various sources, including feedback. Furthermore, though the notion of prediction error has become prominent within the theory of predictive coding, the evidence reviewed here implies that apical amplification and attenuation are concerned with regulating the salience of neuronal signals, not with changing what they code for, as argued further in Section 9.2.

Regional variations in the relative densities of the different classes of inhibitory interneuron strongly suggest that cooperative context-sensitivity is of even greater importance at higher than at lower levels of the cortical hierarchy, as outlined in Section 9.8.

3.6 Research on Cooperative Context-sensitivity Is in Its Infancy

The infancy of research on cooperative context-sensitive neurons is clear in the many unresolved issues noted throughout this book. One simple consequence is that the full extent of that class of neuron is not yet known. It is provisionally defined here as neurons that can cooperate by using one subset of their inputs to amplify or attenuate the transmission of information extracted from another subset of their inputs. This leaves it open for future research to discover more precisely which classes of neuron do or do not have that capability. As so many criteria can be used to distinguish different classes of pyramidal cell, including cortical layer, region, species, and stage of development, it is not feasible to settle that issue by direct observation for every possible class of pyramidal neuron. So, until that becomes feasible (if ever!), we will have to rely on inferences from cases where that capability has been directly demonstrated. Thick-tufted neurons in layer 5b of the neocortex are the paradigmatic example of neurons those having this capability. A mechanism by which context-sensitivity can operate in those cells is BAC firing. Much of the direct evidence for this comes from layer 5 cells of sensory and prefrontal regions of rodent cortex. Studies of rodent visual cortex shows that layer 5 pyramidal cells are likely to have two functionally distinct points of integration if their apical trunks are longer than about half a millimetre (Figure 3.7). Many pyramidal cells in layer 5 of mature cortical regions in many species meet that simple criterion. There is also evidence that apical amplification occurs in some pyramidal cells of layers 2 and 3, though via mechanisms that may differ from those in layer 5 cells (Section 3.3), so the issue of the full extent of the class of neuron that can function as context-sensitive cooperative neurons remains open.

Even if apical amplification were to occur only in layer 5 cells, it would still have a central role in neocortical information processing, because layer 5 cells are in a feedback loop with pyramidal cells in other layers of the neocortex, either directly or indirectly via higher-order non-specific thalamic nuclei, so cells in all layers of the cortex are presumably affected by the context-sensitivity of layer 5 cells.

3.7 Summary and Rapid Growth of This Research Field

This chapter has focused on ways in which neocortical pyramidal cells cooperate by having apical dendrites that are sensitive to context. Section 3.1 discussed the need for temporary relaxation of doubts concerning all attempts to relate mental life to processes that occur within individual cells.

Section 3.2 outlined the soma, axon, dendrites, and synapses that characterize pyramidal neurons. The soma is the cell body housing its DNA, etc., and it generates the sequence of all-or-nothing action potentials that are conveyed to other neurons via an axon that has many bifurcations. The axon projects to the dendrites of other neurons, which are complex branching structures through which the cell receives much of its input. The spike train affects the dendrites to which it projects by releasing a neurotransmitter into the narrow synaptic gap that separates them. These neurotransmitters bind to specific receptor molecules embedded in the post-synaptic membrane, thereby initiating high-speed electrical and slower biochemical events within the postsynaptic cell.

Section 3.3 showed that, for many pyramidal cells, the distinction between their apical and basal dendrites is crucial to their function. This distinction is most obvious for the layer 5 pyramidal cells (Figure 3.3) The section also covered the simple, but radical, hypothesis that some pyramidal cells may function, not as single-point processors, but as two-point processors. Activation of the apical integration zone that has little or no effect on output by itself can greatly increase response to basal activation occurring at about the same time. Far more work has been done on the effects of coincidence between apical and basal activation than outlined here, but, overall, it indicates that a major mode of apical function is to amplify response to basal activation. Later chapters discuss implications of these different modes of apical function for mental life and its disorders.

Section 3.4 outlines pyramidal cell diversity and how these cells are adapted for different purposes in different species, cortical regions, and layers. Many, but not all, can function as context-sensitive two-point processors. They are more likely to be able to function in that way if their apical trunk is longer than about half a millimetre, as are those of many neocortical pyramidal neurons, especially in humans.

Section 3.5 outlined apical inhibition and disinhibition. Apical and basal dendrites are inhibited by separate classes of inhibitory interneuron, which provides further grounds for distinguishing between basal and apical inputs. Locally selective disinhibition of the effects of apical activation is viewed as a mechanism for amplifying the cell's output only when it is particularly relevant to external circumstances and internal states and intentions.

Section 3.6 defined cooperative neurons as pyramidal cells that can use input to one subset of inputs (e.g. those to the apical dendrites) to amplify or attenuate the transmission of information extracted from the other inputs (e.g. the feedforward inputs to the basal dendrites) when there is coincident depolarization (excitation) of both subsets. It notes that which subtypes of pyramidal cell can function as cooperative neurons is only partly known.

Finally, why do I use 'cooperative' to describe pyramidal cells that are sensitive to context? One simple reason is that they operate in reliable, mutually supportive, collectives called population codes (left panel Figure 3.3), although they could do that whether or not they were sensitive to context. The more important reason is that, by enhancing the transmission of information about their basal excitation when it coincides with excitatory apical input, they enhance the coherence and effectiveness of the system's overall activity. This context-sensitive cooperative mode of operation greatly enhances the effectiveness and efficiency of the joint enterprise in which those neurons are engaged.

Though many fundamental issues remain to be explored, research on issues central to cellular psychology and the neuroscience on which it depends is now growing rapidly, as demonstrated by several major review papers, of which only a few examples are given here. Reviews by Larkum (2013), Major and colleagues (2013), and by Ramaswamy and Markram (2015) show that layer 5 thick-tufted pyramidal neurons have two functionally distinct points of integration. Schuman and colleagues (2021) show that apical dendrites in layer 1 are the main route by which top-down and other contextual input reaches pyramidal cells. That makes it likely that at least some cells in layers 2 and 3 can also operate as context-sensitive cooperative neurons because in many regions of many species those cells have apical dendrites in layer 1 and apical trunks longer than about half a millimetre. Aru, Suzuki, and Larkum (2020a) and Shepherd and Yamawaki (2021) clearly and convincingly review evidence that the thalamocortical loops with a key role in conscious experience depend on apical dendrites in layer 1. Larkum and colleagues (2018) review studies relating the neurophysiological evidence for context-sensitive two-point neurons to ultra-high resolution functional neuroimaging of human neocortex. Nelson and Bender (2021) show convincingly how impairments of apical dendritic function have a key role in some common neurodevelopmental disorders, including autism spectrum disorders. They show how these apical dendritic mechanisms are rooted in their genetic foundations and identify specific genetic mutations that impair these fundamental cellular mechanisms. Finally, Tantirigama and colleagues (2020) and Shine and colleagues (2021) review evidence showing unequivocally that changes in brain state (e.g. those from sleeping to waking or from low to high arousal) depend on the neuromodulatory regulation of apical function in pyramidal cells. Chapter 4 explores the far-reaching implications of that neuromodulatory regulation of apical function.

A relevant new technology with great potential is two-photon calcium imaging (2PCI). This can image local post-synaptic activity within many cells simultaneously and with a spatial precision that distinguishes individual dendrites and the spines on them, and with a temporal resolution of 1 millisecond or less (e.g. Szalay et al., 2016; Kerlin et al., 2019). Many of the unresolved issues raised in this book can be studied using 2PCI, particularly if it is combined with the computational modelling and three-way mutual information decomposition that is outlined in Chapter 8.

Notes

1. Ryan and Grant (2009) review evidence on evolutionary changes in post-synaptic complexity and relate them to changes in behavioural capabilities.
2. Bartlett Mel and colleagues have long been leading advocates of advancing beyond the over-simplified point neuron assumption (e.g. Jadi et al., 2014; Tzilivaki, Kastellakis, & Poirazi, 2019; Poirazi & Papoutsi, 2020).
3. Rolls (2014) defines the integrate-and-fire assumption precisely and provides a voluminous and representative example of the extent to which it has dominated twentieth-century theories of relations between brain and mind.
4. Magee and Cook (2000) reported evidence for a 'dendritic democracy'. However, that evidence was predominantly concerned with pyramidal cells in the hippocampus, and not with cells in neocortex.
5. LeDoux (2002) presents a lucid introduction to evidence that synapses have a central role in creating the person that we become. In addition to relating it to learning and memory, LeDoux relates many aspects of mental life to the synaptic level, including developmental changes, working memory, consciousness, emotions, motivation, and reward. He interprets psychosis, depression, anxiety, and addiction as forms of 'synaptic sickness', and uses these interpretations to explain the effects of various pharmacotherapies.
6. For reviews of the early evidence that some classes of pyramidal cell can function as two-point neurons, see Larkum (2013) and Major, Larkum, and Schiller (2013).
7. Cauller and Connors (1994) and Cauller (1995) were among the first papers to see that apical dendrites in layer 1 may have fundamentally different functions from basal dendrites. About 90% of the input to layer 1 consists of long-range connections from distant parts of the neocortex and subcortical nuclei, with only about 10% coming from nearby neurons. The incoming axons arriving at layer 1 are mostly excitatory and connect directly to the apical dendrites of pyramidal cells. Some connect to inhibitory interneurons, but whether that inhibits or disinhibits the apical dendrites depends on which type of interneuron they connect to (see Section 3.5).
8. Williams & Stuart, 2002.
9. Biel and colleagues (2009) provide a broad overview of HCN ion channels and their functions. On the basis of simultaneous whole-cell current-clamp recordings in the apical trunk and apical branches, Harnett, Magee, and Williams (2015) conclude that ion flow through HCN channels has an excitatory effect at somatic and proximal apical trunk sites but reduces the effects of apical input on the cell's output.
10. Poirazi and Papoutsi (2020) show that the field of dendritic computation is growing rapidly with a major role for the distinctive functions of apical dendrites.
11. Rubio-Garrido et al., 2009.
12. Ledergerber and Larkum (2012) showed that cells in different layers of rodent somatosensory cortex have different sensitivities to precise timing.

13. Palmer and colleagues (2014) showed that NMDA receptors have a role in coupling the apical branches to the soma in layer 2/3 cells. Amplifying effects of apical depolarization that probably operate by mechanisms other than BAC firing are reported by Larkum and colleagues (2007), Ledergerber and Larkum (2012), and by Boudewijns and colleagues (2013).

14. Palmer and colleagues (2014) studied anesthetized rodents. Murayama and Larkum (2009), Boudewijns and colleagues (2013), and Xu and colleagues (2012) studied the function of apical dendrites in awake rodents.

15. Schulz et al., 2021.

16. Luebke, 2017; Radnikow & Feldmeyer, 2018.

17. Haga & Fukai, 2018.

18. Douglas & Martin, 2008.

19. Fletcher & Williams, 2019.

20. Ramaswamy and Markram (2015) provide a comprehensive review of all these properties of thick-tufted layer 5 pyramidal neurons. Baker and colleagues (2018) provide an in-depth review of the main subtypes of pyramidal neuron in layers 5 and 6.

21. Crick, 1994.

22. There are many reviews of the main classes of inhibitory interneuron and their subtypes. Those that I have found especially helpful are Harris and Shepherd (2015), van Versendaal and Levelt (2016), and Tremblay and colleagues (2016). The most recent, and most clearly supportive of the conception of context-sensitive neurons with two points of integration, is by Schuman and colleagues (2021).

23. This direct physiological demonstration of the effect of inhibitory interneurons on apical function was by Larkum, Zhu, and Sakmann (199).

24. Psychophysical phenomena occurring on fast time-scales and closely related to apical function are reviewed in depth by Bachmann (2015).

25. Palmer and colleagues (2013) review the role of apical dendrites in inhibitory interactions between the neocortical hemispheres.

26. Schulz & Larkum, 2021.

27. For relations between HCN channel current and apical function see Harnett, Magee, and Williams (2015).

28. Karnani et al., 2014.

29. From the beginning of their research on apical function Larkum, Zhu, and Sakmann (1999) correctly assumed that apical disinhibition has a central role in neocortical information processing.

30. Several papers review evidence that apical disinhibition is a central theme of inhibitory microcircuitry (see, for example, Wang et al, 2004; Harris & Shepherd, 2015; Wang & Yang, 2018; Hertag & Sprekeler, 2019; and Schuman et al., 2021).

31. Wall and colleagues (2016) present an extensive review of the sources of input to all classes of inhibitory interneuron. Letzkus and colleagues (2015) review much of the evidence on disinhibition. Zhang and colleagues (2014a) show that surround suppression depends on SST interneurons, whereas centre facilitation depends on VIP interneurons. Hertag and Sprekeler (2019) report computational investigations of the functional consequences of interactions between SST and VIP interneurons. They conclude that the inhibitory–disinhibitory motif is region and task specific, that inputs to the neurons that disinhibit apical dendrites are highly diverse with strong contributions from cholinergic

and serotonergic systems, and that activation of SST inhibitory interneurons reduces the contribution of apical activation to the cell's output, whereas activation of VIP inhibitory interneurons increases it.

32. As part of their physiological and computational argument for a disinhibitory motif in neocortex, Wang and Yang (2018) review evidence showing that there are large regional differences in the relative proportions of SST and VIP cells and offer a computational rationale for these differences.

33. Schulz et al., 2018.

4

Cooperative Neurons in Various States of Mind and Brain

This chapter discusses the differences between wakefulness, slow-wave sleep (SWS), and the rapid eye movement (REM) sleep in which dreams are more likely to occur. It concludes that context-sensitive pyramidal cells operate in different ways in these different states. Transitions between states are regulated by modulatory neurotransmitters, for example, acetylcholine, noradrenaline (NA), serotonin, and dopamine (DA). NA is also often called norepinephrine (NE), and these variations in terminology tend to obscure the central issues with which we are concerned. In addition to overcoming such terminological difficulties we must also distinguish between different kinds of receptor for each of the neuromodulators.

One of the main ways in which neuromodulators affect neocortical activity is by controlling the mode of apical function. In addition to the amplifying and driving modes of function outlined in Chapter 3, there is a third mode called 'apical isolation'. When awake, apical input in perceptual regions usually operates in amplifying mode. As the level of arousal increases, so too does amplification of the selected activities, and the selection criteria become more narrowly focused. Apical drive is the extreme mode of function in which apical input alone is strong enough to generate pyramidal cell responses, for example, in dreaming or thought. Apical isolation is the mode of function in which apical input has little or no effect on the cell's output, for example, as in deep sleep (SWS). Anaesthesia is shown to provide further evidence that mental state depends on apical function. Finally, Table 4.1 shows that dreaming is like wakeful states in many ways as well as like dreamless sleep in many ways, so, these similarities and differences cast doubt on intuitive conceptions of 'consciousness'.

Physical activity, heart rate, breathing, cortisol production, and many other physiological variables change as arousal increases, and as these various physiological changes tend to be highly correlated it is commonly assumed that, to a first approximation, the overall level of physiological arousal can be quantified as a single variable. However, the various states of mind that we

The Cooperative Neuron. William A. Phillips, Oxford University Press. © Oxford University Press 2023.
DOI: 10.1093/oso/9780198876984.003.0005

are trying to understand cannot be adequately represented by the value of a single variable, for example, the level of arousal. Hobson (2009), who was a renowned expert on sleep and dreaming, characterizes differences in mental state using three dimensions on which brain state varies: activation (A), input–output gating (I), and modulation (M). (A) is roughly equivalent to the overall level of arousal. (I) determines the extent to which cortical activity is focused on internally generated thoughts, rather than being focused on sensorimotor interactions with the external world. (M) is the relative extent to which arousal depends on the aminergic neuromodulators NA, serotonin (5-HT), and histamine (HA), rather than on cholinergic arousal. From that point of view, brain state at any moment can be thought of as a particular point in a three-dimensional AIM space. During dreaming, for example, the neocortex is highly active, that activity is mostly disconnected from sensors and muscles, and there is high cholinergic but low aminergic arousal.

Although I have been contributing to the psychological and neurobiological sciences for several decades, the notion that pyramidal cells operate in fundamentally different ways in different mental states seemed very strange to me initially. That notion first arrived in my mind as an alien from an unknown domain. It now seems to be crucial to the foundations on which our radically new understanding of mind and brain is being built.

4.1 States of Wakefulness and States of Sleep

Wakefulness, deep sleep, and dreaming involve distinct states of muscle tone and of electroencephalographic (EEG) activity. When we are awake muscle tone is high and EEG activity has low amplitude and high frequency. When we are in dreamless SWS, muscle tone is low and EEG activity has high amplitude and low frequency. When we are dreaming there is a complete loss of muscle tone, EEG activity is much like that when awake, and there are usually rapid eye movements. It is often assumed that there are only a few distinct states, for example, waking, sleeping, or dreaming, and that transitions between these states are global, sudden, and well defined. However, 'altered states of consciousness' seem to be far more diverse than those basic distinctions suggest. Furthermore, although transitions between states can be abrupt, they can also be gradual, with properties that distinguish the different states being mixed to varying extents in the intermediate states.

Notions of arousal from the 1950s onwards were dominated by evidence for a network of nerve fibres that project from the brain stem to the neocortex both directly and via intermediary sites. A reticular activating system (RAS) that ascends from subcortical nuclei in the brain stem to all regions of neo-cortex was thought of as specifying a single overall level of arousal. However, we now know that the subcortical regulation of neocortical state is more dif-ferentiated than that, and that there are several different subcortical nuclei in the brain stem, which interact with each other as well as with the neocortex in complex ways, about which much remains to be discovered.[1]

The subcortical nuclei that induce sleep do so by actively opposing the arousing systems that promote wakefulness. Timing, depth, and duration of sleep depend on time of day, amount of prior wakefulness, and many other things. As our sleep debt (time spent awake) increases, so does our need to sleep; sleep debt is not cyclic, but continues to increase until paid off by ad-equate sleep. Though the functions of sleep are still not well understood, it is known to be common to mammals in general. From a metabolic point of view that is no surprise because wakefulness makes high demands on energy expenditure. Although the brain constitutes only 2% of body mass, its use of oxygen and glucose account for about 20% of all energy use when awake. Sleep reduces brain energy demands, resulting in a 44% reduction in glucose metabolism and a 25% reduction in the use of oxygen, although that does not explain why conscious experience must also cease for several hours a day.

As caffeine suppresses the effects of sleep debt and increases arousal, tea and coffee drinkers are well acquainted with their effects on mental state . Although caffeine is one of the most widely used of all psychoactive sub-stances, it is far from clear when its short-term benefits outweigh its long-term costs.

During REM sleep subcortical input arouses the neocortex in some ways but not in others, and it is during that kind of sleep that dreams are most likely to occur. Other typical phenomena of REM sleep include muscle atonia, in which the body goes limp, together with patterns of cortical EEG activity that seem more like being actively awake than being in slow wave sleep (SWS). Strong activation of limbic regions and of the amygdala during REM sleep is consistent with a strong emotional component in the origin and contents of dreams. The genetic and neural bases of wakefulness, SWS, and REM sleep are all strongly conserved throughout mammalian evolution, so we can assume that each of these three naturally occurring states have important functions.[2]

The neurobiological reality of these distinct brain states has been shown by prolonged observation of the relation between behaviour and electrical local field potentials in different parts of the brain. Local field potentials (LFPs) are like EEG measures but reflect activity in within locally specific popula-tions of neurons. This activity varies on a wide range of timescales, from rapid temporary phasic fluctuations lasting for only a few seconds or less to slower more sustained tonic levels that may last an hour or more. Figure 4.1 shows an example of measures of brain state based on LFPs, and relates a rat's behaviour to the two most informative aspects of LFPs recorded in four different parts of the brain: the neocortex, thalamus, hippocampus, and striatum (which is involved in the regulation of motor behaviour). Each tiny dot in Figure 4.1 plots the value of these two variables calculated from a one-second window on the LFPs. They are colour coded according to the observed behaviour at that moment. Densely occupied areas of the two-dimensional LFP graph show brain states in which much time was spent.

Although they overlap, the behavioural states categorized as SWS, REM, quietly awake, or actively awake are clearly related to distinct locations in the two-dimensional space defined by specific patterns of neocortical activity (Figure 4.1). The patterns distinguishing quiet from active waking as well as from REM and SWS are reliably seen in different individual rats. Though neuronal activity during active exploration is like that during quiet waking on the two measures of Figure 4.1, these two states are seen to be categorically distinct on measures of the coherence, or synchronization, of activity across sites. Synchronization of high frequency rhythms (>30 Hz) is weak during active exploration and SWS, moderate during quiet waking, and strong during REM. Synchronization between the neocortex and hippocampus at frequencies of 5–9 Hz was strong during both active exploration and REM, but weak

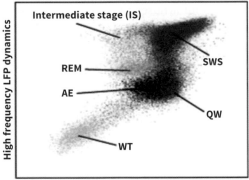

Figure 4.1 Relations between a rat's behaviour and electrical measures of neocortical activity reliably distinguish commonly recurring states and the transitions between them. The axes are two highly informative, but complex, variables defined on the electrical local field potentials (LFPs) recorded in the neocortex, thalamus, hippocampus, and striatum.

Modified from Gervasoni et al., 2004, as approved by Miguel Nicolelis.

during quiet waking and SWS. Thus, quiet waking is more like REM sleep than active waking in some ways, and more like SWS than active waking in other ways. The whisker-twitching state was not reliably seen in all individuals, and sometimes occurred together with LFP dynamics closer to the intermediate stage between SWS and REM sleep. The transition from SWS to REM always occurred via a stage intermediate between SWS and REM. Overall, some transitions between states were common, for example, between active and quiet waking, between quiet waking and SWS, between SWS and REM, and from REM to quiet waking. Other transitions, such as those directly from the awake states to REM, occurred rarely, if at all.[3] Though details of these states and transitions vary to some extent across as well as within species, EEG recordings show that state-dependent variations in the overall electrical activity of the neocortex are much the same for mammals in general.

The overall level of arousal varies continuously when awake and can do so rapidly. These changes are coupled with overt movements such as locomotion, but can also occur when not moving but simply attending intently, planning movements, or otherwise just 'thinking'. This net level of arousal can be predicted with high accuracy by the diameter of the pupil and its rate of change, both of which are coupled with the state of the autonomic nervous system (ANS). Neuronal responses to external stimulation change in at least four ways as the overall level of autonomic arousal increases: the amplification of relevant signals increases; signal to noise ratio improves; temporal precision of neuronal responses is increased; and their variability from moment-to-moment is reduced. In many tasks, and particularly in those that require prefrontal cortical (PFC) function, there is an inverted U relationship between the level of arousal and performance, such that performance is best at intermediate levels. The impairment of some cognitive functions at exceptionally high levels of arousal reflects a third state of wakefulness that arises during highly stressful states as shown in Figure 4.2.[4]

Although we can remain in a particular state for many minutes, or even a few hours, we can also be in transitional states in which properties of two or more of the prototypical states are mixed. One example of a mixed state is the intermediate state (IS) between SWS and REM sleep, but there are also other mixed states, particularly in the transitions between different levels of arousal when awake and in the different levels of arousal between quiet waking and SWS. More exotic mixtures can also occur. For example, lucid dream experiences combine dream content with self-awareness in the sense that, while it is a dream-like experience, the dreamer knows it is a dream. Narcolepsy is another example of a mixture, in which the loss of muscle tone characteristic of REM sleep can occur when awake. The reverse of that also occurs when actions that are part of the dream are not suppressed but performed, resulting in REM behavioural disorder. Courts of law considering illegal acts carried-out in such states cannot avoid making judgements concerning personal responsibility for those acts.

4.2 Modulatory Neurotransmitters Regulate Transitions between Mental States

The excitatory neurotransmitter glutamate and the inhibitory neurotransmitter GABA operate at synapses connecting neurons with high spatial specificity, so they are often described as being point-to-point. Neuromodulators are less spatially specific. When a neuromodulator is released, it diffuses over a greater distance than that occupied by a single synapse, so it affects many neurons around the release site. Neuromodulators also tend to operate over longer timescales than the excitatory and inhibitory inputs whose effects they modulate. The excitatory neurotransmitter glutamate and the inhibitory neurotransmitter GABA operate on the timescale of a few tens of milliseconds, whereas the neuromodulators fluctuate on timescales that range from a few seconds or less to many minutes or more.

The main neuromodulators by which subcortical systems affect neocortical function are acetylcholine (ACh), NA/NE, serotonin (5-HT), histamine (HA), orexin, and dopamine (DA). I refer to them collectively as neuromodulators, and individually as cholinergic arousal, adrenergic arousal, and so on (Figure 4.2). All are important, and much is known about them all. The primary focus here is on the cholinergic and aminergic arousal systems because they have a leading role in modulating overall arousal.[5] Though not directly concerned with the regulation of arousal, dopamine has a crucial impact on the contents of our subjective experience via its central role in motor control, decision making, and reward.

4.2.1 Acetylcholine Increases Neocortical Arousal

Acetylcholine has a prominent role in regulating arousal, vigilance, and attention. It is used by the parasympathetic division of the ANS, where its functions can be caricatured as rest and digest, that is, it relaxes bodily energy consumption by opposing energetic activities and enhancing more vegetative functions. In the neocortex it has arousing effects. Smokers are well acquainted

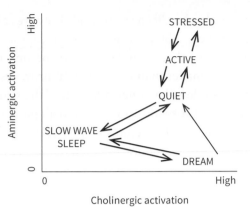

Figure 4.2 A qualitative depiction of levels of cholinergic and aminergic arousal during quiet, active, and stressed wakefulness as compared with those during dreaming and slow wave sleep. Aminergic arousal is the net result of adrenergic, serotonergic, and histaminergic levels of activity. There is no pretension of quantitative precision, so the axes are in arbitrary units. Levels of arousal are notional but range from the lowest to the highest levels likely to occur. Transitions are graded and can occur either gradually or abruptly. Levels of both cholinergic and aminergic arousal fluctuate during quiet, active, and stressed waking, with adrenergic fluctuations tending to be on a faster timescale than cholinergic fluctuations. Although high cholinergic arousal is combined with minimal aminergic arousal in dream states, there are no obvious examples of high aminergic arousal combined with low cholinergic arousal.

with some of its effects because nicotine enhances them. Cholinergic activation contributes to overall arousal by increasing cortical activation and enhancing cortical rhythms typical of wakefulness. When we are mentally or physically active there are large increases in cholinergic activation.[6] During dreaming an exceptionally high level of cholinergic activation is combined with an exceptionally low level of adrenergic arousal (Figure 4.2), so dreams lack the contribution of adrenergic arousal to mental state.

4.2.2 Adrenergic Activity Increases Neocortical Arousal

NA is used by the sympathetic division of the autonomic nervous. In the limit its arousing effects on mental state can produce an adrenaline-rush. Beta-blockers are used to manage cases where adrenergic activation becomes counter-productive because it increases anxiety. Most beta-blockers are aimed at the heart, but some are designed to cross the blood-brain barrier to reach the neocortex and reduce its over-arousal. They are called beta-blockers because they block the beta subtype of adrenergic receptor.

The subcortical nucleus that transmits NA to the neocortex is the locus coeruleus, which is far smaller than neocortex. In primates it contains about 15,000 neurons, which is less than one-millionth of the neurons in the brain. Nevertheless, though tiny, it sends projections to all parts of the central nervous system and spinal cord. It operates at a baseline level during wakefulness, but its activity increases temporarily when required by ongoing stimulus processing, thought, or action. Unpleasant stimuli such as pain, difficulty in breathing, or extremes of heat or cold all generate large increases in neocortical NA. Extremely unpleasant states such as intense fear or intense pain are associated with exceptionally high levels of adrenergic arousal. As adrenergic arousal increases, the effects of attention increase and become more narrowly focused. Adrenergic arousal is low during sleep and virtually absent during the REM state in which dreams occur.

As discussed further in Chapter 5, NA affects cognition in several ways. At moderate levels it enhances perception, attention, working memory, learning, and the executive control functions of the PFC. Drug-induced suppression of the locus coeruleus has a powerful sedating effect. The situations that arouse the neocortex by activating the locus coeruleus have much in common with those that activate the sympathetic nervous system. The locus coeruleus uses NA to arouse the neocortex, while the sympathetic division of the ANS uses it to prepare the body for action. In keeping with this, NA also suppresses the subcortical nuclei that promote sleep.[7] The effects of adrenergic arousal on the operation of neocortical pyramidal cells are complex, depending on many things including the receptor and cell types involved, cortical region, species, and level of arousal, among others. The simple theme emphasized here is that adrenergic arousal tends to enhance the effects of apical depolarization, and thus of context. This is a simplified view, however, and basic issues that it leaves unresolved are outlined in Section 9.4.

Measures of pupil size and its dynamics provide convenient and sensitive ways of monitoring the level of arousal. They can be used in a wide range of species, and at various ages and states of mind. These and other measures indicate that levels of both cholinergic and adrenergic activation can vary greatly from moment during wakefulness. Changes in cholinergic level tend to be more sustained, whereas adrenergic levels fluctuate at a higher rate. Sustained changes in the activity of the cholinergic system when we begin to walk are reflected by sustained dilations of the pupil. Faster changes in adrenergic activation are reflected by faster fluctuations in pupil size.[8]

Pyramidal cells throughout the neocortex are affected by adrenergic arousal, though with less homogeneity across regions than has long been assumed. It is also known that the PFC has a direct and major role in regulating the activity of cells in the locus coeruleus. As the PFC synthesizes activity from much of neocortex, it provides a route by which cognitive activity at high levels of abstraction can modify the operational mode of the context-sensitive neurons on whose activity cognition depends. This suggests that different states of mind are associated with different modes of apical function, as discussed in Section 4.3.

It is important to note that the effects of adrenergic activation on cellular processes are especially complex. Its effects are only partly known, though it seems clear that when maximally activated it can have effects that are the opposite of those that it has when moderately activated. Readers can safely assume that much remains to be discovered about relations between adrenergic activation and mental state.

4.3 Neuromodulators Regulate Mental State by Modifying Apical Function

Communication within pyramidal cells depends on ion flow through several classes of ion channel. That ion flow is dynamically regulated by neuromodulators, such as those of the cholinergic and adrenergic systems, which modify current flow through various kinds of ion channel in complex ways. In neocortical pyramidal cells some kinds of ion channel are distributed evenly across all their dendrites, but some other kinds of ion channel are far denser in apical dendrites than elsewhere (Migliore & Shepherd, 2002). Figure 4.3 shows the main kinds of ion channel. Densities of some of those ion channels in apical dendrites differs profoundly from that in basal dendrites and depends greatly on distance from the soma.

It is well-known that the classical neuromodulators (e.g. ACh, NA, and others) have profound effects on apical function specifically, but until now, their effects on apical function have not been prominent in accounts of how the neuromodulators regulate mental state. For example, a 100-page review of the neural bases of mental state that is impressively comprehensive in other ways fails to mention apical function other than to say that apical dendrites are the main contributor to the EEG signals that are a major source of evidence on these issues![9] This is now beginning to change, and newer major

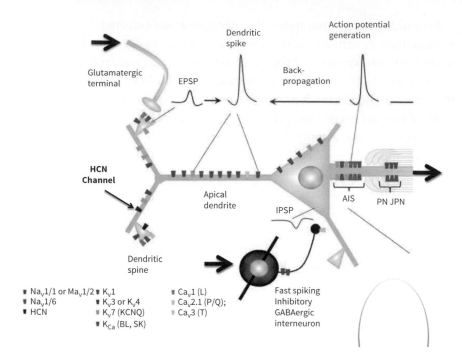

Figure 4.3 Voltage-dependent ion channels in the apical dendrites of neocortical pyramidal cells. One excitatory glutamatergic synapse is shown (EPSP, top left). In the neocortex there are several thousand per pyramidal cell. One inhibitory GABAergic synapse is shown (IPSP, bottom right). In the neocortex there are about one or two thousand per cell. Though there are important differences between the various types of voltage-dependent ion channel shown, the key points here are that these channels are plentiful, interspersed between the synapses, regulate summation of inputs to those synapses over time and space, and are strongly affected by the neuromodulatory systems. Sodium channels are prefixed by Na, potassium channels by K, and calcium channels by Ca. The density of HCN channels increases greatly with distance from the soma. They are most dense in the apical dendrites. The axon initial segment (AIS) is the site where the cell's outputs (i.e. action potentials) are triggered for propagation to other neurons via the axon shown by the arrow and for back-propagation into the cell's own dendrites. For the color coding used to distinguish different kinds of channel see the original figure of which this is a modified version.

Modified from Child and Benarroch (2014) as approved by Eduardo Benarroch, with permission from Wolters Kluwer Health.

reviews make it clear that much of neuromodulation operates via the apical dendrites in layer 1 (Shine et al., 2021).

Synaptic receptors that are metabotropic, operate more slowly, for longer, and with less local point-to-point specificity than those that are ionotropic. There are good grounds for supposing that when combined with a special class of G protein-gated ion channel they provide a mechanism by which cells become sensitive to context, especially to temporal context. It has been proposed that these mechanisms are central to the holistic adaptive capabilities of brain function (Nikolić, 2015, 2022). As that proposal resonates strongly with the evidence for cooperative context-sensitivity it could be further strengthened by relating it explicitly to apical function.

There are some obvious grounds for supposing that apical function is closely related to mental state. Apical isolation seems likely to be involved in deep sleep as there is then no need to disambiguate sensory signals or to amplify them because they are relevant to current goals. Furthermore, apical dendrites are an obvious candidate for involvement during dreaming because they provide many of the synapses via which neocortical pyramidal cells receive input from internal sources. Evidence supporting and clarifying these suppositions are summarized in the remainder of this section.

4.3.1 Cholinergic Activation Enhances Apical Function

In addition to the synapses by which pyramidal cells receive excitatory and inhibitory dendritic input, there are ion channels that restrict integration of that input over time and across different compartments of the dendrites. Prominent amongst these are the voltage-gated HCN and potassium channels discussed in Chapter 3. They are located between synapses of apical dendrites (Figure 4.3) and leak current across the dendritic membrane. When activated, these channels increase compartmentalization and counteract departures from the resting membrane potential. Thus, they restrict integration of the synaptic input over time and along the dendrite. This helps prevent the overactivation seen in epilepsy and other pathologies.[10] The HCN ion channels that restrict spatiotemporal summation are of particular importance here. They are most dense in the apical dendrites and are strongly regulated by arousal.

HCN and voltage-dependent potassium channels (labelled K_v in Figure 4.3) severely restrict the effects of apical input on output. Ion flow through HCN channels is called the I_h current, which, as it reduces the extents of spatial and temporal integration within tuft dendrites, also restricts the effects of apical depolarization on the cell's output. Thus, reducing flow through HCN and/or K_v ion channels enhances the effect of tuft input on the cell's output, but has little or no effect on the output produced by basal inputs alone.[11]

Cholinergic activation increases the effects of apical input on the cell's output by suppressing ion flow through these restrictive ion channels. The density of cholinergic axons and release sites is highest in layer 1 of the neo-cortex, where the apical dendrites and restrictive ion channels are located.[12] Evidence shows that cholinergic arousal enhances the effects of apical input on the cell's output while having little or no effect on its response to direct activation of the soma. These effects are mediated by a class of cholinergic re-ceptor that operates on a longer timescale than those mediated by nicotinic cholinergic receptors. Cholinergic release for only 4 ms can have effects that last for one second or more.[13] In the limit, if strong enough, cholinergic acti-vation can even allow apical input to generate action potential output in the absence of more direct activation of the soma.

Thus, there are at least four ways in which cholinergic activation regulates apical function within neocortical pyramidal cells: by enhancing apical in-tegration; by controlling transmission of information from the apical inte-gration zone to the soma, by disinhibiting input to the apical dendrites, and by its effects on the higher-order thalamic nuclei that project to the apical dendrites.[14]

4.3.2 Adrenergic Activation Enhances Apical Function

Adrenergic activation increases apical effectiveness by reducing the effects of the HCN and potassium ion channels that restrict spatiotemporal summa-tion, as does cholinergic activation.[15] The net result of adrenergic and cho-linergic activation is to suppress response to isolated excitatory inputs to the apical dendrites while enhancing the effects of a coherent burst of synaptic inputs. Variations in adrenergic activation are mainly responsible for the fast fluctuations in levels of alertness when awake, but they also contribute to the overall level of longer-lasting background arousal.

Direct physiological observation in awake mice and in computer models of intracellular processes both show that activation of a particularly sensi-tive class of adrenergic receptor increases the effect of apical input by sup-pressing current flow through the restrictive HCN and potassium channels. Adrenergic arousal enhances apical amplification by increasing the excit-ability of distal apical dendrite.[16]

We can be confident that regulation of mental state varies both across and within species. Nevertheless, there is direct evidence that, because their gen-etic, anatomical, biophysical, and neurochemical bases are so widely shared, basic properties and mechanisms of these neuromodulatory systems are largely conserved across species. Pharmacologically induced variations in the level of adrenergic activation enhances the subjectively reported human awareness of faint visual stimuli and also improves their ability to detect them.[17] Adrenergic activation also increases the reliability with which visual input evokes EEG potentials and enhances blood oxygen-level-dependent (BOLD) fMRI activations in high-order visual cortex.

Adrenergic arousal plays a crucial role in the ability of primates to attend, think, and control impulses. When actively awake, but not too highly stressed, a sensitive class of adrenergic receptor enhances these abilities by suppressing I_h and other ion currents that restrict spatiotemporal summation of inputs to apical dendrites in the PFC. During highly stressful events behaviour becomes more impulsive and action becomes more reflexive than reflective. Levels of adrenergic activation during emergencies can become so great that less-sensitive types of adrenergic receptor in the PFC are activated, further impairing attention, working memory, and impulse control. Performance depending on those cognitive capabilities therefore improves with initial increase in adrenergic activation but worsens as it increases even further, producing an inverted-U relation between arousal and performance known as the Yerkes–Dodson law.[18]

4.3.3 Apical Function Is Also Enhanced by Histamine, Serotonin, and Orexin

These neuromodulators affect neocortical arousal in various ways. They have complex and partially overlapping roles, but, overall, they tend to increase arousal together with NA and ACh (Figure 4.2). For example, histamine (HA) increases neocortical excitability in response to stress or immediate danger, which is why some kinds of antihistamine can increase drowsiness. Axons from the subcortical sites in which HA is synthesized are especially dense in layer 1, which implies that they project to apical dendrites and/or to the inhibitory interneurons that inhibit or disinhibit activation of apical dendrites. HA also depolarizes pyramidal neurons by reducing a background voltage-independent 'leakage' potassium current, which further implicates apical function in the effects of HA because it makes cells more electrotonically compact, thus making them function more like point neurons.[19]

Serotonergic axons are especially dense in the PFC where they modulate neuronal activity via various kinds of serotonergic receptor. Vasoactive intestinal peptide positive (VIP) inhibitory interneurons are rapidly depolarized by serotonergic as well as by cholinergic and glutamatergic arousal, which implicates apical dendrites because it is they that are most disinhibited by VIP interneurons. Interneurons expressing serotonergic receptors are localized mostly in layers 1–3, indicating that they have a role in modulating inputs to the apical branches.[20]

The 5-HT2A class of receptors for serotonin are especially relevant because they are most dense on apical dendrites and are highly potent causes of psychedelic experiences when activated by agonists such as LSD (acid) and psilocybin (magic mushrooms). Why they have such extraordinary and sometimes harmful effects is discussed at the end of this subsection. Here we consider mechanisms by which they have those effects. Activation of this class of receptors is moderately arousing but 5-HT opposes high levels of arousal by inhibiting cholinergic and orexinergic activity (Brown et al., 2012). Activation of 5-HT2A receptors shifts the balance of cooperative cell activity toward greater dependence on apical activation by opposing I_h. In brief, this aspect of 5-HT function can be described as the promotion of quiet imaginative thought, although many unresolved issues underlie that simple description. The extent to which 5-HT affects cooperative cell activity depends on cortical region (being greater in the PFC than elsewhere), cell class (being greater in the PT than in the IT cells of layer 5), and species (they are greater in rats than in mice, for example).[21]

Orexin (also called hypocretin) has a far more important role than is usually realized because it sustains wakefulness by activating the other subcortical nuclei that have arousing effects on neocortex. Orexin is a peptide hormone synthesized in the hypothalamus of all mammalian species, and it coordinates wakeful arousal by simultaneously activating the cholinergic, adrenergic, histaminergic, and serotonergic systems. In addition to those indirect effects on neocortical state, orexin also has direct projections to the neocortex, where it increases the excitability of pyramidal cells. It is probable that those effects involve apical function because orexin directly blocks flow through HCN channels, that is, I_h, in layer 1 of the mouse's equivalent of the PFC.[22]

The reason why orexin has such widespread effects on the cortex and cognition becomes apparent upon examination of the inputs to the hypothalamic orexin cells. These inputs come from various sources, including information about the time of day, and the times at which meals are usually eaten. Orexin-producing cells are inhibited by high blood sugar levels, and by hormonal signals that decrease hunger. They are activated by hormonal signals that increase hunger. On a faster timescale they are also highly sensitive to signals from the amygdala that carry information about emotional events, and can be rapidly suppressed by strong emotions, particularly if positive. Overall, orexin levels tend to be highest during active waking, low to moderate during quiet waking, and low to zero during SWS and REM sleep. Substances that antagonize the effects of orexin help keep sleep continuous by suppressing the impact of microarousals during sleep. All these variables and their relations to specific cognitive processes are open to psychological investigation.[23]

In contrast to the other neuromodulators, dopamine reduces the effect-iveness of apical depolarization and shifts the cell's bias towards dependence of action potential generation only on feedforward basal/peri-somatic de-polarization. The other neuromodulators decrease the effectiveness of basal/ peri-somatic input and increase the effectiveness of apical input by decreasing I_h. Dopamine does the opposite. It increases the effectiveness of basal/peri-somatic input and decreases the effectiveness of apical input by increasing I_h. Mäki-Marttunen and Mäki-Marttunen (2022) review the physiological evi-dence for this and explore its consequences for cellular activity using highly detailed models of layer 5 pyramidal cells. How that relates to the key roles of DA, for example, as in signalling reward, is one of the main issues awaiting ex-ploration within the field of cellular psychology.

4.3.4 The Relationship between Neuromodulatory Regulation of Apical Function and the Reliability and Flexibility of Neocortical Dynamics

A rigorous and wide-ranging dynamic systems perspective on evidence from multiple methodologies concludes that neuromodulation dynamic-ally upregulates, and thus flexibly integrates, subsets of disparate cortical regions that would otherwise operate more independently, thus contrib-uting to basic cognitive capabilities (Shine et al., 2021; Munn et al., 2021). That perspective emphasizes anatomical studies showing that the cholin-ergic system's cortical projections are less diffuse than that of the adren-ergic system. Consequently, the cholinergic system is seen as being more concerned with enhancing reliable local processing, whereas the adren-ergic system is seen as being more concerned with the flexible integration of overall cortical processing. It can be seen that apical function has a central role in that perspective by noting that adrenergic activation predominantly enhances apical influences, whereas cholinergic activation enhances both basal and apical influences on the cell's output. Thus, the effects of apical input on the cell's output increase as the ratio of adrenergic to cholinergic activation increases. This is clearly consistent with the great reduction in both amplification and adrenergic activation during deep sleep , when amp-lification would be counterproductive.

Close comparison of this dynamic systems perspective with that focused on context-sensitive cooperative computation shows them to be mutually supportive in fundamental ways. For example, they agree that neuromodulatory systems strengthen the connection of the apical zone to the soma by suppressing ion flow through HCN ion channels. They also agree that amplification involves converting a single action potential into a brief burst of two to four action potentials. Nevertheless, comparison of these two perspectives also raises a few issues.

The first issue that arises when comparing these two perspectives concerns terminology. Shine and colleagues (2021) use 'integration' to refer to interactions that make processing in distinct regions more interdependent. Here, we use the term in the sense of the integral calculus and as used in the 'integrate-and-fire' conception of point neurons, that is, it refers to summing or pooling a set of inputs to compute a single value about which information is transmitted, either from one cell to another or from the apical zone to the soma within cells. 'Integration' as we define it is contrasted with 'modulation', but as used by Shine and colleagues, it refers to any interaction whatever. So, from their perspective, modulatory effects are a kind of integration. That more general notion of 'integration' can be defended on the grounds that summation can be nonlinear. That terminology is ambiguous, however, because it does not distinguish between summative and modulatory forms of interaction.

This and other terminological ambiguities arise because the field is still so young. If empirical explorations are to be usefully guided by theoretical conceptions, the sooner these terminological differences are resolved, the better. For example, it is agreed that pupillary dynamics provide empirical methods to investigate and differentiate the consequences of cholinergic and adrenergic activation in a wide range of conditions and species. Thus, our theoretical terminology must become more consistent and more precise to facilitate the design and interpretation of such empirical studies.[24]

The second issue that arises when comparing these two perspectives is whether integration and segregation of macroscopic regional interactions are opposed or complementary. Shine and colleagues (2021) sometimes imply that integration (which they associate with flexibility) and segregation (which they associate with reliability) are opposed, but at other points, and more consistently, they state that neural activity in the brain must be simultaneously flexible and reliable. This issue would be resolved if it were shown that a bias towards flexibility occurs when the ratio of aminergic activation to cholinergic activation increases. Furthermore, that ratio is at a minimum during dreaming (Section 4.4) but the opposite extreme, in which aminergic activation is maximal and cholinergic activation is minimal, does not seem to occur naturally. It is not expected to, because aminergic arousal activates the cholinergic system, but cholinergic arousal does not activate the aminergic system.

Thirdly, the integration and segregation of interregional interactions (as studied within dynamical systems perspective of Shine and colleagues) must not be confused with Gestalt grouping and segregation in perception. Gestalt grouping operates within regions of the thalamocortical system on locally specific spatial and temporal scales (Chapter 5). For example, grouping in contour integration, which is one of the most rigorously quantified examples of Gestalt organization, both psychophysically and neurobiologically, operates at small and precise spatial scales within visual cortex (as shown in Figure 5.3, for example). Furthermore, in contrast to the slower timescale on which neuromodulation operates, perceptual segregation operate son a timescale of about 10 ms.[25] Cross-modal contextual interactions are similarly precise and operate via glutamatergic synapses within the thalamocortical system (Chapter 5). That is, Gestalt grouping and segregation operate via high-resolution contextual interactions within the neocortex; one of the functions of neuromodulatory systems is to regulate those intracortical interactions.

Fourthly, cooperative context-sensitivity must also be clearly distinguished from gain modulation (Salinas & Sejnowski, 2001) and neural gain (Aston-Jones Cohen, 2005). Gain is the slope of the quasi-linear rising section of the function that relates neuronal output strength to synaptic input strength. Much evidence validates and popularizes emphasis upon that slope as a way of summarizing relations between the input and output of a neuron or local microcircuit. Building on those highly influential views, Shine and colleagues (2021) focus on changes in that slope as a major way in which neuromodulatory systems regulate cellular biophysics and responsiveness without changing receptive field selectivity. An emphasis upon gain control was also clear in our earlier notions of context-sensitive gain control.[26] It now seems clear, however, that identifying context-sensitivity with gain control is misleading, and Chapter 8 rigorously shows ways in which they are very different. This involves distinguishing between synergistic components of transmitted information that are due to context-sensitivity and those that are intrinsic to the information transmitted. Here, that distinction is presented more intuitively. An increase in slope alone reduces response to weak inputs and increases response to strong inputs. In stark contrast, the effect of cooperative context-sensitivity is to increase response to weak inputs while having little or no effect on response to strong inputs. Furthermore, Salinas and Sejnowski (2001) do not mention context; rather, the paradigmatic example of gain modulation they give is coordinate transformation, which is clearly concerned with transmitting information about relations between two classes of input. That must be clearly distinguished from using one class of input (e.g. that to the apical dendrites) to amplify or attenuate transmission of information about another class of inputs (e.g. that to the basal dendrites). Apical amplification does not necessarily imply an increase the slope of the cell's response to its driving input. The highly detailed multicompartmental model of the effect of apical activation within individual pyramidal cells reported by Shai and colleagues (2015) shows that it can greatly increase the cell's responsiveness by lowering the threshold above which the cell has some response, but without any change in slope. Other models of this kind show that, if there is a sufficient reduction in the threshold, then apical amplification can even involve a reduction in that slope, which thus increases the dynamic range over which apical amplification can operate.[27] None of this implies that the neuromodulators do not regulate the balance between reliability and flexibility, which they do in various ways, including differential effects on interneurons that predominantly inhibit either apical dendrites or locations closer to the soma. What it implies is that an increase in gain, defined as the slope of the input–output function, may not be crucial to the neuromodulatory regulation of context-sensitivity.

Finally, an issue of potentially major importance concerns the role of layer 5 pyramidal neurons in adaptive, slightly 'subcritical' network dynamics.[28] A key role for apical dendrites in or near layer 1 is to provide feedback to pyramidal cells that closes various positive feedback loops (as outlined in several sections of this book). These positive feedback loops are shown to be crucial to basic cognitive functions, but runaway overexcitation is an obvious danger for any system with so many positive feedback loops. Levels of positive feedback in which runaway overexcitation could easily be triggered is an example of 'criticality'. Critical neocortical states can be thought of as those poised between rapid increases in either order or disorder and characterized by long-range correlations in space and time and also by cooperative coalitions of a wide range of sizes.[29] From that perspective, neuromodulation aims at setting the level of apical amplification high enough to achieve current goals while avoiding malfunctional overexcitation. Furthermore, this provides a way in which the distinctive capabilities of cooperative neurons might be empirically related to Freud's metapsychology of the ego, or self; to the psychedelic effects of drugs, such as psilocybin, that enhance the effects of serotonin receptors that are most dense on the apical dendrites of layer 5 pyramidal cells; and to primary states of mind that are both more ancient and predominant during infancy.[30]

The various neuropeptides are important to many aspects of mental life. For example, oxytocin is involved in parental care, pair bonding, and attachment; the endogenous opiates (e.g. endorphins and enkephalins) are involved in many things including pain perception, reward, eating, and food preference. There are approximately 50 different kinds of neuropeptide, and we know little about their interaction with the context-sensitive mechanisms of neocortical pyramidal cells. This lack of information opens another huge area for future research.

Chapter 7 outlines the difficulty of setting and maintaining a healthy balance between apical amplification, and thus flexible sensitivity, while avoiding the harmful apical overamplification or overdrive that occurs in many pathologies. Future studies of relations between criticality and apical function may therefore have fundamental implications for both basic and clinical issues.

4.4 Three Modes of Apical Function: Amplification, Drive, and Isolation

Within neocortical pyramidal cells the current mode of apical function can vary greatly during a normal day, as does mental state. Mental state varies from deep sleep, to dreaming, to quiet or active wakefulness with occasional highly stressful emergencies which greatly change priorities and mental state. Variation in mental state is more complex than can be adequately described using just a single measure, such as overall level of arousal. Nevertheless, variations in just two dimensions defined on the electrical activity of four different brain regions can reliably distinguish active and quiet wakefulness, from each other and from both dreaming and deep sleep (Figure 4.1). Furthermore, these different states are reliably related to cholinergic and aminergic activation (Figure 4.2). Thus, we can infer ways in which these states relate to apical function using what is known about the effects of the neuromodulators on apical function and basic cognitive processes.

First, consider wakefulness. When awake we use internal knowledge, such as intentions, fears, and hopes, to focus on relevant information from our bodies and the external world. That must usually be done, however, without the internal information that specifies relevance becoming a self-fulfilling prophecy. Chapter 3 shows how apical input is used to amplify the transmission of information about input to the basal dendrites of a selected subset of pyramidal cells. Thus, apical amplification is a prominent mode of apical function during both quiet and active wakefulness.

Next, we consider dreamless sleep, in which we expect there to be little or no need to amplify signals that are relevant to current intentions and actions. The low levels of cholinergic and aminergic activation during dreamless sleep support that expectation. The low level of adrenergic activation restricts spatiotemporal summation of inputs to the apical branches and the low level of cholinergic activation prevents apical activation affecting the soma. This suggests that isolation from the soma is the prominent mode of apical function during dreamless sleep.

There may be some forms of long-term memory consolidation during dreamless SWS, nevertheless. Firstly, though restricted, there is some summation of inputs to the apical branches, which could be involved in changes in the strengths of apical synapses independently of its effects on action potential generation. Secondly, though not amplified by apical input, there may still be some transmission of feedforward information from lower to higher cortical regions, which could also be involved in some form of memory consolidation during SWS.

Now consider dreaming. The neocortical activity generated from internal sources during dreams is in some ways like that during awake states, although it is not identical because the electrical activity of the forebrain and its neuromodulatory input during REM states are clearly distinct from that during the awake state (Figures 4.1, 4.2).

During dreaming, imagined percepts are prominent. Neuroimaging using EEG shows that they involve the activation of pyramidal cells in perceptual regions in the neocortex, and as these pyramidal neurons receive their input from internal sources predominantly via their apical dendrites, this indicates that there are conditions in which apical input is sufficient to generate output from those cells. This implies that information that guides perception when awake can be used to generate pseudo-perceptual experiences when dreaming (Figure 4.4).[31]

Michael Spratling, one of the first to see the importance of distinct apical functions, pointed out to me that, in addition to the three modes of function distinguished in Figure 4.4, we can assume at least one other: a mode of function in which, although the apical integration zone is not biophysically isolated from the soma, it receives little or no contextual input and so has little or no effect. He suggests that such a mode of function may be common during normal perception, so that raises yet another issue to be explored.

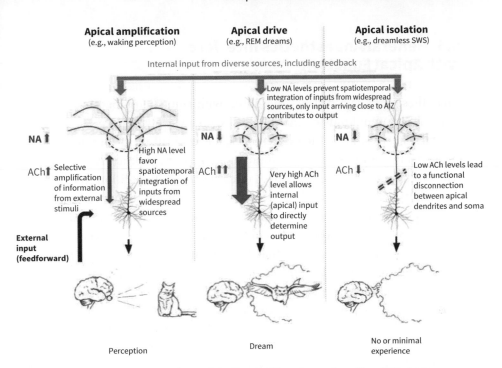

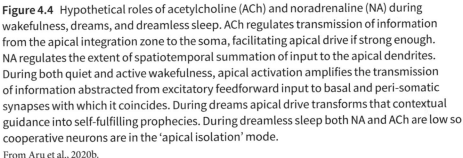

Figure 4.4 Hypothetical roles of acetylcholine (ACh) and noradrenaline (NA) during wakefulness, dreams, and dreamless sleep. ACh regulates transmission of information from the apical integration zone to the soma, facilitating apical drive if strong enough. NA regulates the extent of spatiotemporal summation of input to the apical dendrites. During both quiet and active wakefulness, apical activation amplifies the transmission of information abstracted from excitatory feedforward input to basal and peri-somatic synapses with which it coincides. During dreams apical drive transforms that contextual guidance into self-fulfilling prophecies. During dreamless sleep both NA and ACh are low so cooperative neurons are in the 'apical isolation' mode.
From Aru et al., 2020b.

The notion of apical drive does not necessarily imply some wholly novel mode of function. On the contrary—from an evolutionary point of view, that may be the more ancient mode of pyramidal cell function. In the three-layer cortex, from which the six-layered neocortex evolved, the main driving input to pyramidal cells is received via their apical dendrites (discussed in Chapter 6).[32] Thus, dreaming may involve reversion to a more ancient form of pyramidal cell information processing. However, dreaming may not be the only state in which apical drive occurs—it may also occur under special conditions when awake and when either thinking or highly stressed (discussed further in Chapters 5 and 7).

4.5 General Anaesthetics Interfere with Apical Function

Anaesthesiology is a distinct discipline within medicine because there are so many different kinds of anaesthetics, with a variety of different effects on mental state. Despite all their differences, however, all affect conscious experience, so it is likely that they have fundamental commonalities. A review of this issue in the journal *Anesthesiology* concluded that, in addition to enhancing the activity of subcortical sleep-promoting centres while suppressing that of arousing centres, most general anaesthetics also interfere with apical function (Figure 4.5).[33] Thus, those studies of the basic mechanisms of general anaesthesia provide further evidence that mental state depends on apical function.

One unresolved puzzle in the evidence relating anaesthetics to apical function concerns their effects on the I_h current. Meyer (2015) reviews much evidence showing that various kinds of general anaesthetic enhance communication between the soma and the apical integration zone by blocking I_h (Figure 4.5D), which, if true, implies that anaesthetics prevent selective amplification by amplifying the outputs of all pyramidal cells. However, more recent investigations conflict with that hypothesis, and provide direct evidence that general anaesthetics do not enhance communication between the two integration zones, but rather block it.[34] It is not yet known how this apparent conflict with the earlier data can be resolved. Nevertheless, we can be confident that apical function has a central role in the effects of many anaesthetics on mental state, as shown by Meyer (2015).

4.6 Mental State and Conceptions of Consciousness

The function and neuronal bases of conscious experience are major unsolved mysteries. The problems to be solved have not yet been adequately specified, however, so this section is essentially philosophical in that it attempts to provide conceptual foundations for empirical studies of the functions and neurobiological bases of conscious experience. In some crucial ways, the search for the neural correlates of 'consciousness' may be a search for something that does not exist in the form assumed by intuition. In the early days of physics, much effort went into a search for phlogiston, a supposed fire-like element released during combustion. The science of thermodynamics was revolutionized when, instead of searching for a substance, it related the phenomena of

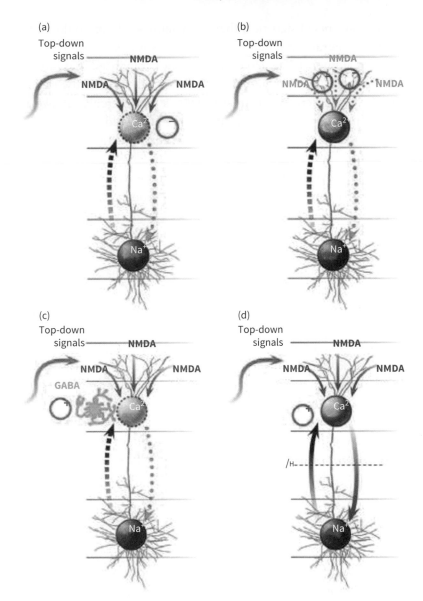

Figure 4.5 Four ways in which anaesthetics interfere with apical function. (a) Some anaesthetics directly suppress the dendritic calcium potentials that carry signals from the apical integration zone to the soma (e.g. urethane, pentobarbital, isoflurane). (b) Some suppress active potentials that carry signals from the distant parts of the apical dendrites to the apical integration zone (e.g. ketamine, nitrous oxide). (c) Some enhance the effects of interneurons that inhibit the apical integration zone (e.g. propofol, barbiturates). (d) Some interfere with the hyperpolarization-activated current, I_h, which flows though HCN ion channels (shown here is I_H) (e.g. propofol, ketamine, isoflurane, halothane, pentobarbital). That is a leak conductance that reduces the extent to which activity is summed over time and along the dendrite.

GABA, γ-aminobutyric acid.

Figure from Kaspar Meyer (2015) and used with his approval, and permission from Wolters Kluwer Health, Inc.

heat to the concepts of statistical thermodynamics. I have no doubt that the search for the neural correlates of consciousness is trying to solve a problem of fundamental importance. However, I am not convinced that intuitive notions of 'consciousness' provide an adequate conception of the phenomena to be understood. Here, our primary focus is on differences between sleep and wakefulness. Chapter 5 provides further discussion of ways in which processes of which we are aware differ from those of which we are not aware when awake.

As noted, I have often engaged in research on these issues, both as a subject and as an experimenter. I have worked with neuropsychological and psychiatric patients whose states of mind often seemed very different from mine, as well as from each other's. Furthermore, teaching an advanced course on drugs and the mind for several years taught me that states of mind are highly variable, and subject to many neurochemical and pharmacological influences. Finally, many hours of mindful mediation in recent years have led me to directly experience new states of mind that I had not experienced in the previous seven decades. Therefore, I proceed on the assumption that there are diverse states of mind and brain that range from those described as 'primitive phenomenal experience' to those described as 'reflective self-consciousness'.

There are many definitions of 'consciousness'. The following definition contains elements common to many of them: 'to see, to hear, to feel, or otherwise to experience something is to be conscious, irrespective of whether in addition one is aware that one is seeing, hearing, and so forth'.[35] This is representative in implicating three different things: experiences themselves, the things experienced, and the thing having the experience. It is also representative in explicitly including sensory and perceptual experiences, which loom large in the history of thought on these issues, from ancient Greek philosophy until now. It is also representative in explicitly stating that self-consciousness is a possible, though not a necessary, aspect of conscious experience.

Before outlining my doubts concerning some common assumptions underlying the notion of consciousness, I must first make clear that I agree with many common assumptions concerning relations between the brain and the conscious mind. No neuron can be a mind. When discussing relations between states of mind and neurons, I am discussing relations between macroscopic properties of a system and its microscopic components. The density of water is greater than that of ice because of the very special, and perhaps unique, properties of H_2O, but no single molecule of H_2O can be water or ice. Subjective experiences are system properties, and endlessly various. It implies a 'subject' who has the experiences, and subjective experiences usually present themselves as conveying information about something other than themselves, for example, the chair on which I am sitting, or a pain in my butt, or a past event that I remember. In that sense, some experiences can be said to be 'of' something other than themselves. Experiences are fundamentally different from whatever it is that the experience is 'of', if anything. Although my perceptions of physical things do indeed convey information necessary to survival, physics tells us that physical things have many properties that are wholly unknown to direct subjective experience. In some ways, those properties even contradict what direct subjective experience tells us.

I do have many doubts about intuitive conceptions of 'consciousness', however. First and foremost, I doubt the value of certainty. Openness is one of the greatest gifts of mind. Closing doors with certainty diminishes that gift. The value of openness is particularly great when thinking about the nature of our own experience. It is tempting to assume that beliefs about our own direct experiences are infallible, as the philosopher Descartes seems to have supposed. In fact, many common, intuitively obvious, beliefs about our own subjective experience are probably false. This includes the illusion of the sensory mosaic, which is the belief that we can narrow our attention to the smallest sensory element of which we are aware (discussed more in Chapter 5). There are many other such examples that, together, convince me that we can, and often do, hold false beliefs about our own direct experience. For many years I taught an undergraduate class on mental imagery in which students were shown a drawing of a simple overhand knot and were asked to reproduce the drawing immediately after it was removed. They also rated the clarity with which they could hold the drawing in mind during that short interval. It turns out that this task is surprisingly difficult. Though only a few lines are involved, it requires imagining a structure in three-dimensional space. Most students were unable to produce anything close to an adequate version of the drawing. Nevertheless, many of those rated the clarity of their temporary mental image of it as being comparable to that when seeing the actual drawing. There was no correlation between their ability to draw the knot and the clarity ratings for their images of it, however. This cannot be explained by their inability to draw the knot because all were able to copy the original drawing accurately if it remained visible. Therefore, I doubt their introspective assessments of the 'clarity' or 'vividness' of their own internal images. Life-long experience has taught me that, when I try to express it, what feels like inner clarity is often found to be vague and sometimes incoherent. While discounting neither my own direct introspective experiences nor the introspective reports of others, I do treat them with considerable caution because they are not always what they purport to be. Thus, when dreams are described as 'vivid', for example,

I do not assume that the experience was equivalent to really perceiving things in all their sensory detail .

I also doubt five other common assumptions concerning 'consciousness':

1. That all experiences are 'of' something other than themselves.
2. That the veracity of many of those experiences are 'of' something other than themselves.
3. That we have an adequate notion of the 'self' or whatever it is that *has* the experience.
4. That all direct experience must be either conscious or unconscious.
5. That the information in the experience can be identified with the conscious experience of that information.

4.6.1 Are All Direct Experiences 'of' Something Other Than Themselves?

I doubt that all experiences are 'of' something other than themselves. Though most sensory and perceptual experiences are of physical things that exist independently of the mind, some of them are not, for example, colour and pain. We experience colour, which conveys information about real properties of external objects, but that experience depends on relations between the observer and the observed. It does not depend only upon the physical reflectance properties of the perceived objects.[36] We certainly experience pain, but that does not prove that, in addition to the experience, there is a pain to be experienced. That applies to all pain, not only to phantom-limb pain, which is certainly not 'of' the pain in the missing limb. Much has been made of demonstrations that some decisions may be detectable in the brain before the subject knows of them.[37] It has also been argued in depth, however, that most of our decisions are made in the process of thinking them through.[38]

Though influenced by many things not experienced, thoughts are not always the experience of something already decided before we knew it. Consider the following conundrum. Many thoughts are internal speech, but how can I say things to myself if I don't know what is to be said? However, if I do know what is to be said, then why do I need to say it to myself? This conundrum is resolved by assuming that saying these things to myself creates the thought experienced. Verbal thought expresses and explores the implications of the hard-won knowledge of grammar, and of much else besides. Thus, that may be how explicitly expressed thoughts give to airy nothing a local habitation and a name. Therefore, I conclude that, although some aspects of some experiences are indeed 'of' something other than themselves, some thoughts are created in the act of thinking them. William James, the intellectual giant on whose work much of twentieth-century psychology was built, spent many years objectively studying the varieties of religious experience, of which there are many, including experiences that are felt to be revelatory.[39] For some people such experiences are the most important things in their lives. It could be argued that if all experience is 'of' something external to itself then there must be something other than themselves that those religious experiences reveal. Alternatively, it could also be argued that some experiences are formed in the process of experiencing them, which implies that they are not experiences 'of' something other than themselves. This is consistent with evidence indicating that by waking up and becoming conscious we can do a whole host of things that we could not do when asleep (covered in Chapter 5).

4.6.2 Can We Rely on the Veracity of Our Own Direct Experiences?

It is possible to doubt the veracity of experiences even when they are 'of' something other than themselves. Many aspects of sensation and perception are indeed highly trustworthy reporters of things other than themselves—which is why they evolved—but some aspects of perception are less trustworthy. The shape and location of the physical things that I experience around me usually corresponds well to my experience of them, but as the thing perceived becomes more abstract, the greater the potential divergence between what is experienced and what it presents itself to be an experience 'of'. Though often of great importance, inferences concerning the minds of others are exceptionally difficult to validate. Their linguistic capabilities enable humans to cooperate in ways that would not be possible otherwise. However, that cooperation comes at a cost because language can also be deceptive, either intentionally or unintentionally. One of the maxims inferred from the study of human conversation was that people usually try to say things that are true. That may usually be the case, but, even when it is, that does not provide the listener with a pure uninterpreted insight into the speaker's mind. Indeed, I doubt that speakers have uninterpreted insight into their *own* mind. In general, there is no easy way for us to disentangle aspects of our experiences that validly convey information about external things from those aspects that come from ourselves.

Indeed, some aspects may come from neither, although they depend on both (as discussed in Chapter 8 from an information theoretic point of view).

4.6.3 What Is the Subject or 'Self' That Has the Experience?

I doubt the adequacy of our conception of what *it is* that *has* the experience. The phrase 'subjective experience' is useful in distinguishing the 'subject' from the 'experience'. In the explicit statement that a *subject* has the experience, however, the phrase implies that if we are to understand the nature of subjective experience, we must possess an adequate notion of how we define the *subject*, or '*self*'. Of course, there is continuity of the physical body of the person who has the experiences, but it is not the physical body that has the experience. It is the mind and brain, which are multifaceted, dynamic, changeable, and highly sensitive to context. A mistaken belief in a single, continuous, self or subject that is the same in all contexts, and to which all experiences must be related, may be part of the problem. I am not convinced that we yet have an adequate conception of the 'self' that has subjective experiences. I reconsider this issue in Chapter 10 from the viewpoint of cooperative context-sensitive computation.

4.6.4 Are States of Mind Binary? Must They be Conscious or Not?

'Consciousness' is a seventeenth-century word. Shakespeare asked the fundamental questions about knowledge and doubt, about self, and about purpose in human life without ever referring to either 'consciousness' or 'awareness'. His plays are replete with thoughts, premeditated actions, and dreams, but in none do I spy implications of a 'consciousness ' or an 'awareness'. In 1890, James devoted large sections of his famous book *The Principles of Psychology* to consciousness. In 1904, however, he published a paper asking: 'Does consciousness exist?, and declares that 'for twenty years past I have mistrusted 'consciousness' as an entity ... It seems that the hour is ripe for it to be openly and universally discarded'. He made clear that he did not doubt the reality of subjective experience, however, and argued that the cognitive functions assumed for 'consciousness' must still be performed somehow or other.[40]

As some may argue that a binary choice between consciousness and nonconsciousness is a logical necessity, I note that what are sometimes referred to as 'altered states of consciousness' are highly various. I am not convinced that it is helpful to squeeze all states of mind into the simple binary choice between being either conscious or not. Consider the comparisons between wakefulness, dreaming, and dreamless sleep shown in Table 4.1. The neuronal dynamics during REM are clearly distinct from the awake state as well as from dreamless sleep. As Figures 4.1 and 4.2 show, the REM state is not in any simple sense 'intermediate' between wakefulness and SWS. Dreaming has many similarities to both wakefulness and dreamless sleep, which differ greatly from each other. The dream state is intermediate between them in some ways, but it is not in other ways, for example in levels of ACh, NA, and muscle tone.

These objective comparisons provide no grounds for concluding either that dreams are conscious because of their similarities to wakefulness or that dreams are unconscious because of their similarities to dreamless sleep. We have memories of dreams if we waken soon after dreaming, but that does not tell us whether they were experienced during the dream or not. Those memories also do not tell us by what part of the brain they would have been experienced during the dream—if they were. On asking myself whether I experienced the many dreams of which I have no recollection while they were happening, my answer is 'I don't know'. I see no way of finding out, other than by having objective indicators that something is being consciously experienced. If I ask 'Do "I" experience my unremembered dreams?', then I am inclined to say that 'I' do not—because, as far as 'I' know, they are no part of me. Furthermore, I do not know whether the information in the dream was created in the act of dreaming, as inner speech is when awake, or whether the dream experience is in some sense 'of' something other than itself. Although many people insist that they were conscious of their unremembered dreams while they were being dreamed, many (e.g. Freudian psychoanalysts) do not.

I have one final question for those who insist that they are conscious of their dreams while dreaming them: how could we possibly distinguish processes that occur *consciously* when dreaming from those that occur *unconsciously* when dreaming? Many paradigms have been invented to distinguish conscious from nonconscious processing when awake, but I know of none that have been applied to dreaming, and until one appears, then views on this issue seem doomed to remain a matter of vague opinion.

Table 4.1 Similarities and differences between three distinct states: wakefulness, dreaming, and dreamless slow wave sleep (SWS). Properties in **bold** are firmly established; the others are less well established. Properties in blue are those that dreaming shares with wakefulness. Properties in red italics are those that dreaming shares with slow wave sleep.

	AWAKE	DREAMING	SWS
ACh levels	**Moderate-High**	Maximum	*Minimum*
Resting potential of pyramidal cells	**Depol (-61mV)**	Depol (-63mV)	*Hyperpol (-75mV)*
Down states	**Rare**	Rare	*Common*
Low freq EEG power	**Low**	Low	*High*
High freq EEG power	**Highs**	High	*Low*
Complexity of EEG/fMRI activity	High	High	*Low*
Regional interdependence	High	Partial	*Low*
Specific experience	Always	Always	*Never*
NA/Serotonin/Orexin/Hist. levels	**Moderate-High**	*Minimal*	Low
Ventrolateral Preoptic activity	**Low**	*High*	High
Responsiveness to sensory input	**High**	*Minimal*	Low
Muscle tone/EMG	**High**	*Low*	Low
Voluntary control/Legal agency	**Yes**	*No*	No
Reduction of dissonance/ incoherence	Yes	*No*	No
PFC activity/ Self-reflective insight	Yes	*No*	No
Memory for experience	Variable	*Brief*	None
Default mode of apical function	**Amplification**	Drive	Isolation
Integration in the apical tuft	**Expanded**	Restricted	Minimal

4.6.5 Can the Information *in* Direct Experience Be Identified *with* That Experience?

If dreams have specific, if incoherent, information content, it could be argued that they must have been experienced by the dreamer. This argument is of doubtful validity, however. Some philosophers have argued that the phenomenal content of experience is separable from its being consciously experienced, and they show that this is compatible with neurobiological theories of consciousness.[41] Even when we are awake, and attending carefully, abstract information can be extracted from sense data without our knowing it. For example, a paradigm that I designed and in which I was a subject showed that briefly flashed words that we are not aware of can greatly facilitate the solving of anagrams of which we *are* aware. As this is the case for function words such as 'be' but not for content words, such as nouns, verbs, adjectives, and adverbs, the level of subliminal processing must have been at a highly abstract level within the perceptual hierarchy. As I was a subject in those experiments myself I can assure the reader that those effects occurred under conditions where I was unaware of whether the briefly flashed words were being presented or not. As there is plenty of other evidence for subliminal processing of information to a high level of abstraction, I conclude that abstract information content of many experiences is computed in the neocortex independently of its being experienced. This can be so, even if in some cases it is created in the process of experiencing it, as argued previously in relation to verbal thought. Thus, any theory of the neural bases of consciousness, including those considered here and in Chapter 5, will have to provide an adequate account of why and how it is that some abstractions can be computed without any conscious experience of them.

4.6.6 Apical Inputs: Effective When We Are Awake, but Not When Deeply Asleep

The evidence reviewed here indicates that, because of changes in the neuromodulatory climate, the mode of apical function depends upon whether we are awake, dreaming, or in SWS. There should be nothing deeply mysterious about this—it makes simple sense, given long-standing assumptions about the functions of conscious experience, and our emerging understanding of the functions of apical input. James argued in 1890 that selection is a cardinal function of consciousness, where selection is between different stimuli, different interpretations of them, different thoughts, and different actions. He considered that

> the mind is at every stage a theatre of simultaneous possibilities. Consciousness consists in the comparison of these with each other, the selection of some, and the suppression of the rest [...] The mind, in short, works on the data it receives very much as a sculptor works on his block of stone [...] Other minds other worlds from the same monotonous and inexpressive chaos.[42]

James' view of this was strikingly prescient. The main advance that we can now offer is to show how the various possibilities are created in the neocortex and how selection between them is made in the context of current input to the apical dendrites of pyramidal cells. This makes apical function an obvious candidate for a central role in the long-sought 'neural correlates of consciousness', which is examined further in Chapter 5.

4.7 Summary

Quiet, active, and highly stressed substates of wakefulness can be distinguished from each other as well as from dreaming and from deep dreamless sleep (SWS). Transitions between states are regulated by interactions between the neocortex and subcortical brain stem nuclei, such as those that release the cholinergic and adrenergic neuromodulators in all regions of neocortex.

Section 4.1 outlined the neurobiological reality of these distinct mental states, and Section 4.2 showed that transitions between them are regulated by cholinergic, adrenergic, serotonergic, and other subcortical neuromodulatory systems. Section 4.3 showed that they do so via various types of ion channel in the cell's membrane that are interspersed between the synapses, and which are abundant in the apical trunk and branches. These neuromodulators increase the effects of apical input on the cell's output by closing ion channels that restrict the spatial integration of excitatory input when they are open. This includes HCN ion channels that are especially sensitive to the neuromodulatory regulators. HCN channels are therefore of far greater functional importance than is commonly realized. Current flow through these channels, I_h, is reduced as arousal increases from low to moderate levels, thereby enabling apical input to have greater effects on the cell's output. Most neuromodulators decrease the effectiveness of basal/peri-somatic activation alone and increase the effectiveness of input to apical dendrites. Thus, they increase the difference between feedforward signals that are amplified because they are coherent or relevant in the current context and those that are not amplified because they are currently irrelevant. They do so by decreasing I_h, which is an electrical ion current that opposes activation of apical dendrites. An increase in adrenergic activation from moderate to exceptionally high, however, may increase, rather than decrease, Ih. If so, then in that case information transmission is likely to be more impulsive and less sensitive to thoughtful context-sensitivity. In contrast to the other neuromodulators, dopamine (DA) increases I_h, so it decreases the relative effectiveness of input to apical dendrites, thus increasing the relative effectiveness of basal and peri-somatic activation.

Section 4.4 argued that there are three distinct modes of apical function: apical amplification (the normal mode of operation in perceptual regions when awake), apical drive (which operates during dreaming when asleep and during imagery when awake), and apical isolation (which prevents both apical amplification and apical drive during dreamless SWS). Section 4.5 showed that general anaesthesia also prevents the normal operation of inputs to the apical dendrites. Finally, Section 4.6 related the evidence for cooperative neurons to conceptions of consciousness and argued that the neural bases of conscious human experiences are a broad class of macroscopic thalamocortical events in which the outputs of a large, dynamically selected subset of cooperative neurons are amplified or generated by inputs to their apical dendrites. It also argued that the difficulty of deciding whether dreams are 'conscious' or not during the dream is one of several reasons for supposing that some intuitive assumptions concerning 'consciousness' may be misleading. As apical dendrites receive subcortical input from the amygdala, ascending signals concerning emotional state could be involved in dreaming.

This perspective on apical function has a striking resemblance to Hobson's AIM model of mental state (summarized at the beginning of the chapter). Overall arousal, seen as the main diagonal of Figure 4.2 (that from low to high levels of both cholinergic and aminergic activation), is equivalent to Hobson's dimension of activation (A). The proportion of apical drive to apical amplification overlaps with his dimension of input-output gating (I). The diagonal of Figure 4.2 from high aminergic and low cholinergic to low aminergic and high cholinergic, is analogous to Hobson's dimension of modulation (M). This convergence between Hobson's notions and ours is remarkable and was unplanned. That suggests that there is some validity in both Hobson's view of variations in the state of the system as a whole and in our view of apical function within individual pyramidal neurons.

Notes

1. Robbins and Everitt (1995) differentiate cholinergic, adrenergic, dopaminergic, and serotonergic components of arousal.
2. Walker (2017) provides a lucid introduction to the latest research on sleep and dreaming. Brown and colleagues (2012) provide a comprehensive review of the neural control of sleep and dreaming. Rasch and Born (2013) review the role of sleep in memory consolidation. Both reviews were written before apical function was widely seen to be important.
3. Gervasoni and colleagues (2004) report these detailed relations between local field potentials in four brain regions and behavioural state in rats.
4. Figure 4.2. presents my own simplified view of these issues. For more detailed research on them see McGinley et al., 2015; Robbins & Arnsten, 2009; Arnsten, Wang, & Paspalas, 2012.
5. Zagha and McCormick (2014) review relations between cholinergic activation and behaviour.
6. For more on rapid changes in mental state when awake see McGinley et al., (2015) and Reimer et al., (2016).
7. Brown and colleagues (2012) and Robbins and Arnsten (2009) review relations between adrenergic activation and mental state.
8. McGinley and colleagues (2015) and Wainstein (2021) show in detail how pupil size can be used to study rapid variations of arousal when awake.
9. Brown et al., 2012.
10. Child & Benarroch, 2014.
11. Berger et al., 2001, 2003; Larkum et al., 2009; Harnett et al., 2015.
12. For example, cholinergic activation reduces I_h in cells of layers 2/3 in the medial entorhinal cortex (Tsuno, Schultheiss, & Hasselmo, 2013).
13. See Williams & Fletcher, 2019; Suzuki & Larkum, 2020. Reducing I_h increases the effects of apical input in layer 5 cells of somatosensory cortex (Berger et al., 2003; Harnett et al, 2015). Suppression of voltage-gated potassium channels, which are dense in apical dendrites and restrict spatiotemporal summation, greatly enhances the effects of apical input on neuronal output (Harnett et al., 2013). Having shown that the effect of apical input on output depends on ACh, Williams and Fletcher (2019) conclude that cholinergic signals dynamically disinhibit apical dendrites of L5B in order to facilitate the context-dependent modulation of perception.
14. Cholinergic activation decreases inhibitory input to the apical dendrites (Brombas et al., 2014; Letzkus et al., 2015). Arousal systems also modify apical function via higher-order thalamic nuclei, which are far more active during wakefulness, and have been shown to convey diverse contextual information to layer 1 of the neocortex (Roth et al., 2016).
15. Phillips and colleagues (2017) review evidence relating adrenergic activation to HCN ionic currents and conscious experience.
16. Labarrera et al., 2018.
17. Gelbard-Sagiv et al., 2018.
18. Arnsten et al., 2012.
19. Haas and colleagues (2008) provide a thorough review of the effects of HA in the neocortex.
20. Zagha and McCormick (2014) review evidence on neuromodulation in general. Celada and colleagues (2013) review evidence on serotonin.

21. For reviews of current knowledge in the area, see Celada et al., 2013, Carhart-Harris et al., 2014, and Elliott et al., 2018.

22. Sakurai (2007) provides a comprehensive review of orexin, which sustains prolonged wakefulness by activating NA, HA, 5-HT, and ACh cells. It activates LC and 5-HT via OX_1Rs and HA via OX_2Rs. Li and colleagues (2010) show that orexin directly blocks I_h in layer 1 of the mouse equivalent of PFC. They note that orexin A increases excitability by reducing postsynaptic I_h, whereas orexin B increases excitability via pre-synaptic effects on higher-order thalamic terminals. Both effects implicate apical function specifically in wakefulness.

23. The psychologists Aston-Jones and Cohen (2005) hypothesize that phasic adrenergic activation facilitates 'exploitation', whereas tonic activation facilitates 'exploration'.

24. Kuipers and Phillips (2021) use pupillary dynamics to assessing levels of arousal in humans during an episodic memory task.

25. Hancock et al., 2008.

26. Phillips & Silverstein, 2013; Phillips, 2017.

27. Bruce Graham (pers. comm.) has performed several highly detailed multicompartmental simulations like those of Shai and colleagues (2015) of pyramidal cells. He finds that the slope of the function relating the cell's output to feedforward basal input is increased by apical depolarization in some cases, but reduced in others. Irrespective of any effect on slope, however, the effect of apical depolarization is to strengthen the cell's response to coincident basal depolarization by lowering the threshold at which it produces some response. Closer study of this issue is therefore likely to be highly relevant to ways in which the classical neuromodulators regulate apical function in context-sensitive neocortical neurons.

28. Munn et al., 2021.

29. Wilting and Priesemann (2019) show how a critical state of neocortical activity characterized by high sensitivity and long-range correlations in space and time can be rigorously distinguished from a state in which neuronal firing across different regions is predominantly asynchronous and independent.

30. Carhart-Harris and colleagues (2014) present a novel and broadly based account of neocortical dynamics that relates criticality to primary and secondary states of consciousness, to the default mode network, and to serotonin receptors, which are most dense in the apical dendrites of layer 5 pyramidal cells. They also show how that opens the door to closer interactions between neuroscience and Freudian notions of the ego and primitive states of mind. Their account also has the merit of indicating how research on the neuromodulatory regulation of context-sensitive cooperative computation could be expanded beyond a focus on cholinergic and adrenergic neuromodulatory systems. However, studies of criticality in neural systems have so far focused on systems composed only of 'integrate-and-fire' point neurons. The study of criticality and subcriticality in systems that also include context-sensitive two-point neurons may therefore reveal many gems that are as yet undiscovered.

31. Hobson, Hong, and Friston (2014) conclude that, when awake, the brain uses its internal predictions to interpret its sensory input, and that when dreaming, the internal predictions are used to generate perceptual experiences. Aru and colleagues (2020b) also conclude that during dreaming, the output of some pyramidal cells in perceptual regions of the neocortex is generated by apical input.

32. Shepherd, 2011.

33. Meyer, 2015.

34. Suzuki & Larkum, 2020.

35. Merker, 2007.

36. Whether colour exists independently of perception or not is debated from many perspectives by Byrne and Hilbert (2003) and their many commentators.

37. Ray et al., 1999.

38. Newell & Shanks, 2012.

39. *The Varieties of Religious Experience* by William James (1902) provides an objective account of the great variety of experiences that can be had without resorting to psychoactive substances. James throughout maintained an open mind concerning what they were experiences 'of', if anything.

40. James, 1904.

41. Polák & Marvan, 2019.

42. James, W. (1890). *The Principles of Psychology*, Vol. 1 (pp. 288–289). Macmillan and Co.

5
What Cooperative Neurons Do for Mental Life

This chapter relates the distinctive capabilities of context-sensitive pyramidal cells to basic cognitive functions. Revolutionary advances in neuroimaging techniques over the past few decades have identified what information is processed in each of the many different neocortical regions of humans and other species. The greater the amount of functional specialization within a system the greater the need for coordination, however, so the activities of individual cells are coordinated within and between neocortical regions such that they operate effectively together as a whole. The focus here is on how all that highly distributed processing is effectively coordinated via the basic cognitive capabilities of contextual disambiguation, selective attention, working memory and imagery, emotional prioritization, cognitive control, and learning.

Section 5.1 shows that perception, language, and rationality all depend on sensitivity to context. Section 5.2 shows how context-sensitive pyramidal cells in perceptual regions contribute to that by selectively amplifying coherent patterns of activity arising from sensory data. Section 5.3 outlines evidence that conscious experience when awake depends on context-sensitive pyramidal cells. Sections 5.4 to 5.8 outline evidence implicating their activities in selective attention, short-term memory (STM) and imagery, prioritization of emotionally significant events, cognitive control, and learning. As these various cognitive functions are interdependent, there is some overlap between the different sections. Section 5.3, on conscious experience when awake, overlaps with all the others because, from the perspective advocated here, conscious states are not something distinct from all those other more specific cognitive functions. They are states characterized by the operation of all or most of those cognitive functions.

Short term memory, working memory, and thought in general are examined in depth. Throughout our lives it is important to know who is thinking what. That knowledge is rarely, if ever, certain, however, and this book cannot reduce those uncertainties. What it tries to do is help you understand what

The Cooperative Neuron. William A. Phillips, Oxford University Press. © Oxford University Press 2023.
DOI: 10.1093/oso/9780198876984.003.0006

thought is, what it depends on, how it is achieved, and why unintended unin-
vited thoughts appear so often in our minds.

5.1 The Coordination of Mental Processes Depends on Cooperative Context-sensitivity

In this section we first focus on evidence that perception involves the use of
context to search for coherent interpretations of sensory input. That is then
shown to apply to other aspects of mental life, such as dissonance reduction,
bounded rationality, and language.

5.1.1 Perception Depends on Contextual Disambiguation That Seeks Coherent Interpretations

Perceptual interpretations of the rich sensory input available to us at each moment occurs within a complex and ever-changing context that includes other
parts of the current and previous sensory input together with current emotions, intentions, and our state of arousal. Many psychophysical paradigms
show that various components of that spatial and temporal context are used to
resolve ambiguities in the sensory data that we receive.[1] Though ambiguity is
inherent in all sensory data, its resolution using CONTEXTUAL constraints is
so effective in daily life that it usually goes unnoticed. Contextual disambiguation is crucial to what you are doing right now, for example. Your reading of
this text depends on contextual disambiguation at several levels of abstraction, from perception of the individual symbols of which it is composed, to
interpretation of its meaning. For example, when reading the capitalized word
in the above sentence, the second symbol is unlikely to be seen as being ambiguous. It is ambiguous, nevertheless, as you can see by noting that when it
occurs in the context of digits it is unlikely to be interpreted as a letter, particularly if it refers to a historic date, such as the falling of the twin towers on
September 11, 2001. The logic of contextual disambiguation can be inferred
by noting that an 'O' is missing from 'C NTEXT'. This shows that context is
neither necessary nor sufficient to see the symbol, and that the symbol itself is
both necessary and sufficient.

The words 'ambiguity' and 'context' are themselves ambiguous, however,
and I intend them to be interpreted broadly. By 'ambiguity' I mean ambiguities of presence, interpretation, or relevance to current goals. By 'context'

I mean that which is used to reduce ambiguity by strengthening relevant signals and weakening irrelevant signals. On this interpretation, relevance to current goals is a major form of context. Alternative interpretations of individual symbols are more relevant if proofreading than if reading for meaning, for example. Although these examples focus on the ambiguity of a single element, contextual disambiguation is usually cooperative in the sense that the individual elements help disambiguate each other, which is obviously needed at the level of letter identification when reading hand-writing. It is also cooperative in the sense that different levels of abstraction cooperate to help disambiguate each other. For example, interpreting hand-written letters depends on interpretation of the message being conveyed as well as on interpretation of the symbols. The extent to which perception depends on context is so great that some philosophers, psychologists, and cognitive neuroscientists argue that there are no such things as 'facts', only interpretations.[2]

The use of context to interpret the world within which we live implies increasing the coherence between our beliefs and the evidence of our senses, and also between our intentions and the outcomes of our actions. Figure 5.1 gives an example of the effectiveness of coherence, and of the persistent at-tempts to reduce incoherence. Your visual system has good reason to interpret each side of the figure as depicting part of a three-dimensional object. That does not lead to a stable percept, however, because the interpretations of the left and right sides of the figure are incompatible. The persistence of the un-stable perceptual experience produced by such pictures shows that inferences drawn from all the local coherences are not blocked by the global incoher-ence. That produces the persistent experience of conflict between the partial perceptual interpretations. Though such striking examples of the persistent

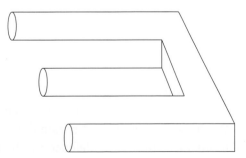

Figure 5.1 The devil's pitchfork shows that when there is substantial local coherence the visual system persists in trying to find a globally coherent interpretation that incorporates those local coherences.

search for coherence are not common in perception, they have much in common with the search for coherence in higher cognitive functions, where persistent indecision is more common.

The persistence of strong local coherence and the search for ways of incorporating them into a broader coherence is of crucial importance to far more than visual perception. It also applies to our goals, our beliefs, and our knowledge of ourselves. We must all choose between conflicting goals, reconcile our beliefs with each other and with the evidence of our senses. We must also find ways to live with self-knowledge that is not what we would prefer it to be. Events in the life of the writer George Orwell provide dramatic examples of how difficult that can be. He tried exceptionally hard to be honest about the conflicts, or dissonances, in his own life, but was unable to resolve them. Though well-aware of the horrors of violence, he volunteered to fight in the Spanish civil war. Though he was a life-long socialist, he wrote damning critiques of state socialism (*Animal Farm* and *1984*). He was also an Etonian scholar who sided with the down and outs in Paris and London. He died in 1950 at the age of 46, leaving his dissonances unresolved, but leaving us with warnings of enduring value, for example, beware of propaganda, surveillance, disinformation, and dishonesty.

Our common need to increase coherence and reduce dissonance in our mental lives is at the centre of one of the most influential and lasting theories in social psychology. First proposed in 1957 by Leon Festinger, the theory of cognitive dissonance reduction still has much to offer contemporary psychology. Festinger's theory of cognitive dissonance reduction argues that we are intrinsically motivated to reduce conflicts and seek harmony between the many different things that we know about ourselves, our behaviour, and our surroundings. He distinguished four different ways in which dissonance can be avoided or reduced, that is, by changing our behaviour, by changing our surroundings, by changing our beliefs, and by avoiding situations in which dissonance is salient. Though proposed in the early days of cognitive psychology, the theory of cognitive dissonance has many resonances with currently influential theories of neocortical function, and with the theory of predictive processing in particular.[3] The evidence for cooperative neurons indicates that the search for coherence and the avoidance of dissonance are so important that cellular mechanisms have evolved to facilitate them. This also raises the possibility that the context-sensitivity of pyramidal neurons could provide cellular foundations for some of the defence mechanisms assumed in Freudian psychoanalysis.

5.1.2 Context-sensitive Perception Can Be More Valid Than the Sensory Data

The devil's pitchfork shown in Figure 5.1 was devised such that local context guides interpretation towards interpretations that are globally incoherent. Usually, however, local context guides perception to a global interpretation that is both coherent and valid. Indeed, Ben Craven has devised a demonstration showing that context can guide interpretation towards an overall percept that is even more valid than the raw data itself! Figure 5.2 shows his demonstration, which is a variation on Rene Magritte's painting of a pipe above a caption saying, in French, 'This is not a pipe'. The point of Magritte's painting is to draw our attention to the difference between a pipe and a picture of a pipe. Ben combined that with the checkerboard illusion that was devised by Edward Adelson in 1995 using computer-generated imagery. Ben created a similar effect of context, except that he took a photo of a real checkerboard partly shadowed by a pipe. Though you may not believe it, the patch of light from the white square at the centre of the shadow in Figure 5.2 is darker than the patch from the black square at which the arrow points, as shown by the inset in Figure 5.2. The visual system allows for the shadow, however, and overrides sensory data that would be misleading if considered locally. That use of context creates a percept that is closer to the distal reality than is the raw data itself. These effects of context presumably operate via a combination of cooperative and competitive context-sensitivity, as outlined in Section 5.2.6.

The original painting by Magritte on which Figure 5.2 is based draws attention to four very different kinds of information in human conscious experience. First, there is the fleeting sensory-motor information on which our direct interactions with things in the world are based. Second, there are abstract perceptual representations of those things that can be activated by the things themselves, or by either pictures or thoughts of them. Third, there are abstract symbolic linguistic representations. Finally, there is information in strategic control systems concerning current and long-term goals. Abstract perceptual representations have an internal structure that echoes that in the things represented. They have an internal structure that can be meaningfully transformed in ways learned from the real world to produce novel but meaningful percepts, as in the processes of mental rotation or imagined combinations, for example. They are therefore

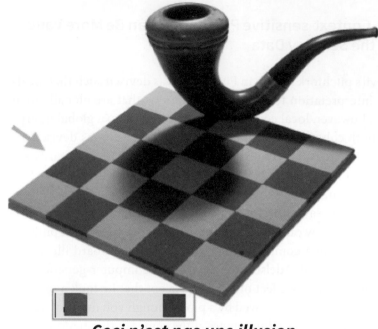

Ceci n'est pas une illusion

Figure 5.2 A photograph taken to demonstrate that context-sensitive interpretation can make the percept more valid than the raw sensory data. As the square at the centre is in shadow, the absolute amount of light reflected from it is less than the arrowed dark square, as can be seen by the rectangular inset below showing patches copied from those two squares and in the same relative position as above, but with the surrounding context removed. The brightness of the square on the right of the inset is identical to the central square. The perceptual inference that allows for the shadow in a way that correctly shows the brightness of the central square operates non-consciously to produce what we consciously experience. We are unaware of the ambiguity that it resolves, and we are unable to voluntarily prevent that inference. By comparing the patches shown out of context in the inset with those same patches in context above, you can see that in this case context operates mainly by amplifying the relative brightness of the central square, which is in shadow.

Adapted with permission from a demonstration by Ben Craven.

descriptive and restricted to the sensory domains from which they are abstracted. Words do not have an internal structure that echoes the things represented by those words. Therefore, they are categorical and in principle able to represent anything representable. As cooperative cells are present in all cortical regions, they presumably operate on all four kinds of information.

5.1.3 Language and Rationality Depend on Sensitivity to Context

Context-sensitivity and the search for coherence are also crucial at higher levels of abstraction, such as those involved in sentence production and comprehension. Consider '*To celebrate the end of the financial crisis he held a ball in the bank*'. This is full of ambiguity. It conveys no adequate information about who 'he' is. Meanings of pronouns are specified by context, as are the meanings of many common words, such as 'this' and 'that', for example. Furthermore, the words 'held', 'ball', and 'bank' are all ambiguous, as shown by comparing their meanings in the above sentence with their meanings in '*He held a ball in his hand, then rolled it down the bank*'. Some key principles of contextual disambiguation and the search for coherence can be inferred from these simple examples. First, though interpreted in the context of the whole, the parts are not merged but remain distinct from each other. Second, mutual disambiguation of the parts seeks coherent interpretations of the whole. Third, the whole thus formed can be familiar, as in the case of the word 'CONTEXT', for example, or novel, as in the previous italicized sentences. Fourth, the effects of context on word interpretation can be so strong that they override the effects of large differences in the probability with which default meanings are ascribed to ambiguous words. Possible, but improbable, meanings that fit the context are selected, while more probable meanings that do not fit are suppressed. Much humour depends upon these ambiguities and their various resolutions, as in the Victorian music hall song about the country girl who 'sits amongst the cabbages and peas', for example.

Effective and efficient mechanisms of the context-sensitive search for coherence are important prerequisites for the evolution of linguistic capabilities because language is replete with local ambiguity that must be resolved holistically to create and comprehend novel but coherent messages.[4] Edelman (2008) reviews a wide array of arguments and evidence indicating that mental life depends on sensitivity to context, with that dependence being especially strong in the case of language. For example, he notes that (on average) the 1,000 most common words in English have an average of 3.5 different meanings! So, without contextual disambiguation much of what we say would have so many different possible meanings that it would be of little use for interpersonal communication or for thought.

Psycholinguistic work on sentence interpretation may help us understand some of the more advanced capabilities that have evolved in cooperative context-sensitive neurons. Four maxims summarize the assumptions on which effective and efficient conversations are based. Summarized in four words they state that people usually try to say things that are true, concise, clear, and relevant. These maxims can be broken, as when lying, for example, but effective communication depends upon adherence to them being the rule, rather than the exception. These maxims are even more applicable to communications between pyramidal neurons in neocortex, where we can assume that they have evolved to cooperate effectively and efficiently in the pursuit of common goals. Though neocortical neurons can interact in ways that lead to misinformation, as in illusions, for example, we can assume that they have evolved such that they usually transmit valid and useful information. We can also assume that, in contrast to humans, pyramidal cells never lie in the sense of transmitting information that they know to be false or misleading. Therefore, I assume that all four of these maxims are applicable to communication between neurons, as well as to conversations between humans. Of these four maxims it is the injunction to be 'relevant' that has the most extensive ramifications, as shown by its place at the centre of what is known within psycholinguistics and social psychology as relevance theory.[5]

There are also grounds for supposing that the context-sensitivity that supports cooperative selection is crucial to the rationality of conscious thought. An assumption of rationality is commonly made and given empirical support in several areas of psychology and the social sciences. Nevertheless, much doubt has been cast on that assumption by the systematic irrationality observed in various psychological investigations, especially those concerned with judgements of probability and decision-making. Vlaev (2018) argues that human decisions are usually rational if interpreted within the context in which they were made, with the amount of contextual information that can be considered being strictly bounded. He shows that rationality assumptions typically hold if interpreted as operating within a well-specified context. This conception of the contextually bounded rationality of human judgements is supported by evidence that what operates as context is highly selective and dynamic. In part this is because it is guided by attended cues in the current stimulus input or in working memory. These contextual biases can be so strong that they can even affect our judgements and beliefs about ourselves. A surprising consequence of this is that currently available stimulus cues can in some cases lead us to think that judgements that we made a few seconds earlier were the opposite of what they really were![6]

5.2 Context Guides Perception via Apical Dendrites

Section 5.1 argued that neocortex continually seeks to maximize coherent meaning in our sensory input by perceiving things in context. It also argued that higher cognitive functions such as language and rationality are also highly dependent on context. This widespread sensitivity to context in mental life is matched by widespread context-sensitivity of pyramidal cells in perceptual and other regions of neocortex.[7] Excitatory contextual input to apical dendrites can reduce the range of feedforward sensory inputs to which pyramidal cells respond by strengthening the response of some cells but not others. That makes the information that they transmit more precise, but it usually makes little or no contribution to specification of the feedforward input to which pyramidal cells in perceptual regions are most sensitive, and thus to what they are interpreted as transmitting information about.

5.2.1 Physiological Studies Implicate Context-sensitive Apical Dendrites in Figure–Ground Segregation and Figural Synthesis

Many of these studies have been of the primary visual cortex, V1, which is at the base of two hierarchies of abstraction known as the 'what' and the 'where' visual pathways. Pyramidal cells in V1 are selectively tuned to various combinations of elementary properties such as the orientation of lines or edges, their size, and direction of motion. In higher cortical regions selective tuning is to more complex things, such as faces and many other things. The strength with which the cell responds to the input to which it is tuned depends on a wide variety of contextual inputs. These include input transmitted to the cell from within the same region, or from other cortical regions at similar levels in the hierarchy of abstractions, or from higher regions. Input from higher regions is sometimes referred to as feedback, implying that the recurrent activity was initiated in lower regions. In contrast, it is also sometimes referred to as 'top-down', implying that it was initiated in higher regions.

Amplifying effects of context are fundamental to figure–ground segregation. It has long been known that the sustained components of the response of pyramidal cells in V1 are amplified if the input to which they are tuned is part of the figure rather than of the ground. Far more has been discovered about the role of contextual amplification in figure–ground segregation and figural synthesis since then. These more recent discoveries confirm and clarify the distinction between the feedforward pathways that specify tuning and the various inputs that amplify response when it is part of the figure. For example, the sustained response to elements within a figure is amplified by feedback to V1 from higher regions. It is greatly reduced when micro-stimulation suppresses output from V4, implying that it depends in part on feedback from higher levels. Responses to elements that are part of a figure rather than of the ground are amplified by long-range intraregional and feedback inputs to apical dendrites in layer 1 of V1. This amplification depends on NMDA receptors, a distinct class of receptor for the excitatory neurotransmitter glutamate. Blocking those receptors greatly reduces the selective amplification of responses to figures but has little or no effect on responses of cells to their feedforward sensory input. This modulatory effect of NMDA receptors is as expected given that their activation is dependent upon prior activation of the cell from other sources. This evidence indicates that NMDA receptors have a crucial role in integrating inputs to the apical integration zone, and thus in influencing the cell's output via calcium spikes in the apical trunk.[8] The extent to which the effect of apical input depends upon prior generation of back-propagated action potentials as well as upon apical NMDA spikes, is not yet clear, and may depend upon the length of the apical trunk, and thus on the cortical layer in which the cell's soma resides.

Selective amplification of pyramidal cell responses to their feedforward receptive field input when they are part of a figure has also been clearly demonstrated in paradigms that study contour integration by the Gestalt cue of good continuation, as shown in Figure 5.3. Responses of cells in V1 to the oriented edges or lines to which they are selectively tuned is stronger if they are part of a straight or smoothly curving contour or straight line than if they are not. Contextual amplification is even stronger if the line or edge forms a closed contour, confirming its role in figural synthesis. Contour integration is a direct demonstration of contextual effects that amplify the salience of signals that cooperate to form a figure without corrupting the feedforward message that those signals convey.[9]

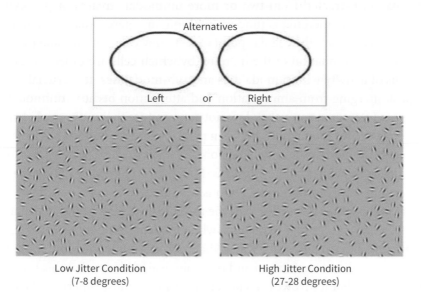

Figure 5.3   Contour integration as used in human psychophysical experiments to investigate the ability to group elements in a way that depends on the extent to which line elements are aligned to form a smooth contour. Elements that together form the smooth egg-shaped contour are more salient though less informative than the random background elements. Detectability of the figure depends on quantifiable parameters, such as the approximation to co-linearity of the elements in the figure and the density of the elements in the display. For example, when deviation from smoothness is low (7–8 degrees), as in the display on the left, the contour is more detectable than when it is high (27–28 degrees), as on the right. The egg-shaped contour in the display on the left is just above the threshold of detectability so is not easy to see. That in the display on the right is below the usual threshold of detectability, so it will be detectable by few, if any, readers.

Figure from Butler et al., (2013), as approved by Pamela Butler.

5.2.2 Physiological Studies Directly Implicate Apical Dendrites in the Cross-modal Amplification of Unimodal Signals

Via their own specific thalamic nuclei, the distinct visual, auditory, and somaesthetic modalities project to primary sensory regions of cortex that are referred to as V1, A1, and S1, respectively. The modality specific information extracted by those primary sensory regions is then transmitted to higher modality specific regions where other information is extracted. Multimodal regions at higher, more abstract, levels in the perceptual hierarchy then merge information extracted from two or more unimodal streams of processing. This multimodal merging is fundamental to many perceptual and cognitive phenomena.[10] From the cellular point of view, however, multimodal merging is simply a continuation of the merging by which cells are tuned to specific patterns of activity within modalities and sub-modalities. It is crucial to distinguish merging from amplification and attenuation because unimodal regions can interact in a way that does not compromise their unimodal identity. This evidence for interactions between primary sensory regions has led some to suggest that perhaps unimodal regions do not exist, despite the vast amount of evidence showing that they do. This dilemma is resolved by noting that the interactions between unimodal regions modulate transmission of their unimodal information. That preserves the unimodal identity of the information that they transmit to higher regions, while implementing cross-modal amplification of the strength with which that information is transmitted (Figure 5.4). There is direct anatomical and physiological evidence that this is indeed the case, and that it involves apical dendrites in the most superficial layers of the cortex. Though the following discussion is focused mainly on vision in auditory context, there is ample evidence that analogous interactions occur between all pairwise combinations of V1, A1, and S1.[11]

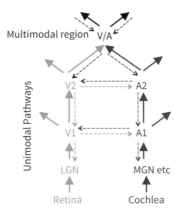

Figure 5.4 Contextual interactions between unimodal sensory regions. Unimodal visual regions depicted here are primary (V1) and secondary (V2) visual cortex. Unimodal auditory regions are primary (A1) and secondary (A2) auditory cortex. V/A is a multimodal region. V1 and A1 transmit unimodal information to the higher unimodal regions in their modality, but the strength or effectiveness with which they do so can be amplified by cross-modal interactions. Feedforward sensory inputs from which information is extracted for further feedforward transmission are shown as solid lines. Modulatory interactions are shown as dotted lines. Thus, the cross-modal interactions do not corrupt the unimodal information transmission that they amplify.

LGN, lateral geniculate nucleus; MGN, medial geniculate nucleus.

Responses of pyramidal cells in mouse V1 to the visual input to which they are tuned are strongly amplified when the onset of that input coincides with the abrupt onset of loud sounds. That occurs only in cells that are selectively sensitive to the current visual input, however. This amplification is due to direct connections from auditory cortex to pyramidal cell dendrites and to inhibitory and disinhibitory interneurons in layer 1 of V1. The dynamics of the resulting interactions are complex, and not yet adequately understand. Their net effect, however, is to enhance the cell's selective sensitivity by amplifying responses to its most preferred inputs while suppressing its response to less preferred input. In the dark their net effect is inhibitory, thus ensuring that auditory stimulation alone does not generate activity in V1. As this cross-modal amplification is more pronounced at lower levels of visual contrast, it suggests that faint images of predators in a dim environment are more likely to be detected when they coincide with abrupt sound onsets.[12] In general, these cross-modal interactions reduce in strength as the unimodal feedforward information from the sensors increases in strength. This is known as the principle of inverse effectiveness, which characterizes cross-modal interactions as studied by psychological methods.

Sensory signals are also perceived in the context of our own actions. Pyramidal cells in regions of neocortex concerned with speech perception, for example, respond more strongly to other people's voices than to the sounds that we generate ourselves when speaking. Similarly, pyramidal cells in mouse visual cortex respond more strongly to movements in the visual image that are generated by movements of things in the external world rather than by the mouse's own movements. Information distinguishing external from self-generated changes in the visual image is computed in higher-order thalamus and transmitted to the apical dendrites in layer 1 of the cortex. There it amplifies response to feedforward input from the lateral geniculate nucleus of those events that are not generated by the mouse's movement. Its effect is clearly amplifying rather than driving. Output from those cells requires sensory input and preserves the cell's feature specificity and high spatial sensitivity, rather than conveying information about the much larger part of the visual image from which the cells in higher-order thalamus extract information.[13]

Intermodal interactions in humans can produce illusions, such as the 'double-flash' illusion in which a single flash is seen as two if accompanied by two brief sounds. This is thought to reflect higher temporal resolution in hearing than in vision. Conversely, vision has a higher spatial resolution than hearing, which is thought to underlie the ventriloquist's illusion in which visual input guides perception of the location from which sounds are perceived as arising. Another example of intermodal interactions in humans may be provided by synaesthesia, which involves sensory input in one modality inducing sensory experience in another modality, as when a particular sound is experienced as also having a particular colour. This may be a consequence of a modified form of the anatomy and physiology outlined above. It could occur if, instead of modulating response to sensory input in the target modality, intermodal pathways generate activity within that modality by themselves.

The evidence for interactions between unimodal regions and for multimodal regions in which they are merged validates the ancient notion of a *sensus communis*, or common sense, used by philosophers such as Aristotle. In current psychological terminology that notion is an example of a hypothetical construct, but one for which we are now beginning to see the physical realization in networks of cells that include cooperative neurons.

5.2.3 High-resolution Brain Imaging Implicates Layer 1 in the Context-sensitivity of Perceptual Regions of the Human Neocortex

Most of the evidence on cooperative context-sensitivity at the cellular level has come from studies of species other than humans. Direct evidence is now also provided by neuroimaging of contextual effects in humans. High-resolution fMRI imaging shows that information received from a visible surround about an occluded part of a scene is greatest in the superficial layers. Other things that have been discovered using that partial occlusion paradigm include the following. First, contextual input from the surround can enhance the processing of weak or ambiguous feedforward sensory data when it is available. Second, the effects of the contextual surround generalize across different spatial frequencies of the feedforward input. Third, they are well modelled by assuming that the surrounding scene generates line sketches of the occluded part of the scene. This paradigm is also now being used to clarify many other issues, concerning the role of context in scene perception. As fMRI signals predominantly reflect synaptic activity, rather than action potentials, and include inhibitory as all as excitatory synaptic currents, these neuroimaging findings are consistent with modulatory functions of the apical input. Thus, this high-resolution neuroimaging is consistent with other evidence that apical dendrites are sensitive to context in humans as well as in other species. The exact conditions in which that contextual input is used to fill in missing feedforward data rather than to amplify weak feedforward data remain to be clarified.[14]

5.2.4 Object Recognition Depends on Disambiguating Effects of Context

Many psychophysical studies in humans show that object recognition is facilitated when objects are presented in the context of scenes in which they are likely to occur. Neuroimaging data collected during these experiments indicate that the orbitofrontal cortex a major multimodal association region, provides contextual information that is used to guide visual object recognition by the inferotemporal pathway. Magnocellular cells rapidly convey low spatial frequency information from V1 to the orbitofrontal cortex. There it is combined with other information to compute possible interpretations of that coarsely grained information. These possible interpretations are then projected to inferotemporal cortical regions where they are used to guide interpretation of both finely grained and coarsely grained information arriving more slowly from the secondary visual areas. The initial guesses produced by orbitofrontal cortex facilitate recognition by sensitizing the inferotempora pathway to the most likely candidate objects. This facilitates object recognition by amplifying those interpretations that are more likely given the contextual input from orbitofrontal cortex.[15] The role of apical dendrites in these effects of context on object recognition remains to be explored.

5.2.5 Apical Disinhibition Is a Mechanism for Cooperative Context-sensitivity

Figure 3.8 shows how VIP cells disinhibit apical dendrites by making small holes in the inhibitory blankets cast over them by SOM/SST cells (Karnani et al., 2014).[16] If those apical dendrites also receive adequate excitatory input, then the cell's response to its feedforward input will be amplified. It has now been shown that apical inhibition and disinhibition have central roles in mediating suppression and contextual facilitation in visual regions of mouse neocortex. If a visual stimulus is presented within a surround sharing many of the same features, then the salience of information about that stimulus is reduced by the inhibitory effect of SOM/SST interneurons. If the features of the stimulus differ from those of its surround, however, then locally specific VIP interneurons reduce surround suppression by inhibiting the SOM/SST inter-neurons that contribute to it.[17]

As mentioned, the context within which sensory processing operates also includes current motor activities. Sensorimotor integration and active sensing depend on fast and effective two-way communication between sensory and motor regions of neocortex. So, sensory regions receive input from motor cortex as well as the sense data to which they are selectively sensitive. Motor regions that move a mouse's whiskers are connected to pyramidal cells and VIP interneurons in the somatosensory cortex that receives sensory signals from those whiskers. When mice move their whiskers, selective amplification of the information that somatosensory neurons transmit about sensory input is disinhibited by VIP interneurons, and this information is used to estimate the position of objects sensed by moving the whiskers.[18]

5.2.6 Neocortical Context-sensitivity Is Both Cooperative and Competitive

Divisive normalization is the paradigmatic example of competitive context-sensitivity. It is a widespread canonical computation that has been seen in many different neural systems. It can be understood intuitively by noting that a tall cat is not as high as a short horse. That would make no sense if 'tall' and 'short' were interpreted as referring to absolute height. It makes sense because they are im-plicitly interpreted as being scaled relative to the average heights of the kind of thing that they describe. Normalization is often used within statistics to trans-late sets of measurements made in various ways to a 'neutral' or 'standardized' scale. It has been shown to be a common operation in biological neural systems.

Some key properties of divisive normalization contrast sharply with those of cooperative context-sensitivity. As the numerator in the division is never larger than the divisor its primary effects are suppressive, not amplifying. Divisive normalization depends on pooling a narrow set of local activities, not a wide and highly diverse set of inputs as does cooperative context-sensitivity. It is competitive in that any reductions in suppression of some local processors in the pool must be balanced by more suppression of others, analogous to that in zero-sum games. Thus, the rich get richer, and the poor get poorer, which is often described as 'winner takes all'. A basic function of normalization is to convert information into a common standardized scale, whereas the basic function of cooperative context-sensitivity is to select the information that is currently relevant. Divisive normalization reduces the correlations between signals, whereas cooperative context-sensitivity increases them by seeking coherence. Finally, divisive normalization is most prominent at sensorimotor stages of processing, whereas cooperative context-sensitivity is more crucial at higher than at lower levels of the cortical hierarchy. Carandini and Heeger (2012) provide an authoritative review of divisive normalization as a canonical computation in neural systems.

Jim Kay has confirmed that, though contrasting with cooperative context-sensitivity in several ways, divisive normalization is also a form of context-sensitivity. He applied the information theoretic measures outlined in Chapter 8 to physiological data on divisive normalization and found that divisive normalization in neocortex does indeed modify the strength of neural signals without corrupting the information that they transmit about their receptive field inputs. Normalization transmits little or no information specifically about the normalizer.

Given all these differences it is no surprise that cooperative and competitive context-sensitivity depend on different mechanisms. Neocortical mechanisms of divisive normalization are thought to include the inhibitory effects of interneurons that target basal and peri-somatic locations of the cell as well as those that target the apical dendrites. Basal and peri-somatic input to the soma is normalized by the parvalbumin (PV) basket cells that receive feedforward input and inhibit basal dendrites and soma but not apical dendrites (Figure 3.8).[19] Inhibitory SOM/SST interneurons, such as Martinotti cells, that target the apical dendrites also contribute to divisive normalization, including surround suppression. As these cells are tuned to orientation in V1 that explains the greater suppression there by similarly oriented surrounds. These suppressive effects do not completely block the cell's output. They simply reduce its salience. The effectiveness of normalizing activities by inhibiting apical dendrites depends on their being activated and connected to the soma, whereas input normalization via PV inhibitory interneurons does not.[20]

Interactions between somatosensory cortices in the left and right hemispheres are an example of suppression due specifically to inhibition of apical dendrites. Interhemispheric suppression in the case of somesthesis was outlined in Section 3.5. It operates by inhibiting the apical dendrites of layer 5 pyramidal cells. This interhemispheric suppression does not prevent the cell from responding to its feedforward receptive field input, however. It simply reduces the amplifying effects of apical activation on action potential output. The inhibition that it produces is 'silent', in the sense that it has no effect at the soma unless paired with feedforward input to the soma. Thus, competition between the left and right hemispheres is not due to any simple summation of excitatory and inhibitory inputs. The inhibitory interneurons by which it operates include neurogliaform cells, and much is now known about the cascade of intracellular molecular events by which they suppress excitation of apical dendrites. Competitive interactions between the two cortical hemispheres are seen in various psychophysical, electrophysiological, and pharmacological studies, as well as in various pathologies. These interactions have now been related in detail to intracellular biophysics.[21]

We can therefore assume that the operation of neocortex depends upon both cooperative and competitive forms of context-sensitivity. Overall, the net effect of context-sensitive interactions is likely to be inhibitory because more activities are usually suppressed than are amplified. This has been directly observed in the case of context-sensitive interactions between primary sensory modalities.[22] It has been known since at least 1995 that both surround suppression and amplification by contour integration affect pyramidal cell activities in neocortex.[23] The amazing demonstration shown in Figure 5.2 of the context-sensitivity that underlies conscious experience presumably involves both forms acting in concert, as usual.

Several theories exist in which these two forms of context-sensitivity are either explicitly or implicitly combined; only a few are considered here. They are explicitly distinguished in the computational models of Brosch and Neumann (2014a, 2014b). Those models show in detail how they can operate effectively together. Recurrent contextual signals are shown to be able to select and amplify the relevant feedforward information by disinhibiting apical dendrites that are suppressed by normalizing influences.[24] Models of selective attention that combine cooperative with competitive context-sensitivity have also been developed by Mike Spratling's lab in London.

Heeger and Zemlianova (2020) present a theory that combines divisive normalization with recurrent amplification. Though there is much similarity between their theory and the perspective of cooperative context-sensitivity, there are also a few differences. Both depend upon amplifying as well as upon divisive operations. Both emphasize modulatory processes that preserve the reliability of feedforward information transmission. Both assume a common local cortical microcircuitry in which there are functionally distinct subsets of inhibitory interneurons. Amplification in both is stronger for weak than for strong inputs. Both imply that neocortical pyramidal cells, but not inhibitory interneurons, have not one but two points of integration, with one summing the feedforward drive and the other summing recurrent information received from other parts of the network.

One way in which Heeger and Zemlianova's (2020) model of recurrent amplification differs from the perspective advocated here is that it analyses the microcircuit's temporal dynamics in far greater detail. They note that the hypothesis that synchronized oscillations provide a way of dynamically grouping neocortical activities remains controversial and suggest a role for it that is more than its critics allow but less than its advocates assume. That view resonates with our emphasis on apical dendrites as a mechanism for cooperative context-sensitivity and is compatible with the temporal dynamics of apical function as modelled by Siegel, Körding, and König (2000). A major task for the future, therefore, is to explore the possibility that the cellular anatomy and physiology of cooperative neurons as outlined here could provide cellular foundations for the recurrent amplification shown to be based on combining cooperative and competitive context-sensitivity.

The implementation of normalization by inhibitory interneurons that are distinct from those that inhibit apical dendrites has crucial implications for its relation to apical function. First, as input normalization does not depend on the cells that inhibit the apical dendrites, the feedforward signals that are amplified by apical disinhibition are subject to normalization independently of apical function. Second, neural modelling shows that normalization magnifies the consequences of small differences in salience. This is because normalization operates in a winner-takes-all manner such that it transforms a small advantage over the others in the population over which the normalization is being performed into a large difference. Thus, a small but selective amplification at one level of a feedforward hierarchy can be turned into all-or-nothing selection at the next. Third, because divisive normalization is widespread and competitive, amplification of the outputs of a few dynamically selected pyramidal cells by cooperative context-sensitivity implies indirect attenuation of the many outputs of those cells with which they compete.[25]

As this book focuses on cooperative interactions between cells, it is necessary to acknowledge that competition is also crucial. Indeed, to avoid the pruning of brain cells that occurs most prolifically in early stages of development, they must compete or die. That conclusion must be complemented, however, by the well-established conclusion that they must cooperate to live. The more numerous and diverse their collaborators the richer the organism's mental life.

5.3 Conscious Experience

William James (1890) argued that a cardinal function of consciousness is selection from a set of alternative possibilities (see Section 4.6), that is, choosing between alternative percepts, thoughts, and actions. That argument still seems valid, so this section examines the possibility that context-sensitive pyramidal cells contribute to conscious experience by amplifying the output of selected cells. First, however, it is necessary to note that loss of consciousness is the most likely result of a widespread amplification of pyramidal cell activity in general, as indicated, for example, by the epileptic loss of consciousness (reviewed in Chapter 7), which suggests that conscious experience depends on restricting amplification to a few selected targets.

Levels of cholinergic and adrenergic arousal are minimal during slow wave sleep so apical inputs to pyramidal cells then have little or no influence on their outputs (Chapter 4). During wakefulness these arousal levels are higher but fluctuate from moment to moment depending upon various aspects of the current context. As these neuromodulators regulate the effects of apical input on pyramidal cell outputs those effects will fluctuate along with arousal levels. In contrast to Chapter 4, which is concerned with differences between wakefulness and other states of mind, this section is concerned with why and how we are aware of some things but not others when awake. It is more concerned with the functions of conscious experience and the neuronal mechanisms by which they are implemented than with what is often called the 'hard problem of consciousness', that is, why things 'feel' the way they do.

As the focus here is on the mammalian thalamocortical system, I must first acknowledge that there are grounds for supposing that there may be some kinds of conscious experience that do not depend on the thalamocortical system. For example, there are grounds for supposing that there may be a primitive form of 'consciousness' in the brain stem, and that this may include some form of 'pre-reflexive self-awareness'. As the brain stem is ancient, that helps justify the injunction to treat other species as being not only conscious, but also as possibly having some form of self-awareness. Whether there is conscious experience outside of the thalamocortical system or not, however, there is widespread agreement that in humans the thalamocortical system is the main stage on which conscious experience occurs, even though a host of processes behind the scenes are necessary to make that possible.[26]

This section considers the role of context-sensitive apical dendrites in processes that are crucial to prominent theories of the neurobiological bases of conscious experience. One of those theories is based on recurrent interactions within and between cortical regions. One is based on recurrent corticothalamic interactions. One is based on broadcasting of information within the neocortex. Another is based on the concept of integrated information. Finally, many views of consciousness focus on fluctuations in the levels of neuromodulatory arousal when awake.

5.3.1 Recurrent Interactions between Cortical Regions Are Implicated in Neuronal Bases of Conscious Experience

Several theories associate conscious experience with recurrent loops formed by feedback from higher to lower levels, for as in the ventral 'what' or dorsal 'where' hierarchical pathways in vision, for example. Though there are no direct connections between primary sensory regions and frontal regions in primates, feedback from the highest to the lowest hierarchical levels is mediated by a chain of more local feedforward–feedback loops. Thus, recurrent loops within and between the levels of hierarchical abstraction could provide a neural basis for 'phenomenal' awareness of detailed sensory information. Recurrent loops linking the lowest and highest levels via a chain of local loops have been described as providing a neuronal basis for attentive or 'access' awareness of sensory information.

Recurrent feedback from higher to lower hierarchical levels provides an important part of the context within which the extraction of information from the feedforward sensory data proceeds, but that context also includes other recurrent connections. There is ample evidence for recurrent connections between cells that process information about nonoverlapping parts of the sensory input within regions and between regions at the same hierarchical level. Such connections have been called 'lateral', 'horizontal', or 'association fields'.

Figure 5.5 summarizes an influential theory of the dependence of conscious perceptual experience on these recurrent connections, which argues that visual awareness involves major transitions from being fully or subjectively invisible to being visible, and then from being unattended to being attended. It argues that the distinction between visible things that we attend and those of which we are aware, but that are unattended, echoes that between working memory and iconic sensory memory. As these two forms of memory are categorically distinct that implies two categorically distinct forms of visual awareness. Sensory awareness can convey a huge amount of information, but depends upon the presence of the sensory input, outliving it for only about one tenth of a second, if that. Only a tiny amount of that sensory information can be attended at any moment, however. Major functional consequences flow from the distinction between these two forms of memory or knowledge. Some highly selected information can long outlive the sensory input, and have lasting consequences, but only if attended, either voluntarily or automatically. According to recurrent processing

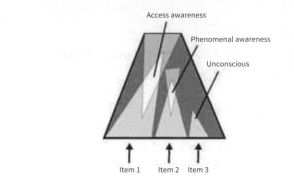

Figure 5.5 Distinct forms and stages of perceptual awareness from the viewpoint of recurrent processing theory. A: Item 1 is attended so it is part of access awareness. Item 2 becomes part of phenomenal awareness but it is not attended. Item 3 is processed to some extent, but the subject has no awareness of it. Recurrence is depicted as the overlap between the upward pointing and the downward pointing triangles.
B: Perceptual processes that occur at each of four stages of awareness. All occur when visible, whether attended or not. Only feature extraction and categorization occur when fully invisible. Interference and inference occur to some extent when subjectively invisible.

A: Lamme, 2004b. B: Lamme, 2020. Use of these figures approved by Victor Lamme, with permission from Elsevier.

theory, local feature extraction, feedforward categorization, some other forms of inference, and some forms of interference such as masking, occur whether the information becomes part of conscious experience or not. The theory contrasts such operations with those that depend strongly upon the information becoming part of conscious experience, and thus available to selective processes such as attention.

These specific operations include those concerned with perceptual organization such as figure-ground segregation and figural grouping, both within and across hierarchical levels.[27] This can be understood intuitively by noting that selective attention requires the specification of entities from which attention can select. Figure 5.3 provides an example of organizational processes, such as figural synthesis, that occur pre-attentively. The pop-out of such figures from the background does not depend upon first attending to the figures. This may explain why we are unable to voluntarily prevent such operations, as shown by what is referred to as the 'cognitive impenetrability' of many perceptual phenomena.

Thus, in essence, recurrent processing theory implies that perceptual information is part of conscious experience if and only if it is available to selective attention, which resonates with William James' arguments for selection as a cardinal function of consciousness. The perspective on conscious experience shown in Figure 5.5 is concerned specifically with visual perception, though it seems likely to have a more general relevance.

5.3.2 Apical Dendrites Are Implicated in Interregional Recurrence

Cooperative context-sensitivity is implicated in recurrence within and between regions on the grounds that if each link in a recurrent loop were sufficient to generate activity in the next by itself then there would be the danger of generating runaway overactivity. Furthermore, recurrent loops in which all connections are strong enough to activate the post-synaptic cell would operate as a population code for a single message in which any part implies all the other parts. Those problems are reduced by including a link in the recurrent loop that operates as an amplifier of response to input from outside the loop. There is clear anatomical evidence that many long-range recurrent inputs to neocortical pyramidal cells do indeed involve apical dendrites, which can operate in that way.

For these and other reasons, several theories propose that apical dendrites have a key role in conscious experience.[28] They are supported by direct physiological evidence for the causal role of apical dendrites in enabling mice detect small whisker deflections. The strength of calcium currents in the apical dendrites of a subset of pyramidal cells in layer 5 of mice's primary somatosensory cortex is strongly correlated with the probability that they detect weak whisker deflections. Furthermore, that detection probability can be raised or lowered by enhancing or opposing active currents in the apical dendrites, thus demonstrating that they have a causal role in perceptual detection.[29]

5.3.3 Apical Dendrites Are Implicated in Recurrent Feedback from the Higher-order Thalamus to the Neocortex

It has long been thought that higher-order thalamus has a crucial role in conscious experience. If that is so, then it implicates apical dendrites in conscious experience because higher-order thalamus projects strongly to layer 1 of the cortex, where it connects directly to the apical branches and also to the interneurons that inhibit them.[30] That view has now been supported and further developed by direct evidence that in both somaesthetic and visual regions of neocortex a major function of the higher-order thalamus is to regulate the coupling between the apical zone and the soma. These new discoveries concerning apical function have led to the dendritic integration theory of conscious experience (Aru, Suzuki, and Larkum, 2020). It proposes that conscious experience depends on coupling the apical integration zone to the soma to form both recurrent cortico-cortical and recurrent corticothalamic loops. The evidence reviewed here supports several aspects of that theory, including its proposals concerning the effects of anaesthesia, cholinergic arousal, and on the distinct role of the apical integration zone in forming recurrent corticothalamic loops. Dendritic Integration Theory puts the central emphasis on the role of higher-order thalamus in regulating the coupling of the apical integration zone to the soma.[31] Though the perspective advocated in this book agrees with several fundamental aspects of that theory, there are a few important differences. First, there is the simple matter of terminology. The phrase 'apical amplification' makes clear that the perspective advocated concerns apical dendrites specifically, not dendritic computation in general. Second, amplification contrasts with integration in that the key point of the notion of apical amplification is that apical input can function in a way that keeps its effects separate from those of basal inputs, rather than being summed with them as in integrate-and-fire point neurons. Third, the perspective advocated here emphasizes several subcortical inputs to apical dendrites that includes but extends well-beyond the thalamus. Fourth, the perspective advocated here explicitly argues that context-sensitive selection between alternatives is a cardinal function of conscious experience.

As coupling the apical integration zone to the soma will have no effect on output if the apical integration zone receives no input, coupling is a factor that enables apical input to affect the cell's output, but it is not usually sufficient to produce an effect of that coupling. It is therefore important to note that higher-order thalamus does more than regulate coupling between the apical calcium-spike initiation zone and the soma. It also regulates input to the apical zone, including effects that reduce rather than enhance the salience of response to selected feedforward sensory signals. For example, input to layer 1 of the neocortex from higher-order thalamus reduces the salience of feedforward visual signals generated by the animal's own movements.[32]

Recurrent interactions between the prefrontal cortex (PFC) and the higher-order thalamus are particularly complex, even in mice. The higher-order thalamus is that which receives most of its input from diverse internal sources rather than from sensory receptors as do the specific thalamic nuclei. Pyramidal cells in lower layers of PFC transiently activate two distinct higher-order thalamic nuclei, one of which sends both excitatory and inhibitory signals back to the most distant tips of the apical tree whereas the other activates synapses closer to the apical integration zone. In both cases this feedback has an amplifying rather than a driving effect on the pyramidal cells affected. That avoids strong loops that could lead to over-excitation that would corrupt the selective sensitivity of cortical cells. It has been directly shown that reverberant activity can be maintained in these corticothalamic loops via strong direct excitatory connections from the thalamic nuclei to neurons in layers 2 and 3 of the cortex, which then activate the cells in layer 5, which activate the thalamic nuclei.[33]

Among the many findings concerning relations between the higher-order thalamus and the neocortex, at least four are especially relevant here. First, cells in the higher-order thalamus provide input to a much larger population of pyramidal cells in neocortex than that from which they receive input. Second, some connections from the cortex to the thalamus are driving, and some are amplifying. Third, cells in higher-order thalamic nuclei receive inputs from a wide diversity of cortical and subcortical sources, not only from regions of cortex to which they project.[34] Fourth, activity in higher-order thalamic nuclei is more closely related to the subject's confidence in their judgements about sensory input than to the accuracy of their judgements.[35] If confidence is equivalent to salience, it provides further grounds for supposing that input from higher-order thalamic nuclei can amplify cortical response to direct feedforward inputs.

5.3.4 Apical Dendrites Provide a Cellular Mechanism for Reception of the 'Broadcasting' Implicated in Conscious Experience

'Broadcasting' is the transmission of information about neuronal activity in a way that makes it widely available to cells in many other cortical regions. This is central to the Global Neuronal Workspace theory, which is well summarized by Anil Seth in *Scholarpedia* under 'Models of Consciousness'. That theory was inspired by artificial intelligence (AI) algorithms that operate by cooperative interactions between large collections of specialized programs. The idea that conscious experience involves broadcasting in the neocortex is supported by neuroimaging evidence that a sensory input activates more cortical regions if it is experienced than if it is not. Though rarely made explicit, the notion of broadcasting implies that pyramidal cells can be affected by the broadcast information without that being merged with the locally specific information that they extract and transmit. If the cells receiving the broadcast merged all their inputs into the value of a single variable, then their outputs would all be much the same, and of little informative value. This suggests that pyramidal cells can receive the broadcast and be affected by it but without that compromising their individually distinct contributions. The context-sensitivity of apical dendrites provides that capability. Thus, the output of pyramidal cells can be broadcast in the sense that it is used as part of the contextual input to cells in several different cortical regions. That allows for broadcasting to have a wide range of different breadths. Some pyramidal cells could provide contextual input to a few other cells. Some could provide it to many more.

No pyramidal cell could provide apical input directly to all the other pyramidal cells that need to receive the broadcast, but it could do so indirectly via a chain of intermediaries. A crucial property of such mediated contextual interactions is that they will only operate if cells in the mediating connections are currently activated by feedforward input to their basal dendrites. That is in good agreement with evidence from various cognitive paradigms indicating that the effects of context are restricted to cells that are currently active. This is consistent with the possibility that the 'context' within which we perceive, think, and act is not provided by all that we know or believe, but only by currently active percepts, thoughts, and decisions (Section 5.1).

5.3.5 Apical Dendrites Provide Capabilities Implied by the Integrated Information Theory of Consciousness

The integrated information theory of consciousness proposed by Tononi and others is abstract, complex, highly ambitious, and controversial, as well as highly influential. It proposes that conscious experience depends on integrated information, where that implies systems with a special form of feedback or recurrent connectivity. It is formulated using its own version of information theory and implies that neuronal signals convey information about distinct things even when they interact to form a coherent whole.[36] Though the integrated information theory (IIT) of consciousness has some fundamental similarities to the coherent infomax theory outlined in Chapter 8, it cannot be adequately summarized in a few pages, so I make no attempt to do that. Instead, I simply note that the basic goal of the neocortex, as seen by the coherent infomax theory, is to maximize coherence between context-sensitive local processors transmitting messages that remain distinct despite their interaction. IIT refers to this interaction as 'integration'. That terminology is unhelpful in relation to cooperation between pyramidal cells because it does not imply that they have two distinct sets of influences on their outputs with information being transmitted specifically about only one of those two inputs. A basic similarity between IIT and context-sensitive cooperative computation is that they both imply reconciliation between opposing objectives because as organization (whether called coherence or integration) increases then information carrying capacity decreases, so it is impossible for both to be at a maximum. The reality and reconciliation of those opposed objectives implies a dialectical philosophy of evolution (Section 6.1).

5.3.6 Conscious Experience Depends on Fluctuating Levels of the Neuromodulatory Systems That Regulate Apical Function

As outlined in Chapter 4, acetylcholine, orexin, noradrenaline, serotonin, and histamine all tend to produce wakefulness. Although it was originally thought that these neuromodulators affect cortical activity uniformly as a whole, and change only on a slow timescale, we now know that their activity levels vary across cortical regions and can fluctuate from moment to moment when awake.

First, consider cholinergic arousal. Though long assumed to diffusely activate the cortex uniformly as a whole, advances in molecular genetics, quantitative neuroanatomy, and physiology now show it to be far more differentiated. Cholinergic activation can rapidly and effectively regulate specific cognitive processes such as transitions between mental states during sleep. During wakefulness it is implicated in basic cognitive functions such as selective attention and learning. For example, when mice are actively performing an auditory recognition task the activity of most pyramidal cells in auditory cortex is much suppressed, but the activity of a few is enhanced. These inhibitory and disinhibitory processes depend upon cholinergic modulation that increases relevant and suppresses irrelevant pyramidal cell activity by activating all three main types of inhibitory interneuron. This includes the VIP interneurons that specifically disinhibit the apical integration zone and apical branches. Cholinergic activation increases the electrical excitability of apical dendrites via modulation of calcium channels, thus powerfully enhancing apical functions. The effects of general anaesthetics that disconnect apical input from the soma by directly or indirectly blocking metabotropic cholinergic receptors show the dependence of both conscious experience and apical function on cholinergic arousal. The role of cholinergic activation in cognitive function is clearly implied by its role in pathologies as diverse as Alzheimer's disease, schizophrenia, and autism, all of which have major implications for what is or is not consciously experienced (see Chapter 7).[37]

Now consider adrenergic arousal. We have direct evidence that adrenergic activation affects apical function and basic cognitive processes. However, there is also evidence that some interpret as suggesting that adrenergic arousal is not necessary to either perceptual awareness or apical function, so that raises crucial issues to be resolved. The evidence that adrenergic activation affects perceptual experience, thought and learning includes psychopharmacological experiments in humans. For example, drugs that increase adrenergic activation increase people's ability to detect and discriminate weak visual stimuli. They also increase cortical EEG and fMRI responses to those stimuli. Drugs that decrease adrenergic activation have the opposite effect. Apical function is implicated in these effects of adrenergic arousal because that greatly enhances apical function. This has been directly shown by observing the effects of activating adrenoreceptors on apical calcium currents in awake mice. It increases calcium currents in the apical branches and lowers the threshold for the generation of calcium spikes by the apical integration zone. These effects are produced by a reduction in the leak currents that flow through HCN channels in apical dendrites. These findings clearly indicate that adrenergic arousal has a major role in enhancing perceptual awareness, and other basic processes of conscious cognition. They also indicate that it does so by regulating the amplifying effects that inputs to apical dendrites have on the output of pyramidal neurons.[38]

Nevertheless, there is also evidence that is interpreted as indicating that adrenergic activity is not necessary for conscious experience. This comes from clinical observations of patients suffering from cataplexy, which is a common symptom of narcoleptic sleep disorder. Muscle tone is lost during a cataplectic episode, so the person suddenly goes limp and collapses for a few minutes. That seems to involve temporary inactivity of the subcortical nucleus that helps maintain muscle tone, and which sends adrenergic signals to the cortex. People remain conscious during cataleptic attacks, however. So, prima facie, that indicates that conscious experience does not require adrenergic activation. A similar conclusion is suggested by studies of the effects of cholinergic or adrenergic activation in prefrontal and parietal regions of rodents under sevoflurane anaesthesia. Cholinergic activation in the PFC but not the parietal cortex restored a wakeful state, despite the anaesthesia. In contrast to that, adrenergic activation in the prefrontal and parietal regions produced no wakeful behaviour. Further evidence casting doubt on the role of adrenergic activation in apical function and conscious experience is that, although blocking metabotropic cholinergic receptors disconnects the apical input from the soma, blocking adrenergic receptors does not.[39] Thus, these empirical findings cast doubt on the role of adrenergic arousal in conscious experience. These doubts have led some to conclude that the function of the noradrenergic system is primarily to ensure that postural muscle tone is appropriately matched to arousal state, rather than to regulate conscious cognitive functions.[40] However, this conclusion is far from convincing, given the role of adrenergic activation in perceptual experience and in attention and working memory.

How can these apparently contradictory empirical findings be reconciled? One simple way is by noting that, although adrenergic activation plays a major role in extending the integration of inputs to the apical branches over space and time, adrenergic arousal is not necessary for integration to occur because histamine, serotonin and orexin also facilitate apical integration. It is common for there to be multiple alternative routes by which important biological requirements are met, and so it may be for conscious experience. It is known that histamine and serotonin remain active during cataplexy, so that can explain how conscious function can be largely preserved when adrenergic arousal is suppressed during a cataplectic episode, even though a primary function of adrenergic arousal is to enhance conscious cognition. Furthermore, histamine and serotonin facilitate apical function by suppressing the deactivating HCN currents, as does noradrenaline.

In addition to these complexities there are also grounds for supposing that there may be regional differences in the effects of exceptionally high levels of adrenergic activation. At those levels, apical amplification may be suppressed in the PFC, though not in other regions (Chapter 4). Thus, there are several grounds for supposing that fluctuating regulation of apical function by the neuromodulators has a central role in basic cognitive processes, such as attention, working memory, and emotional prioritization that together constitute the current state of mind.

5.4 Selective Attention

Selective attention involves processes by which perception, thought, learning, and action are dominated by a few selected things rather than by many alternative possibilities. It is a broad topic, encompassing a wide range of issues. At the level of pyramidal cells, it involves increased responses to attended stimuli together with reduced responses to other stimuli. These effects occur in primary sensory regions, as well as in higher regions. Both psychological and neurobiological studies show that pre-attentive processing can convey a huge amount of information because it operates concurrently across many streams of processing, whereas selective attention is serial in that the amount of information that can be selected for enhanced processing at any moment is highly limited. Pre-attentive concurrent feedforward processing can rapidly recognize familiar things up to high levels of abstraction, including the recognition of familiar words in humans. Attention is needed to help select relevant signals to be amplified, and to form memorable schematic descriptions of novel things and events.

As the capacity of attention is so limited there is often rivalry between alternative foci of attention. For example, there may be rivalry between the cerebral hemispheres because they tend to draw attention in opposite directions. There is also active suppression of currently irrelevant things. The ability to avoid or overcome distractions varies across individuals, and over time and practice within individuals. Disorders of attention are common and often managed in part by pharmacotherapy.

Psychological studies show that attentive search for a single target can operate simultaneously across many concurrent streams of processing but can find only one target within each quarter of a second or so, producing a phenomenon known as the attentional blink. They also show that attention operates within a spatial framework in that what is amplified is information about the properties of a single coherent object or event located in space.[41]

Selective attention is often conceived of as biassing the competition that underlies divisive normalization (Reynolds and Heeger, 2009). From that point of view competitive context-sensitivity mediated by inhibitory interneurons can be seen as providing a neural mechanism for divisive normalization with cooperative context-sensitivity providing the bias. Furthermore, selective attention can operate via cooperative context-sensitivity by directly activating apical dendrites as well as by disinhibiting them.

5.4.1 Context-sensitive Pyramidal Cells Are Implicated in Selective Attention on Empirical and Computational Grounds

The theory of biased competition, developed to summarize the known psychophysical properties of selective attention, relates in detail to neuronal activity. It notes that there is competition between pyramidal neurons that detect different stimuli within a small region of space. This competition is ubiquitous because it arises from normalization at each level of the abstraction hierarchy (Section 5.2.6). That tends to produce a winner-takes-all outcome, thus converting amplification into selection. This competition can be biased by signals specifying which pyramidal cells are to have their outputs amplified.[42] Various ways in which this amplification could be achieved at the cellular level have been proposed, and apical mechanisms are an obvious candidate.

Availability for selection by attention depends upon processes of figure–ground organization, inference, and interference, as outlined by Lamme (Figure 5.5). Within that large set of perceptible events, some events 'pop out' automatically and are given enhanced processing in a way that is experienced as an involuntary direction of attention. The preceding sections implicate apical function in all those processes. We also have some ability to voluntarily choose what to attend to, however, so it is the capabilities, mechanisms, and limitations of that voluntary attention that are the central concern of this section.

Typically, attention enhances the responses of pyramidal cells to their sensory input without changing the stimuli to which they are most sensitive, that is, their receptive field selectivity. In some cases, attention does enhance the precision of that sensitivity, however. Voluntary selective attention has effects on local processing that are comparable to those of coincident auditory stimulation on the responses of pyramidal cells in primary visual cortex to visual stimulation. Those intermodal interactions are shown by dotted lines in Figure 5.4 and are implemented by intermodal connections to the apical dendrites in layer 1. Furthermore, attention usually has little or no effect unless the cell receives some sensory input, thus showing that it has modulatory effects of the kind that apical dendrites can produce.

Several computational models show explicitly how selective attention could modulate feedforward transmission using the context-sensitivity of apical dendrites in neurons with two points of integration. Sensory input in these models produces output in the absence of top-down bias, whereas attention's modulatory effects produce no output in the absence of sensory input. Some models designed by Spratling and colleagues (among the earliest of this kind) explicitly use neurons that have distinct apical and basal compartments, with cooperation being implemented through modulatory signals arriving at the apical dendrites, and competition occurring at the basal dendrites; their later work shows how those models of selective attention can be combined with predictive coding.[43] These models replicate the facilitating effects of attending to specific spatial locations and the effects of attending to specified features. They also account for many other visual phenomena including the regulation of collinear facilitation by attention. Though these models have been applied primarily to visual data processing, their computational style may well have a far wider significance.

There are other computational models that also use the context-sensitivity of apical dendrites to produce the amplifying effects of attention. They show that the effects of attention are compatible with divisive normalization and are enhanced by it, that the fast dynamics of these effects are compatible with EEG data from studies of attention, and that input to the apical dendrites can switch their mode of operation from being modulatory to being driving if the apical input is strong enough.[44]

5.4.2 Apical Disinhibition Is Directly Implicated in Selective Attention

Apical dendrites and inhibitory interneurons in layer 1 are implicated in selective attention on simple anatomical grounds: they receive input from the higher cortical regions and thalamic nuclei whose activity is increased when attending and which produce deficits in attention demanding tasks when their function is impaired. Selective attention can therefore amplify the outputs from a few selected pyramidal cells, while suppressing that of many others. Choosing which to amplify and which to suppress is difficult, however, because it is far from easy to decide what merits attention and what does not. If relevant signals are ignored, then potentially useful information will be disregarded, as it does in pathological cases where spatial neglect occurs. If irrelevant or misleading information is attended then more information is amplified than can be effectively dealt with, and information overload will impair both current processing and learning, for example, as it does in attention deficit disorders. A *tour de force* of technical virtuosity using multiple simultaneous electrode recordings in slices of rodent brain, together with dual whole-cell recordings in the living animal, has clarified how the balance between amplification and suppression is regulated at the level of pyramidal cells. It shows that inputs to layer 1 from sources, such as those selecting what is to be attended, can amplify the output of selected pyramidal cells, both by directly activating their apical dendrites and by disinhibiting them.[45]

The selective capabilities of apical dendrites have been related in detail to the phenomena of interhemispheric inhibition (Sections 3.5 and 5.2). If events attracting attention to one side of space happen at about the same time as events attracting it to the other side, then one of them may not be noticed. Pathologically increased interhemispheric inhibition is a common symptom of neglect disorders due to parietal lobe damage, called extinction by neurologists. A patient's responses to light touch on one foot are much reduced if preceded by a touch to the other foot. These suppressive effects of preceding stimulation last for a few hundred milliseconds, because they are due to a special class of long-acting inhibitory receptors on the apical dendrites of pyramidal cells. The interhemispheric inhibition has no effect on the cell's output in the absence of its preferred sensory input, showing that it is not simply due to the summation of excitatory and inhibitory input. It does not block the initial part of the cell's response to its preferred input but curtails it by activating the neurogliaform inhibitory interneurons in layer 1 that generate a slowly decaying form of inhibition. This is all as expected of a suppressive effect that reduces the apical amplification of sensory responses.[46] However, it is unclear whether this interhemispheric inhibition suppresses apical contributions to output that make an initially imperceptible response accessible to attention, or whether it does so by suppressing attention to an already perceptible event, or both.

The time course of interhemispheric inhibition in the case of somesthesis is like the 'attentional blink' that occurs when a second stimulus that is to be attended follows too soon after a previously attended stimulus. It has been suggested that this effect arises because of the time required for the operation of recurrent loops in which apical dendrites have a pivotal role, so the possibility that these various phenomena depend on the same or similar cellular mechanisms merits further investigation.[47]

To understand attention at a cellular level it is not enough to know how apical inputs amplify relevant and suppress irrelevant outputs. It is also necessary to know the sources of the apical inputs. Several frontal regions have been identified as major sources of locally specific amplifying input to pyramidal cells in sensory and perceptual regions. In particular, the cingulate frontal region, which has a key role in selective attention, projects predominantly to layer 1 of perceptual regions, with a smaller projection to layer 6. Activating locally specific cells in the cingulate gyrus of awake mice increases the response of cells in visual cortex to sensory input at a specific location while suppressing responses of cells sensitive to the nearby surround. The increase is greatest to the cell's preferred sensory input, which is not changed by the amplifying input from the cingulate. Inactivation of the cingulate gyrus decreases the response of cells to their preferred visual input. Activating it when the mice are engaged in a visual discrimination task improves their performance, thus showing that cingulate input amplifies transmission of selected information about the sensory input. In addition to providing direct excitatory input to apical dendrites, the cingulate gyrus activates the inhibitory interneurons that disinhibit them, thus further implicating apical dendrites in selective attention.[48] Thus, to further clarify what determines relevance (from the neuronal viewpoint), we need to find out more about the inputs to, and operations within, the cingulate gyrus.

Judgements of what to amplify and what to suppress within a visual scene also involve the frontal eye field. This is a prefrontal region involved in target selection and the control of eye movements. Recent studies of the frontal eye fields have been particularly useful in distinguishing two classes of criteria on which selective attention is based. Exogenous, or external, criteria are based on stimulus properties. Endogenous (internal) criteria include current intentions and emotional evaluation. Both classes of criteria have major effects on attention and compete when opposed. Salient stimuli can often capture attention automatically when inconsistent with current intentions, thus showing that, although voluntary choice of what to attend to is important, it is not omnipotent. Nevertheless, selective amplification by some neurons in the frontal eye fields is more dependent on current intentions than on stimulus salience. There is also a large class of visually responsive neurons in the frontal eye fields whose responses at stimulus onset are initially sensitive only to stimulus-based criteria for salience, and not to the internal criteria for current relevance. This dependence on stimulus salience is reduced if subjects emphasize accuracy, rather than speed, however.[49] So, it may be that contextual input to the apical dendrites of cells in the frontal eye fields changes rapidly as processing proceeds, consisting of local purely external stimulus-based components initially, with input from other sources being added later.

As mentioned, the interneurons that disinhibit apical dendrites (i.e. VIP inhibitory interneurons) have a key role in determining which cells have their outputs amplified. Their inputs are highly diverse, including input from higher cortical areas, from higher-order thalamic nuclei, from the cholinergic and serotonergic systems, and from motor cortex during locomotion and other movements. Furthermore, reinforcement signals during auditory discrimination tasks disinhibit apical dendrites in both auditory and prefrontal regions when awake This diversity of input to cells that disinhibit the apical dendrites of context-sensitive pyramidal cells is as expected if the function of those dendrites is to put feedforward processing in a broad context, including task-dependent processes of attention.[50]

As discussed, localized deactivation of cells in higher-order thalamic nuclei, such as the pulvinar in vision, causes severe deficits of attention to the associated location in space. It also produces a localized increase in low-frequency oscillations, such as those that occur across the whole cortex during sleep. This suggests that localized interactions between higher-order thalamus and cortex are required to maintain a selected part or parts of cortex in an active state of attentive awareness, thus again implicating the amplifying capabilities of apical dendrites in selective attention.[51]

5.4.3 Selective Attention and Apical Function Depend on Cholinergic Activation

Attention to selected signals when awake depends on temporary increases in the cholinergic input to specific cortical regions. That enables the intracortical amplification of responses to relevant signals and suppression of responses to irrelevant signals. The signal to noise ratio is thus increased, where 'signal' is defined as relevance to the context, and noise is irrelevant information. That improves the detection of relevant signals as shown by behaviour. Reducing cholinergic input to the cortex has the opposite effects. These temporary increases in cholinergic input can be evoked by properties of the feedforward sensory signals, or by prefrontal regions that specify current goals, or by both, which cooperate to make search for things that have high stimulus salience particularly easy.[52]

Cholinergic activation is also clearly related to the normalization theory of selective attention as biased competition. Normalization occurs at all or most stages of cortical processing and signals that are selected for amplification by processes of attention have a crucial advantage in the normalizing winner-takes-all competition. The normalization theory of attention has now been further developed by noting that the effects of attention on neuronal firing rates, variability, and synchrony match those produced by cholinergic activation, which varies over time and cortical regions to a far greater extent than originally supposed.[53] This enhanced version of the normalization model of attention has several major implications. First, pyramidal cells receive information about both the current stimulus context and the internal context. Second, they can use context to amplify response to their preferred sensory input. Third, this amplification depends on cholinergic inputs to neocortex. As mentioned, the context-sensitivity of pyramidal cells meets these three requirements. It explains the effects of cholinergic activation as directly regulating the amplifying effects of intracortical context by disinhibiting input to the apical dendrites, and by coupling the apical integration zone to the soma. It also does so indirectly via its effects on the higher-order thalamic nuclei that regulate apical function, and it combines effectively with the normalizing processes that in effect convert amplification into selection.

5.4.4 Prefrontal and Temporal Regions Contribute to Selective Attention

Functional neuroimaging in humans shows that prefrontal regions are involved in both the attentional enhancement of relevant stimuli and the suppression of distracters.[54] The activity of pyramidal cells in prefrontal regions is especially dependent on arousal. It is greatly enhanced by orexin, both directly and by orexin's activation of the other arousing neuromodulators. In the PFC, the direct effects of orexin increase responsiveness in all layers, whereas these effects are more restricted in other regions. Orexin increases the responsiveness of prefrontal cells by enhancing apical function in at least two ways. It opposes HCN leak currents in apical dendrites, and it has a presynaptic excitatory action on inputs to apical dendrites from nonspecific thalamus.[55] Thus, these effects of arousal on apical dendrites have a central role in maintaining the contributions of prefrontal cells to higher cognitive functions such as selective attention.

Prefrontal regions have a key role in maintaining the focus of attention and suppressing distractions, but they also have a key role in switching the focus when needed. The implicit judgements required to classify signals as distractions to be suppressed are far from trivial. Assessment of the need to switch the focus of attention is even more difficult, so it is no surprise that both aspects of selective attention depend on prefrontal regions whose dynamics depend upon cooperative interactions with many other regions.

The maintenance and switching of attentional focus have also been related to different levels of adrenergic activation in prefrontal regions. When adrenergic activation in prefrontal regions is low goal-dependent selective attention has little or no effect. When adrenergic activation is moderate, the focus of attention selected by prefrontal cells is maintained by activation of low threshold adrenergic receptors, which enhances apical function by opposing HCN currents. This amplifies pyramidal cell responses to task-relevant signals, thus improving performance in tasks that depend upon maintaining the focus of attention. At higher adrenergic levels activation of high threshold receptors enables the switching of attentional focus. That improves performance in tasks requiring shifts of attention but can in some circumstances impair performance in tasks requiring maintained attention and the suppression of distractors.[56] When stress is high, both adrenergic and dopaminergic activation are raised to levels that in effect take the more recently evolved functions of the PFC 'off-line', while strengthening the functions of more primitive circuits, thus producing behaviour that is more reflexive than reflective.[57]

During binocular rivalry, or when viewing ambiguous figures, attention may be drawn alternately to one winning local coalition after another. When there is no coherent overall winner, for example, as when viewing impossible figures such as the devil's pitchfork (Figure 5.1), then attention is sequentially drawn to partially coherent local coalitions. The continual conflict that is experienced between them shows that the short-term dynamics, from which perceptual experience arises, continually seeks coherence.

Section 5.3 argues that selective amplification based on the local stimulus context makes pre-conscious percepts available to attention. So, if signals have already been amplified pre-attentively, what more can be done by voluntary attention? A key property of attention emphasized here is that in addition to increasing the amplification of selected information it extends its duration, as discussed in the following section. Both of these greatly increases the effects of the cell's output on cortical regions to which it projects. As this voluntary selection depends on the PFC, which receives information from many other cortical regions, this form of attention has the dynamics and context-sensitivity of which we experience as the voluntary control of attention.

Although frontal eye fields and parietal regions have been emphasized above and in much of the research on the neurobiological bases of selective attention, regions of the temporal lobe also make a major contribution (Ramezanpour & Fallah, 2022). That is in clear accord with the perspective advocated here because it seems safe to assume that cooperative context-sensitive pyramidal cells are at least as plentiful in temporal regions as they are in parietal regions. Therefore, their role in temporal lobe selective attention invites extensive exploration.

5.5 Working Memory and Imagery

The neuronal bases of STM, and working memory in general, are examined in depth because they are crucial to so many aspects of human mental life. They are usually, though not always, under voluntary control. Searching for their neuronal bases requires us to specify what those processes are in terms that can be explicitly related to neuronal capabilities.

As the findings and conclusions outlined in this section are highly significant but not widely known, they are presented in sufficient detail for their validity to be assessed. As most, though not all, of the available cellular evidence has been concerned with visual forms of STM, which can be studied in many different species, it is the primary (but not only) focus of this section, which begins by outlining some of the main conclusions concerning working memory inferred from studies of behaviour (Sections 5.5.1 and 5.5.2). It then reviews evidence relating them to the properties of cooperative neurons (Sections 5.5.3–5.5.10). Finally, it discusses five major issues that remain to be resolved concerning these fundamental cognitive capabilities (Sections 5.5.11–5.5.15).

5.5.1 Psychological Investigations Show Basic Properties of Working Memory

Working memory has been defined as being concerned with 'a system, or a set of processes, holding mental representations temporarily available for use in thought and action'. It is an exceptionally broad and loosely defined field of research. By 2018, over 11,000 published papers had 'working memory' in the title. The plethora of empirical data provided by this research is so great that a panel of 16 experts concluded that it is unrealistic to expect any single theory to explain all of it.[58] So, working memory is not a single thing—it is a broad field of research that overlaps with research on attention, thought, and imagery.

I use STM to refer specifically to the temporary retention of a small, selected, amount of information that has been abstracted from recent sensory input, where 'recent' is on the time scale of a few seconds. The notion of working memory is broader because it includes information that was not abstracted from recent sensory input but internally generated and maintained by a recycling process, such as that of subvocal rehearsal in the case of the phonological loop. The notion of such a loop suggests that imagining saying a word also involves imagining hearing it being said. The notion of working memory also includes the ability to perform internal operations upon the information that is maintained.

I refer to STMs in the plural for two reasons. First, different subtypes can be distinguished by the semantic domain of the retained information. This applies within modalities as well as between them. For example, the STMs for properties such as shape or colour of a seen object involve cortical regions that differ from those specifying its location. Different semantic domains can also have different computational requirements, particularly if they involve specifying complex relationships, rather than specifying the value of a single variable, such as size or orientation. Second, the information may be maintained in at least two forms. The best known, referred to as the active form, is that in which the cells involved continue to transmit action potentials that persist after the stimulus to be 'kept in mind' has been removed. The other, referred to as the silent form, is that in which information is briefly maintained by temporary changes in synaptic strength.

One way in which phenomena in the field of working memory have been organized is by hypothesizing four basic components, such as the central executive, the phonological loop, the visuospatial sketchpad (VSSP), and the episodic buffer. The central executive directs attention to relevant information, suppresses irrelevant information and inappropriate actions, and coordinates processing at a strategic level. The phonological loop temporarily maintains information about the sounds of words in a form that enables internal implicit rehearsal. Subcomponents of the visuospatial sketchpad maintain information about visual properties such as shape, colour, and spatial locations of things in the scene. The episodic buffer can be thought of as a temporary form of episodic memory (i.e. a temporary multimodal memory for recent events).

Various depictions of the functional organization provisionally inferred from psychological studies have been proposed; Figure 5.6 relates it to perception.

The fundamental differences between STM, sensory storage, and long-term memory (LTM) were clearly established in the 1970s and 1980s, which was the beginning of the cognitive revolution that released psychology from the overly restrictive constraints of behaviourism. It is now widely agreed that visual STMs are categorically distinct from both the transient persistence of sensory information and from visual LTMs.

When I began to explore these cognitive capabilities in the 1960s the existence of verbal STM had just gained widespread acceptance, so the issue on which I worked was whether there is an analogous form of visual STM. That required more than simply presenting people with things to look at because much information about what they see can first be translated into a verbal form at presentation, and then maintained in a verbal, rather than a visual, form. To distinguish visual from verbal STM, we used novel meaningless visual shapes that are not easily described verbally. To enable testing of memory for indefinitely complex inputs using a single simple response we developed the change detection technique, which was inspired by the random poststimulus sampling technique previously developed by George Sperling. We found visual STM to be in several ways wholly distinct from sensory storage and from visual LTM. In stark contrast to the huge amount that can be maintained briefly for much less than a second in the sensory systems and indefinitely in LTM, the amount of information that visual STM can maintain is small. In contrast to LTM, STM does not survive long after attention turns to other things. Our tests of neuropsychological patients showed that

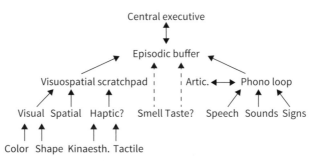

Figure 5.6 A psychological theory of the flow of information from sensory input to the four main components of working memory. 'Sounds' includes music; 'signs' includes both lip reading and reading of text.

VSSP, visuospatial sketchpad; Artic, Articulation.

Redrawn, with his approval, from Alan Baddeley (2012).

closed-head injury and alcoholism have little or no effect on visual STM, although both greatly impair long-term learning. Visual STM is categorically distinct from the fleeting persistence of sensory information in several ways. Fleeting sensory persistence (also called iconic memory or sensory storage) is an example of what is popularly called photographic memory, except that it can contain only one scene at a time and lasts for less than a second. All the many people that we tested had the form of photographic memory that lasts for about one tenth of a second as shown by their ability to detect the addition or deletion of a single dot in displays composed of hundreds of randomly placed dots. We never found anyone with a photographic memory lasting longer than that. We did not expect to because we interpreted sensory storage as reflecting the current state of activity in the sensory cortices.

We assumed that the highly restricted ability to detect small random changes when sensory mechanisms for doing so are blocked applies not only to random dot displays but also to natural scenes. The many demonstrations of what is now known as change blindness show that assumption to be correct. Thus, in contrast to sensory storage, visual STM has a far lower capacity but resists replacement by subsequent sensory input. Visual STM for the properties of specific objects can represent them in a way that generalizes across spatial location. Spatial STM for location can represent it in a way that generalizes across different objects that could be seen at that location. The evidence for sensory storage reflects temporal aspects of processing in sensory regions of neocortex that are topographically precise, whereas evidence for the STM of novel visual patterns reflects the use of higher cortical regions to compute abstract schematic descriptions of the novel things presented.[59]

It is sometimes argued that the temporary activation of LTM is an alternative to the componential conception of working memory. When I was young, experimental psychology was dominated by a behaviourism of which one consequence was deep scepticism of the possibility of distinguishing rapid forgetting in a single memory store prior to its long-term consolidation from a temporary internal memory store. Modern versions of that view are still championed by some influential theorists, but I see it as being wholly unconvincing because there are strong grounds for supposing that there are ways in which information is stored temporarily in a form that is distinct from that of activated LTM. Nevertheless, even though the identification of STMs or working memories with activated LTM is unconvincing, STMs certainly make use of relevant prior knowledge. When interpreting and remembering a new sentence we use our knowledge of words and grammar. When a new word is heard it is represented as a new combination of familiar phonemes, or of the distinctive features that distinguish speech sounds if they are not composed of familiar phonemes. When interpreting and remembering novel scenes we do so by using our knowledge of the visual appearance of familiar things and of ways in which they may be related. In the case of novel random shapes those familiar things may simply be the elementary features of which the shape is composed.

Indeed, there is a sense in which all experience involves use of LTM because the functional organization of the cortical regions within which sensation, perception, and STM occur is dependent on the environment to which the system has been exposed. If kittens are reared in a visual environment that predominantly consists of orientations around the vertical, then their primary visual cortex will develop in such a way as to discriminate only between orientations around the vertical. Furthermore, in contrast to common supposition, that activity dependence applies to prenatal as well as to postnatal development. Prenatal development of a body image in somatosensory and motor cortices depends not only on an abstract genetically specified body-plan, but also on input to the cortex from the body that the embryo does really develop, even if that is misshapen. When information is temporarily maintained by STM mechanisms about a new combination of familiar elements and relations, that new information is signalled in a way that uses prior knowledge of the elements and of the ways in which they may be related.

Modifiability by learning is one of the ways in which 'seeing as' differs from 'seeing', as distinguished by the philosopher Ludwig Wittgenstein. Both are affected by learning, but the sensory 'seeing' tends to become closed to modification by learning after the 'critical period' of development; 'seeing as' continues to be modifiable by learning throughout life.

5.5.2 Short-term Memories Involve a Common Attentional Resource or Central Executive

Evidence for the dependence of some aspects of visual STM on capacities shared with other cognitive functions is clear in my own studies of interference with STM for novel visual patterns, such as those formed by randomly filling about half the squares in a 4 × 4 or 5 × 5 matrix array. We referred to this visual STM as visualization on the assumption that it involves the creation and temporary maintenance of schematic visual descriptions of the patterns to be visualized. We found that people's visual STM for the displayed patterns was greatly reduced by adding five digits that were shown to them while visualizing, but not by merely reading the digits. Presentation modality of the digits did not affect the interference that adding them caused. When the intervening activity involved processing patterns like those being visualized, the amount of interference depended upon whether the intervening task required representations that outlived sensory storage. It caused interference when it involved formation of a maintainable representation, but not when the maintenance required was provided by sensory storage. We concluded that visualization requires capabilities shared by many other attention-demanding tasks such as those provided by a central executive. Though that conclusion has been interpreted by some as casting doubt on the existence of a visual STM that is distinct from a central executive or widely shared resources, that is not necessarily so. What these studies of interference with visualization suggest is that the maintenance of novel visual descriptions in higher perceptual regions depends on central executive processes that presumably involve frontoparietal regions.[60]

Guidance of selective attention is clearly a central function of such executive processes. It is often assumed that uninterrupted attention is necessary to sustain working memories. However, much interest has been generated by recent findings showing that, if selected, information can be temporarily preserved while attention is engaged in other things. There is evidence that this is so in the studies of visual STM that we reported long ago. We found that people can, to some extent, temporarily maintain information about the first of a sequence of three novel shapes while detecting changes in the two that follow if that intervening detection can be performed using sensory storage rather than visual STM.[61]

5.5.3 Cellular Bases of STMs Involve the Distinctive Properties of Context-sensitive Apical Dendrites

Three possibilities are prominent in current theories of the cellular bases of STMs. The first proposes persistent poststimulus neuronal firing due to intrinsic biophysical cellular properties. The second proposes persistent poststimulus neuronal firing due to recurrent reverberatory circuitry. The third proposes temporary changes in synaptic strengths.[62] They are not mutually exclusive.

Though the distinctive properties of apical dendrites are not yet familiar to most psychologists working on STM, neuroscientists who are familiar with them typically assume working memory to be amongst their main functions. There are at least five prima facie grounds for that assumption. First, input of internally stored information to pyramidal cells involved in working memory is predominantly via their apical dendrites. Second, as shown in detail in previous chapters, context-sensitivity is the primary function of apical dendrites, which relates it to STM because STM depends on context, and vice versa. STM for image segments is far better when they are viewed in the context of coherent rather than of scrambled scenes.[63] Third, output bursts of two to four action potentials within about 15 ms due to apical activation produces short-term synaptic facilitation, which could lengthen the time over which recurrent connections can produce persistent firing. Long-lasting calcium plateaux in the apical trunk and branches lengthen the time over which contextual input to apical dendrites influences output.[64] Fourth, STM is dependent on selective attention, which involves apical function (discussed earlier). Last, but not least, recurrence is a major mechanism producing post-stimulus persistence of neural activity, and apical dendrites are key links in many recurrent loops. When discussing the recurrent interaction between information from external and internal sources, leading neurophysiologist Lamme (2004b, p. 580) concludes that:

> Where the two meet, neural activation can be maintained via reverberatory mechanisms, which for a short while can continue to occur independently of the current input or output. In psychological terms, a focus of attentive awareness, or working memory, is formed. Information thus processed receives contextual embedding and is poised for storage into episodic memory.

Though that view does not explicitly emphasize apical dendrites, their anatomical and physiological properties are as required for the reverberatory mechanisms proposed. A role for apical dendrites in STMs does not invalidate any of the three currently prominent hypotheses concerning their neuronal bases. Indeed, it provides cellular foundations for key aspects of each of them.

In addition to these prima facie arguments, there are now direct empirical grounds for supposing that context-sensitive apical dendrites provide cellular foundations for working memory; they are summarized here so that the structure of the argument does not get lost in all the details. Unimodal sensory regions receive persistent post-stimulus modulatory input when there is information in working memory (Section 5.5.4). Visuospatial STM involves persistent activity in the eye fields of prefrontal and parietal regions (Section 5.5.5). The persistence of activity in the PFC depends on its recurrent connections with thalamic nuclei (Section 5.5.6). Recurrent persistence is restrained by the context-sensitivity of links in the loop and by inhibitory interneurons (Section 5.5.7). Information is also temporarily maintained in a silent form via short-term synaptic changes (Section 5.5.8). Temporary maintenance of information depends on the neuromodulators that regulate apical function (Section 5.5.9). Section 5.5.10 summarizes all these subtle arguments.

5.5.4 Unimodal Sensory Regions Receive Persistent Post-stimulus Modulatory Input When There Is Information in Working Memory

Information about the orientation of a briefly presented visual grating composed of several parallel lines has been extracted from fMRI studies of early visual regions several seconds after its presentation. This has led some to conclude that persistent activity in early visual areas can retain information about visual features held in working memory for several seconds after the stimulus has been removed. However, that conclusion has been rejected on several grounds and these findings are more plausibly interpreted as reflecting the persistence of modulatory input from higher regions.[65]

The identification of STM with activity in the primary visual cortex is incompatible with what we know about the persistence of activity in sensory regions following stimulus offset. As explained in 5.5.2, sensory storage has properties that are categorically distinct from visual STM. It is of high capacity, lasts less than a second, is replaced by subsequent input, and does not require selective attention. It was directly demonstrated long ago that this persistence is in part due to the persistence of its input from the LGN. Highly detailed information about a preceding stimulus can persist in visual cortex in the form of 'off' responses, lasting for about 100 ms or so. Counterintuitively, there is evidence that these off responses have sufficient resolution to enable high-level recognition of patterns that were not visible when presented because they were buried in a dense field of random elements. Thus, we can recognize things by the signals that they generate when disappearing, even though we cannot distinguish them from the background when they were present. So, as predicted from the neurophysiology, this is further evidence for things that are seen only when they disappear![66]

This is also relevant to temporal aspects of somaesthetic and motor functions. Layer 5B pyramidal cells in somatosensory cortex have recurrent connections with higher-order thalamic nuclei that modulate cortical activity via thalamic inputs to the apical dendrites of layer 5B pyramidal cells. Some of these are implicated in the persistent neuronal activity associated with the planning of action. Others are involved in the details of sensory perception and execution of the planned actions, so their potential roles in sensory persistence and STM await exploration.[67] Temporal aspects are even more crucial in auditory perception. In the auditory cortex, spike rates of pyramidal cells temporarily preserve information about the frequency of recently heard tones. That form of temporary maintenance seems more relevant to sensory persistence than to STM.

Persistent context-dependent input to apical synapses in layer 1 has been observed in the primary visual cortex of monkeys when they were judging which of several lines in a brief display was connected to the fixation point without moving their eyes—a task known as mental curve tracing shown to involve attention that spreads along the connected curves while ignoring nearby distractor curves. Slightly enhanced activity of the relevant cells in V1 persisted for up to nearly a second following stimulus presentation. That enhancement was interrupted by a briefly flashed mask, occurred only when the line was relevant to the task, was locally specific, and was limited to only one or very few lines. These poststimulus activities were much the same as those that occurred when the monkey judged the connectivity of a line segment in a display that remained present until after the judgement was made. If the display was removed before the judgement could be made, then attention enhanced the sustained activity only of the specific cells representing the target curve. On at least three grounds these findings implicate the effects of some form of STM rather than of either sensory storage or LTM. First, the sustained information outlived sensory storage, such as that in the transient off-response, but was exceptionally short compared with LTM. Second, it can sustain only a small amount of information. Third, it was reinstated following a masking stimulus. These experiments also found that the persistent modulatory effects in V1 were initiated via layers 1 and 5. This indicates that they implicate input to apical dendrites of pyramidal cells in V1 from higher regions such as inferotemporal, parietal, or PFC.[68]

5.5.5 Visuospatial STM Involves Persistent Activity in the Eye Fields of the Prefrontal and Parietal Regions

Neurophysiological and neuroimaging studies show that, in addition to its better-known role in selective attention, the parietal region temporarily contains information abstracted from recent visual input in a form that survives changes in the visual input due to eye and body movements. Information about the shape of familiar objects seen within a few seconds ago can be extracted from multivoxel pattern analysis of fMRI recordings from the superior intraparietal sulcus, but only if those objects are attended. Though those studies were not designed to study apical function, the finding that this temporary persistence depends on task context suggests that apical function is involved.[69]

As parietal regions have a crucial role in guiding attention, persistent activity in those regions during STM suggests that STM may involve continued top-down attention to selected cells in perceptual regions that continues after feedforward sensory inputs to those cells ends. If so, that raises the issue of what selects the information to be given continued attention. As STMs depend on a common attentional resource, or central executive, it has long been argued that prefrontal regions have a central role in selecting information for STM. Neuroimaging studies in humans and direct recordings from pyramidal cells in the PFC of nonhuman primates have often observed post-stimulus PFC activity that distinguishes different stimuli and persists throughout the time for which information about those stimuli is temporarily maintained. That post-stimulus PFC activity may wax and wane in strength during the delay, but usually persists to some extent throughout the whole delay. This persistence has most often been observed in species with larger brains, such as primates. In humans it has been directly observed in intracranial recordings as well as in neuroimaging of prefrontal activity. In rodents, sequential activity spanning the whole delay between a stimulus and response has been observed across a chain of pyramidal cells in the PFC.[70]

This persistent PFC activity provides feedback to apical dendrites in posterior perceptual regions, such as those sensitive to motion, colour, shapes, or to specific kinds of thing, such as faces. This has been shown many times, including studies in which macaque monkeys saw the location of a visual cue and received a reward if they made a saccade to that location after a brief delay. Persistent activity during the delay was directly observed in location-specific pyramidal cells in the frontal eye fields of PFC cells that project back to the perceptual regions from which they receive feedforward input. This feedback from the frontal eye fields amplifies the response of cells in the perceptual regions to their feedforward sensory input (Section 5.4). When that input was no longer present, but the information in it was still needed, cells in the frontal eye field continued to transmit information back to the apical dendrites of the cells in perceptual regions from which those cells received input to their basal dendrites.[71]

As this input to perceptual regions from frontal regions is modulatory it explains why neuroimaging studies in humans (e.g. those using EEG and fMRI measures) often observe persistent activity in perceptual regions during STM, whereas direct neurophysiological studies of the action potentials produced by cells in those posterior perceptual regions during STM rarely observe persistent activity. Neuroimaging reflects the effects of modulatory synaptic currents in apical dendrites even when those currents have little or no effect on action potential output. Therefore, the neuroimaging data can be interpreted as reflecting the modulatory feedback, whereas the cellular data reflects their lack of an effect when there is no relevant feedforward information to amplify.

5.5.6 Persistence of Activity in the PFC Depends on Its Recurrent Connections with Thalamic Nuclei

Pyramidal cells in both L5B and L6 of the PFC send excitatory signals to each of the two higher-order thalamic nuclei, which send excitatory signals back to the PFC, thus forming recurrent loops that can sustain persistent activity. Overall, the combined effect of these recurrent corticothalamic loops is to alter the response of PFC cells to their other inputs, thus sustaining currently relevant cognitive representations. The role of the higher-order thalamus in this short-term persistence in the PFC is not to specify the information that persists, but rather to ensure the persistence of that information within the PFC. When information about either faces or patterns of motion is to be attended and temporarily stored, that differentially enhances connectivity between the PFC and either the fusiform face area, or the visual motion sensitive area in perceptual regions. It is the connections between the PFC and posterior cortical regions that specify the semantic content of pyramidal cell activity in the PFC.

Thus, the higher-order thalamus regulates the persistence of current activity in the PFC without specifying the semantics of the information that persists. As the feedback from the thalamus to the PFC is predominantly to the apical dendrites in layer 1, they are a key link in these recurrent PFC–thalamic loops. Indeed, the thalamic feedback is even clearly stratified within layer 1. One of the two thalamic nuclei in these PFC–thalamic loops functions in a way that has similarities to the feedforward connections in perceptual regions. It provides strong but transient driving inputs to the PFC. Axons from that thalamic nucleus are most dense in the deeper levels of layer 1 so the synapses that they form are close to the apical integration zone. The other thalamic nucleus in these recurrent loops is more like the modulatory feedback in perceptual regions. It does not provide drive, but instead provides modulatory influences that accumulate over time. Axons from that thalamic nucleus are most dense in the upper levels of layer 1, so the synapses formed are further away from the apical integration zone. The full functional implications of this stratification of thalamic inputs to apical dendrites in the PFC are yet to be discovered.[72]

Apical dendrites in layer 1 are also a key link in the recurrent connections between the higher-order thalamus and the premotor region of the PFC. These recurrent loops support persistent frontal activity during motor planning. Persistent activity in this premotor region anticipates specific movements by a second or more prior to their onset. It has been proposed that the capabilities of these recurrent corticothalamic loops are a precursor of the 'thoughts' that are expressed internally but whose external expression is suppressed. It is therefore proposed that such corticothalamic loops may provide cellular foundations upon which much of higher cognition evolved.[73]

5.5.7 Recurrent Persistence Is Restrained by Inhibitory Interneurons and by Context-sensitivity of Links in the Cortico-cortical and Thalamo-cortical Loops

Anatomically it is clear that loops, chains of loops, and loops within loops are common in the thalamocortical system. If unrestrained, those loops, which connect excitory cells would be in danger of producing persistent overactivation. Percepts, memories, and thoughts would then become fixed or repetitive when they should be dynamically changing. That is indeed what may happen in obsessive–compulsive and other disorders with repetitive thoughts and actions. Francis Crick and Christof Koch propose that, in the absence of pathology, there are no strong corticothalamic loops.[74] Persistence due to corticothalamic recurrence must therefore be adequately restrained. This is presumably why the thalamic feedback to cortex is most dense in layer 1, thus having modulatory, rather than driving, effects.

Overactivation in these recurrent loops is also restrained by projections from the thalamic nuclei to inhibitory interneurons in the PFC, as well as to pyramidal cells in that region. As elsewhere, thalamic inputs to the inhibitory interneurons in the PFC are most dense in layer 1, so it is specifically overamplification that these projections to inhibitory interneurons resist. Selected pyramidal cells can then be made more responsive to their driving inputs by activating inhibitory interneurons that disinhibit the apical dendrites of those selected cells in the PFC. Working memory has been shown to depend on such disinhibition. Activating the interneurons in the PFC that amplify the responses of a few selected cells by disinhibiting their apical dendrites enhances STM for the specific information that they transmit. This is further evidence that STM depends on the activity of apical dendrites in layer 1 of the PFC. Indeed, the theoretical proposal of a disinhibitory microcircuit motif was originally motivated by the need to explain how the PFC contributes to the temporary maintenance of selected information.[75]

5.5.8 Information Is Also Temporarily Maintained in a Silent Form via Short-term Synaptic Changes

Persistent activity that outlasts the stimulus is not the only way in which information can be temporarily maintained in neocortex. Most studies of poststimulus persistence have been concerned with STM for a single item during an intervening period that does not require attention to other things. As mentioned, however, we found long ago that uninterrupted attention is not necessary for temporary maintenance. Neuroimaging of cortical activity now indicates that poststimulus persistence of neuronal activity is not the only way in which information can be temporarily maintained. There is a form of temporary maintenance that is 'silent', or 'latent', in the sense that it is only seen in the cortical region's response to further sensory input. In one such study, two randomly oriented grating stimuli composed of many parallel lines were presented, one either side of fixation, and people were asked to remember the orientations of the gratings on both sides. A retro-cue then indicated which item should be the current focus of attention. An impulsive, task-irrelevant, high-contrast 'probe' stimulus displaying concentric circles was then presented at the locations of both gratings while subjects were maintaining information about the orientations presented. Multivariate pattern analysis of EEG recordings over visual cortices of left and right hemispheres found poststimulus persistence of the pattern of activity evoked by the presented gratings, but only when they were the current focus of attention. Nevertheless, information about the orientation that was not the current focus of attention was still temporarily maintained in that region, as shown by response to the irrelevant probe stimulus. Those findings were interpreted as indicating that information can be temporarily stored in the visual cortex via changes in synaptic efficacy, membrane potentials, or extracellular transmitter concentrations.[76]

A 'silent' form of temporary maintenance also occurs in the PFC. Multivariate pattern analysis of PFC activity in paradigms in which more than one stimulus is to be maintained now provide evidence on cellular bases of the temporary maintenance of currently unattended information. The pattern of neuronal activity evoked in the PFC by a cue that guides attention to one of two items begins by being specific to the cue. It then changes to one that specifies a mapping from cue to response. However, the activity specifying that mapping does not always persist throughout the whole interval of temporary maintenance. Information specifying that mapping can be temporarily maintained in a latent, silent, or hidden form that is revealed by analysing the response of the PFC to a probe input that does evoke neuronal activity in that region of the PFC. This probe could be another stimulus, microelectrode stimulation, transcranial magnetic stimulation (TMS), or even input that is artificially generated by brief pulses of light that specifically activate cells that send excitatory signals to them. When tested with any of these probing inputs, the region responds with a pattern of activity from which the information temporarily maintained can be retrieved. The pattern of activity generated in these ways is in some conditions the same as that generated by actual presentation of the information to be remembered. In other conditions it may be a different pattern of activity, but, nevertheless, one that is specific to the remembered item.[77]

Research on silent forms of STM is in its infancy but their context-sensitivity suggests that they probably involve apical function. The neuronal mechanism most often considered by pioneers in the study of silent forms of temporary maintenance is a short-term synaptic plasticity that is conceptually equivalent to long-term maintenance by changes in synaptic strength, except that it is far more temporary and limited to a tiny amount of information. Computational theory and simulations show this to be possible. Though that theoretical work has not yet explicitly considered the role of context-sensitivity in apical dendrites, it is based on recurrent connections and the long time-constants of calcium kinetics, both of which suggest involvement of apical function.[78]

The presence of latent STM information in the neuronal response to TMS provides further grounds for supposing that context-sensitive pyramidal cells are involved. Multivariate pattern analysis has been used to decode fMRI signals received from regions of the visual cortex during STM for faces, words, and seen directions of movement in abstract dot patterns. Temporary maintenance of activity distinguishing different instances of each class was observed within the cortical region specifically sensitive to that class, although that maintained information decayed rapidly when unattended. Nevertheless, a TMS pulse briefly reactivated that information in the fMRI signal, but only when the item was potentially relevant later in the trial. The dependence on task context suggests that apical dendrites are implicated because they are the main conveyer of contextual input to pyramidal cells. Additionally, apical function is also implicated by the ability of TMS to elicit the temporarily maintained latent information. The action of that stimulation at cellular and network levels is complex but it predominantly activates fibres and inhibitory interneurons in the upper cortical layers, particularly in layer 1, thus having large effects on the calcium currents upon which apical function depends.[79]

Thus, in summary, four aspects of the evidence for a silent form of STM indicate that it involves apical synapses in layer 1. First, the temporarily stored but silent information was revealed by observing the region's response to feedforward input, which is regulated by input to the apical dendrites in layer 1. Second, TMS can evoke expression of these synaptic modifications, which predominantly affects dendritic currents in layer 1. Third, as expected, if the synapses involved are those that regulate response to feedforward input, the response to an unrelated probe was not reactivation of the multivariate pattern of activity generated by the remembered item itself. Instead, it was a different, though still distinctive, pattern of activity. Fourth, computer models of these effects rely on recurrent connections and the long-time constants of calcium kinetics, which are both characteristic of apical function.

5.5.9 Temporary Maintenance of Information Depends on the Neuromodulators That Regulate Apical Function

STM and working memory functions in general are highly sensitive to adrenergic, cholinergic, serotonergic, and dopaminergic arousal. Psychologists discovered long ago that cognitive functions such as attention, STM, and thought are impaired if arousal is either too high or too low, leading to inverted-U shaped functions in which performance first rises then falls as the level of arousal increases from minimal to maximal. These classical neuromodulators all have especially large effects on apical function (see Sections 4.3 and 4.4).[80]

A distinctive property of the PFC is that it is reciprocally connected with all the main subcortical neuromodulatory centres. Thus, it helps govern neuromodulatory input to neocortical regions, including itself. Consequently, the levels of these neuromodulators at any time are the result of an ever-changing interaction between different cortical and subcortical influences that wax and wane on different time scales and depend on different conditions. Furthermore, interactions between the neuromodulators include cooperation as well as competition between them. For example, the persistent activity in the PFC on which working memory depends can be enhanced by cooperation between adrenergic and dopaminergic systems.[81]

The effects of neuromodulatory input to the apical integration zone arise from complex interactions between the different neuromodulators. In part, they depend upon the spatial distribution of different types of neuromodulatory receptor on the cell's basal and apical dendritic trees, their efficacy, and their temporal dynamics. Though much remains to be discovered about neuromodulatory regulation of PFC function, we already know enough to be confident that it has a crucial role in working memory. As in other regions, apical function in the PFC depends on adequate levels of cholinergic arousal, which is necessary to disinhibit the apical dendrites in layer 1 and to enable coupling between the apical integration zone and the soma. Layer 5B neurons in the PFC are shifted into a primed state when their long-acting cholinergic receptors are stimulated. When in that primed state, they can respond to a brief suprathreshold input from their feedforward excitatory input with persistent firing that can last for some tens of seconds.[82]

There is ample evidence that working memory functions and the temporary maintenance of information in the PFC are strongly dependent on adrenergic arousal. As in other cortical regions, moderate (but not high) levels of adrenergic arousal block the HCN currents that restrict the effects of apical input to PFC pyramidal cells. That increases the persistent poststimulus activity of pyramidal cells in the PFC.[83] Adrenergic modulation also regulates working memory functions of the PFC by effects on interneurons that specifically inhibit apical dendrites.[84]

Many unresolved issues arise concerning the role of neuromodulators in these higher cognitive functions. For example, their effects at the intracellular level in the primate PFC may in some ways be opposite to those seen in cortical sensory regions and in the hippocampus of rodents. For example, in primates, working memory and other PFC functions can be rapidly suppressed by exposure to uncontrollable stress. These effects are complex, and not yet fully understood. Nevertheless, they are known to involve the adrenergic receptors that are exceptionally dense in apical dendrites. Differing levels of adrenergic activation engage functionally distinct receptors. Moderate levels engage high affinity adrenergic receptors that improve working memory functions, whereas higher levels engage lower-affinity receptors that may suppress PFC functions under certain conditions. In colloquial terms we can interpret that as implying that the strategic planning functions of PFC are temporarily disengaged during emergencies or other highly stressful events where there may be little time for thoughtful contemplation.[85] Furthermore, there is evidence that a difference in adrenergic function is one of the many factors that produce large individual differences in working memory capabilities. In some people adrenergic arousal may be chronically low, such that the frontoparietal network is underactivated, which results in greater default-mode activity and mind wandering, combined with a reduction in the STM persistence that depends on apical function.[86]

5.5.10 Neuronal Foundations of STMs: Interim Conclusions

The weight of evidence clearly indicates that the distinctive capabilities of context-sensitive cooperative neurons have a major role in STM. These findings show that visuospatial STM involves persistent poststimulus activity of cells in frontoparietal regions, and specifically the frontal eye fields. This persistent activity amplifies sensory response to input from one or a few selected locations in space. It does so in much the same way as does attention to selected aspects of current stimulation, which also involves apical function (Section 5.4). Activity is sustained in frontal regions during spatial STM by excitatory frontothalamic loops that can generate reverberant activity lasting several seconds. This ability arises from several properties of the frontothalamic loops. First, local microcircuits in prefrontal and premotor cortex project strongly to thalamic cells that project back to themselves. Second, frontothalamic projections evoke robust firing in the thalamus via synapses that are strongly facilitating, that is, their responses to subsequent inputs in a burst are not depressed, but rather are increased. Third, they do not automatically evoke the strong inhibition that tends to oppose persistence in sensory corticothalamic loops. Fourth, the thalamic feedback to frontal cortex is mostly excitatory and mostly to apical dendrites; so, it can elicit long-lasting dendritic calcium currents. Fifth, the effects of the thalamic feedback depend on neuromodulators that block HCN currents in the apical dendrites to which they project. Thus, reverberation in frontothalamic loops is highly regulated and state dependent. Thalamic feedback specifies which cells should remain active in the PFC, but it does not specify their semantics, as implied by our fundamental distinction between the information transmitted by neural signals and their strength. Finally, in addition to these key properties it is also possible that short-term changes in the strengths of the synapses in these frontothalamic loops can temporarily store information when attention is diverted to other things. Thus, seen as a whole, these findings constitute a major advance in our understanding of the cellular foundations of working memory. They raise five unresolved, but crucial, issues concerning working memory and imagery.

5.5.11 STMs for Abstract Descriptions of Complex Unfamiliar Things

The first unresolved issue concerns relations between STMs for a simple variable, such as position, relates to STMs for abstract descriptions of unfamiliar things. The STM information tested in the delayed response paradigms discussed earlier focused on where to look, reach, or touch. In many cases this involved a simple binary choice and was rarely more than a choice between eight alternatives. So, only between one and three bits of information are required by those tasks. In contrast to that, the visual STM for novel patterns that I studied for many years, both as a subject and as an experimenter, involved creating a description of the structural gist of a novel pattern that generalizes across location, is not erased by unrelated eye movements, and has an information capacity that far exceeds 3 bits, for example, 25 bits in the case of a 5×5 matrix in which half of the locations are filled at random. There is convincing evidence for persistent activity of cells in the frontal eye fields as a basis for spatial STM in mice, but that cannot provide a basis for the visual STM for novel patterns. In any case, demonstrations of STM for spatial location in mice do not show that they can visualize the properties of complex unfamiliar things. Even in macaques, that ability is far less than it is in humans (Chapter 6). The neuronal bases of the kind of visualization that we study in humans are therefore unlikely to be fully revealed by studies of memory for a few bits of information about a single variable by rodents.

5.5.12 Modes of Apical Function Involved in STMs

The second unresolved issue concerns the mode of apical function involved in thalamic feedback to layer 1. We now need to discover what determines whether it has amplifying effects on the cell's response to its more direct somatic inputs, as it does during attention to current percepts, or whether it has driving effects on the cell's outputs, as it does during dreaming. Although there are some similarities between the generation of perceptual experiences from internal resources when dreaming and when retaining information about something perceived a few seconds ago, there remain obvious differences that need clarification. In addition, the possibility that thalamic feedback to the PFC somehow combines aspects of both amplification and drive awaits investigation.

5.5.13 How Visual Imagery and Verbal Thought Are Related to Apical Function

The third unresolved issues concerns relations between apical function, imagery, and other thoughts. By 'imagery' I mean the generation of percept-like experiences in the absence of a current sensory or STM basis for them. Imagining a particular stimulus increases the excitability of cells in visual cortex to which that is the preferred input. This is closely related to holding that stimulus in STM. Imagining a stimulus in a specific location in the visual field increases the probability that TMS of the part of cortex representing that location will generate the experience of flashing points of light, described as 'phosphenes'. This suggests that apical dendrites are involved because it is they that are most affected by TMS. However, imagery is not dependent on primary sensory areas, so I must emphasize that visualization is far from being equivalent to really seeing the things visualized. If it were, there would be no need for the artwork that we hang on our walls or click on our smartphones, nor for any of the other sensual experiences that we so actively seek. Visual imagery is impaired little, if at all, in patients with damage restricted to the occipital cortex, but it is greatly impaired in patients with damage to frontoparietal regions or to the left fusiform gyrus. Meta-analysis of 27 fMRI studies of visual imagery confirms that it is these regions, rather than early visual regions, that are primarily involved in visual imagery. Any effects of imagery on early sensory regions are a secondary consequence of its primary effects on regions that deal with information about more abstract things.[87]

Some imagery involves the creation of new descriptions of familiar things. When subjects imagine a familiar symbol, such as the letter R rotated by a specified amount, the speed, ease, and accuracy with which they can do so increase as the deviation of the angle from the standard upright orientation increases. I assume that mental rotation does not change the orientations signalled by outputs from cells in primary or secondary regions of visual cortex because that is specified by their sensory input. Furthermore, mentally rotating an image of a familiar symbol does not operate on the long-term knowledge of that symbol's appearance. When imaging it in a different orientation, the knowledge of its usual orientation is unaffected and remains as functionally available as when not imagining it rotated. Thus, we can infer that mental rotation involves using long-term knowledge to create new descriptions. The dependence of both imagery and STM on the ability to create new descriptions is also indicated by the finding that some forms of imagery, such as imagining hand-written letters, interferes strongly with STM for novel shapes or patterns.[88] The extent to which studies of cooperative neurons can throw light on these issues remains to be seen.

5.5.14 Distinguishing Imagination from Reality

Although people have long thought deeply about the crucial issue of how imagination or fantasy or lies can be distinguished from reality, it remains unresolved. Consider the famous conversation between Theseus and his betrothed, Hippolyta, in Act V scene I, near the end of Shakespeare's play *A Midsummer Night's Dream*. They discuss the various fallings in and out of love, and other 'dream-like' experiences previously portrayed in the play:

HIPPOLYTA 'Tis strange my Theseus, that these lovers speak of.
THESEUS More strange than true: I never may believe
These antique fables, these fairy toys.
Lovers and madmen have such seething brains,
Such shaping fantasies, that apprehend
More than cool reason ever comprehends.
The lunatic, the lover and the poet
Are of imagination all compact:
One sees more devils than vast hell can hold,
That is the madman: the lover, all as frantic,
Sees Helen's beauty in a brow of Egypt:
The poets eye, in fine frenzy rolling,
Doth glance from heaven to earth, from earth to heaven;
And as imagination bodies forth
The forms of things unknown, the poet's pen
Turns them to shapes and gives to airy nothing
A local habitation and a name.
Such tricks hath strong imagination,
That if it would apprehend some joy
It comprehends some bringer of that joy;
Or in the night, imagining some fear,
How easy is a bush supposed a bear
HIPPOLYTA But all the story of the night told over,
And all their minds transfigured so together,
More witnesseth than fancy's images
And grows to something of great constancy;
But howsoever, strange and admirable.

To the cool reason of Theseus those doubtful of this book's claims could now add:

> The cellular psychologist in quixotic fervour so confined,
> Doth infer from mind to brain, from brain to mind,
> And gives to unfairly biased speculation
> The looks of fine and dandy formulation,
> While leaving fairer judgement far behind.

To which, in a less sceptical frame of mind, we could reply:

> What's in the world that minds may re-cognize,
> Was first conveyed to brains by eyes,
> Where there it waits till its again in view,
> Or, used to generate a thought that's new.

Dramatists and philosophers have long pondered these issues because they are far from being only of theatrical, academic, or poetic interest. Consider Joan of Arc, burned at the stake in 1431 for leading military opposition to subjugation of a part of France by English troops. How could she possibly have known whether the voices telling her to do so were or were not from an external source? The importance of this issue is not restricted to imaginary characters such as Theseus, to historical characters, such as Joan of Arc, or to those in a psychotic state; it is important to us all. I hope and expect that the current blurring of the boundaries between truth and lies, between the real and the virtual, will lead to advances in our understanding and management of these issues at a societal level. Here I consider them from philosophical, psychological, and neurobiological perspectives.

Friedrich Nietzsche argued that all 'facts' are no more than interpretations. We don't have to go that far, however, to see that there is some subjectivity in all realism, and some objectivity in all fantasy. Approximations to realism are subjective in several ways, not least of which is that prior knowledge is used to guide the acquisition of new knowledge. We face the ever-present danger of predictions from current knowledge becoming self-fulfilling prophecies. The reality of that danger is clearly shown by the plentiful evidence for what is known as confirmation bias, which is the tendency to search for, interpret, accumulate, and recall information in a way that supports our existing beliefs. It is pervasive throughout mental life, from simple perceptual decisions to political beliefs, and has been studied by imaging people's brain activity during experiments in which they had the opportunity to use further sensory data to improve their decisions concerning patterns of movement seen in a random dot display. The stronger their confidence in their initial judgements, the stronger their bias towards using new data only when it confirmed their initial judgement, that is, they simply ignored conflicting data. This led the investigators to conclude that confidence acts as a top-down controller that selectively amplifies new information consistent with the observer's expectations, while ignoring any inconsistent data.[89] Self-fulfilling prophecies are both common and difficult to detect. They are the price we pay for our ability to build and use the broad conceptual frameworks upon which our lives depend. Advances in our understanding of the information-processing capabilities of context-sensitive pyramidal cells sheds light on these issues because they selectively amplify new information that is consistent with the context signalled by their apical input. Therefore, I expect that we will soon see intense exploration of relations between confirmation bias and apical function.

Even at this early stage some intriguing possibilities arise. The two effective modes of apical function are amplification and drive. In amplification mode the action potentials by which neurons communicate can be generated by feedforward drive alone but not by cooperative context-sensitivity alone. That preserves the validity of the information transmitted about sensory input. In drive mode, however, apical input from internal sources by itself generates action potentials in perceptual regions, and thus imaginary percepts. We can be confident that something like that happens during dreams (Chapter 4). Perhaps something similar also happens during thought and imagination when awake.

With this in mind, we can now consider the distinction between 'fact' and 'fiction' from a perspective that is meaningfully related to neuronal activity. We can now ask how signals that express internal information using apical drive are distinguished from those that select relevant sensory data using apical amplification. A prior issue raised by that reformulation of the problem of reality and imagination is whether drive and amplification are as dichotomous as that implies. They may or may not be, so we need more direct physiological evidence on that issue. If drive and amplification can indeed be combined in various proportions at the cellular level, then sites to which the cells project would necessarily have difficulty distinguishing between internal and external contributions to the signals that they receive. That is, the distinction would then be quantitative, rather than being a simple dichotomy such as between 'true' and 'false'. Chapter 8 discusses a way in which the precise quantification required to resolve this issue can be obtained.

Furthermore, the initial distinction between imagination and reality at the cellular level may need to be complemented by inferences drawn at a systemic level. That is presumably what happens when we realize that the occasional reversals in our experience of ambiguous figures, such as Necker cubes, are not due to changes in the sensory data, but to changes in our interpretation of that data. That realization presumably involves an intuitive insight into Ludwig Wittgenstein's interpretation of differences between 'seeing' and 'seeing as'.

5.5.15   The Tiny Capacities of STMs

The fifth unresolved issue concerns the highly limited capacities of STMs. One obvious way in which imagination can be distinguished from reality arises from the huge difference in the amount of sensory detail that can be generated from within and from without. There is no doubt that the amount of information that can be stored in working memory is severely limited. However, that limitation does not greatly constrain our daily activity because the moment-by-moment information on which most of that activity depends remains available in the real world, for us to select as needed, without having to depend on STM. Although some people describe their imaginary experiences as vivid, they do not usually confuse them with perception. I assume that that is at least in part because imagined experiences do not contain the wealth of sensory detail that can usually be interrogated at will in direct perceptual experience based on sensory data. My studies many years ago clearly showed the tiny 'capacity' of visual STM for novel patterns. Since then, work on what is known as change blindness has confirmed that the tiny capacity of visual STM applies to normal daily life, as I took for granted in Phillips (1974). One major new contribution of the studies on change blindness is that they clarify the dependence of visual STM on selective attention. Another is that they draw attention to what is known as 'change blindness blindness', that is, the surprise that most people express when they learn of the striking restrictions on STM demonstrated by the evidence for change blindness. This adds to the grounds for doubting the veracity of common beliefs about our own direct conscious experiences (Section 4.6). I assume that it occurs because the sensory experiences of which we are directly aware convey a wealth of information that is often assumed, incorrectly, to be stored in mind for at least a few seconds.

These large differences in the capacity of sensory storage and STM raise two subsidiary issues. How can 'capacity' be adequately defined and measured? Why is the 'capacity of working memory' so limited? Measuring 'capacity' by counting the number of 'items' or 'chunks' that can be imagined or stored in

STM would suffice if those notions are adequately defined, but this has not yet happened. There exist attempts to use information theory to measure working memory capacity, but that approach is in its infancy and it is difficult to judge its potential.[90] Nevertheless, even at this early stage, there are grounds for supposing that an information-theoretic approach to defining and measuring working memory capacity involves context-sensitivity because it relates the accuracy with which information is stored to the amplitude of neuronal responses, which depends on context.

We still do not know why the capacity of STMs is so limited. We do not even know whether it is a necessary computational constraint or a biological limitation. For years I assumed that it reflects a basic computational constraint arising from a combinatoric explosion of some kind, but now, given the Big Data processing capabilities of AI algorithms, I am not quite so sure. Nevertheless, there are still grounds for supposing that working memory and reasoning are limited by unavoidable combinatoric constraints. Prominent among these is the theory of relational complexity,[91] which has been most successfully applied to developmental issues (Chapter 6). Attempts to relate it to neurobiology have not yet advanced far beyond suggesting that STM information is stored in frontoparietal regions whereas reasoning and 'fluid intelligence' are more dependent on prefrontal regions. Another possible perspective on this issue may come from comparing the attention and working memory capabilities of humans with neural network algorithms for natural language processing that were in part inspired by analogies to neurobiology (Vaswani et al., 2017) (see Section 9.7).

5.5.16 Working Memory as Recurrent Amplification Combined with Divisive Normalization

In what may prove to be a major advance, Heeger and Mackey (2019) show how many working memory phenomena can be explained by combining divisive normalization with recurrent amplification. They show that many phenomena of working memory are simulated by a computational model in which they are combined. Heeger and Mackey (2019) also describe how that functional model can also simulate key sequential phenomena of working memory and motor control. Further, they show how, in addition to being temporarily stored, information can be modified by the complex sequential dynamics of this model, thus potentially explaining some feats of the imagination. Here, I first discuss ways in which their model resonates with our perspective on cooperative context-sensitivity, then consider a few important differences.

Both perspectives assume that a common style of information processing underlies neocortical capabilities, but with several possible variations. Both perspectives include context-sensitive local processors (cells) with two functionally distinct points of integration. The recurrent weights in their model are much the same as the contextual fields specified by synapses of the apical dendrites in layer 1.[92] Both combine cooperative with competitive context-sensitivity, and both assume a key role for recurrence in working memory. Both perspectives see that role as being regulated by inhibitory interneurons and assume that the operational mode of those pyramidal cells is strongly regulated by the classical neuromodulators. Finally, amplification in both is greatest when input drive is weak and reduces towards zero as input drive approaches its upper asymptote (see Figure 8.4).

One important difference between our view of context-sensitive cooperative computation and the model of Heeger and Mackey is that sequential temporal structure is much better incorporated into their theory than into our perspective (though that is begun in Chapter 8). Another important difference is that a wider conception of context is developed here than it is in their theory. We do not identify context with top-down feedback from the next level up in the hierarchy. For us, it also includes lateral intraregional connections to account for various intraregional phenomena (e.g. contour integration and many others), input from the higher-order thalamus, and from subcortical nuclei such as the amygdala to account for emotional prioritization, as outlined in the following section.

As currently formulated, these two perspectives have five more minor differences between them. First, the local processors referred to as 'cells' in the recurrent amplification proposed by Heeger and Mackey (2019) are intended to be populations of cells, not single cells, but that is not explicitly incorporated in their model. Second, the outputs generated by the local processors that they propose are quantified as spike rates, whereas the evidence on cooperative context-sensitivity indicates that burst probability is more important, so the timescale of a burst (i.e. 15–20 ms) is more important than in their model. Third, in contrast to the emphasis here, distinct classes of inhibitory interneurons and their distinct patterns of connectivity in their model is not related to the known anatomy and physiology of inhibitory interneurons. Hertag and Sprekeler (2019) offer a model that is more closely based on the evidence for cooperative context-sensitivity with respect to these three differences. Fourth, Heeger and Mackey define amplification as being multiplicative, whereas context-sensitivity (as quantified in Chapter 8) is explicitly distinguished from a purely multiplicative operation as well as from a purely divisive operation. Finally, there is a terminological difference in that what Heeger and Mackey describe as recurrent drive is defined in this book as apical amplification, which is explicitly distinguished from apical drive.

One simple observation emerges from a close comparison of these two theoretical perspectives: there is little overlap in the empirical evidence cited in their support. So, as their inferences are based on independent sources of empirical evidence, it increases our confidence in their commonalities. Convincingly identifying those commonalities will not be easy because the empirical grounds on which each is built are large, and rigorous formulation of each perspective is intellectually challenging. Nevertheless, those skilled in the mathematics of neural integrator dynamics and information theory may soon be able to find essential commonalities between context-sensitive cooperative computation and the model of Heeger and Mackey (2019). If so, that may well be a major further step forward in the development of cellular psychology as a key field of research within the sciences of brain and mind.

5.6 Prioritization of Emotionally Charged Events

Far from being coolly calculating, it is our head, rather than our heart, that provides the stage on which our emotional lives occur. Emotion and cognition are not competing siblings. They are inextricably interconnected, like inseparable conjoined twins. Emotional experiences are characterized by various levels of positive or negative valence that range from delight to despair. They are also characterized by various levels of arousal that range from being highly activated to being so drowsy that we are nearly asleep. Although some experiences may be classified as 'emotional' because their emotional aspects are salient, I assume that all experiences have an emotional tone, even when that is not salient. Although there are various theories of the neuronal bases of the emotional aspects of experience, there is widespread agreement that they involve two-way interactions within and between neocortical regions and subcortical nuclei, such as the amygdala, basal ganglia, hypothalamus, and the various neuromodulatory nuclei of the midbrain and brain stem.[93] There are many anatomical connections between cortical regions and these subcortical nuclei, with most, though not all, of them being reciprocal. Thus, emotional aspects of experience arise from a sequence of interactions between neural centres operating at very different levels of abstraction. For example, these interactions enable the amygdala (a 'danger detector') to influence and be influenced by a wide array of other subcortical nuclei and cortical regions. So, though we may at first suppose a bush seen at night to be a bear, further inspection and thought may assuage any underlying fear prompting that supposition. As the two-way interactions affect the activity of neocortical pyramidal cells without corrupting the semantic content of their outputs, it is likely that they operate via the modulatory capabilities of the apical integration zone. The following summarizes evidence showing that to be so.

The extensive effects of emotional tone on perception, thought, and learning all involve these modulatory interactions. Information about the current bodily state is interpreted by cingulate and prefrontal regions in a way that is heavily dependent on the current context, thus indicating that context-sensitive pyramidal cells are involved in these effects of emotional prioritization. Neocortical regions that make major contributions to emotional experience include the anterior cingulate cortices and medial regions of the PFC.

The cortical contributions to emotional experience are particularly relevant to the voluntary selection of actions to be taken and to the suppression of actions that are inappropriate in the current context. Investigations in many different labs show that events are more likely to be perceived, thought about, remembered, and acted upon if they are emotionally arousing. Neuronal signals that are selected for prioritization because they are emotionally charged are strengthened, whereas those that are not selected are weakened. Cortical and subcortical centres all contribute to selection for prioritization, with the effectiveness of that selection being greater when different subcortical nuclei and cortical regions all agree with each other. This prioritization has been clearly related to adrenergic arousal, which usually enhances apical function by suppressing the ionic currents that reduce the effectiveness of contextual input to the apical dendrites (Chapter 4). Many of the effects of emotional arousal on cognition and action are thus presumably mediated by apical amplification. Furthermore, highly stressful events produce exceptionally high levels of adrenergic activation (Figure 4.2), which changes the mode of apical function such that in highly emotional situations fast impulsive reactions tend to be enhanced at the expense of thoughtful reflection.[94]

Apical function is also implicated in emotional prioritization by locally specific projections to the apical dendrites from the amygdala, which has a central role in sensitivity to fearful situations. Neuroimaging studies in humans show that the amygdala responds strongly to threats and other fearful events. They also show that cortical regions in the ventral stream of processing concerned with object recognition respond more strongly to emotionally charged events. Projections from the amygdala to the visual cortex play a leading role in this amplification of cortical responses to fearful events. This is shown by the absence of that amplification when the amygdala is removed, as it sometimes is in humans for clinical reasons.

Figure 5.7 summarizes the connections between the amygdala and the cortex in macaque monkeys. We can assume that these connections are much the same as those in other primates, including humans. In all these species, and in many others (e.g. rodents), sensory and perceptual regions of the cortex project to the amygdala, which projects to parts of the brainstem that evoke fearful responses (e.g. freezing or fleeing) when frightening events occur. Nuclei in the amygdala also send signals back to the cortex. The key findings of the anatomical study on which Figure 5.7 is based are that these

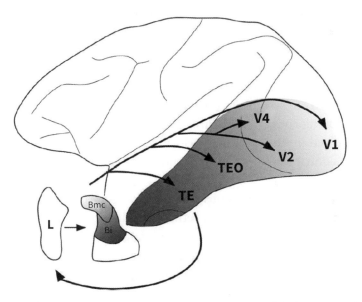

Figure 5.7 Connections in macaques from nuclei of the amygdala (L, Bmc, and Bi) to regions of visual cortex and from them back to the amygdala. Information about current retinal input is first received by primary visual cortex (V1). From there information is fed forward through a hierarchy of regions such as V2, TEO and TE where descriptions of increasing abstraction are computed. All levels of this hierarchy of abstraction receive information about emotional state from the amygdala, which presumably amplifies the transmission of visual information that is currently emotionally significant. That assumption is supported by the apical location of inputs from the amygdala to the cortex. If the inputs were to basal and peri-somatic locations, their effects could not be disentangled from those of the sensory input about which visual cortex transmits information.

From: Freese & Amaral, 2005. Its use is approved by David Amaral, with permission from John Wiley and Sons.

connections from the amygdala to the visual cortex are predominantly to the border between layers 1 and 2 of the neocortex, which is close to the apical integration zone, thus unequivocally implicating apical function in emotional prioritization. The amygdala also sends some projections to layer 5/6 of are TE, which interprets current visual input at the highest level of abstraction. In the primary visual cortex, which represents visual input at the highest level of sensory detail, the amygdala again projects to the border between layers 1 and 2 of the neocortex. From this anatomical evidence it is therefore concluded that, by analogy to feedback connections from higher to lower levels of cortical abstraction, the amygdala is more likely to amplify the response of cortical cells to their preferred sensory input, rather than to generate output by themselves.[95] This conclusion makes sense from a functional point of view, because if the amygdala were sufficient to activate our visual system by itself, then we would indeed be in danger of seeing 'more devils than vast hell can hold'. Even if the effect of the amygdala on cortical processing is modulatory there may be an overemphasis on potential threats. This is because the connections between the cortex and the amygdala form recurrent loops that reinforce a particular way of interpreting the input once initiated. So, the danger of oversensitivity to possible or imagined threats needs to be kept in check. If loops connecting cooperative neurons in the neocortex to the amygdala are indeed involved in this emotional prioritization, then further study of them is likely to contribute to our understanding of various disorders related to anxiety.

The anatomical studies of loops connecting the cortex to the amygdala in macaques show that they preserve retinotopic differentiation. This local differentiation and its ability to adapt to experience is also reported in studies of auditory fear learning. Conditioned fear learning was studied in mice by pairing a brief sequence of harmless and uninformative beeps with a mild electric stimulation to the feet. Physiological experiments combined with electron microscopy showed that this conditioned fear learning involved increasing the number of synapses that directly conveyed excitatory signals from the amygdala to apical dendrites of layer 5 cells. Synapses connecting the amygdala to cells in higher layers were not affected, nor were synapses carrying the feedforward auditory information to those cells. This highly localized strengthening of the direct modulatory connections from the amygdala to the auditory cortex continued to consolidate over a period of at least three days. Thus, locally specific inputs from subcortical centres concerned with emotion to apical dendrites in layer 1 adapts in a way that enhances responses to events perceived as threatening, although it does so without compromising the validity of the information about the sensory input that they transmit.[96]

Godenzini, Shai, and Palmer (2022) showed that the enhanced response of pyramidal cells in the mouse auditory cortex to tones associated with foot shock is due to enhanced response to those tones by apical, but not by basal dendrites. This shows that learning can affect apical dendrites only and that by doing so it changes the extent to which that cell's response to its basal inputs are to be amplified by emotional prioritization.

5.7 Cognitive Control

Cognitive control refers to the ability to strategically guide internal processing and behaviour in accordance with current goals. It helps specify what is and what is not relevant to current goals. It switches selection when goals change, and prevents automatic impulsive actions and reactions that would be inappropriate in current circumstances. Many psychological paradigms have been designed to study differences between controlled and automatic processing. In 1935, Stroop devised one of the best known, which asks people to make responses that conflict with those likely to occur automatically. For example, fluent readers are shown colour names and asked to name the colour in which the words are printed, rather than to say the word itself, which is the more automatic response. When the colour name and the colour in which it is printed are the same, little cognitive control is required, other than letting the automatic response happen. Cognitive control is required when automatic and task-relevant responses are in conflict. Then, in addition to voluntarily choosing the relevant response (i.e. naming the colour of the ink), the automatic response (i.e. reading the word) must be suppressed. Differences in the speed, ease, and accuracy of controlled and automatic responses are interpreted as reflecting the additional operations upon which cognitive control depends. Behavioural studies show several basic properties of cognitive control processes: they are required when habitual responses would be inadequate; they need voluntary effort of some kind; and they tend to operate serially because they are of highly limited capacity. Therefore, as the Nobel Prize winner Daniel Kahneman (2011) argues in detail, control processes require more time than automatic processes, so they are associated with thinking slowly, rather than with thinking quickly. Finally, it has long been known that these control processes depend on various regions of the PFC.

Cognitive control differs from emotional prioritization in that it takes far more into account than emotional state. Nevertheless, at the cellular level it uses similar mechanisms and has similar effects. For example, when a conflict between alternative responses is detected, the dorsolateral PFC selectively amplifies processing of the stimulus information most relevant to the current task. This cognitive control is exerted via connections from the PFC to apical dendrites and inhibitory interneurons in layer 1, so it depends upon apical function and its inhibitory regulation. Although much remains to be discovered about these processes at the cellular level, we know that selective amplification can occur without suppression of task-irrelevant features, and that this is consistent with the amplification arising from both excitation and disinhibition of the apical dendrites of selected pyramidal cells.[97]

Research on cognitive control processes initially focused on the effects of the cognitive control signals from the PFC on processing within perceptual and motor regions. This is now being complemented by research on the neural substrates of cognitive control operations within the PFC. Although this research is still in the early stages, it is already clear that learning is crucial, and that a major part of that learning concerns understanding what activities are appropriate in what contexts. Indeed, the current evidence indicates that the learning upon which cognitive control depends is 'context-control learning', and that this involves recurrent loops connecting the PFC to the caudate nucleus of the basal ganglia. It is only via the thalamus that the caudate loop returns to the cortex, so that is likely to contribute to whatever the thalamus achieves via apical amplification.[98]

Cognitive control can modify automatic emotional prioritization. It is possible to voluntarily increase or decrease the emotions evoked by either pleasant or unpleasant events. The belief that a treatment will reduce pain is by itself sufficient to reduce the pain that is experienced and remembered. These placebo effects involve reduced activity of cortical regions associated with pain, and increased activity of PFC regions involved in cognitive control. Overall, cognitive control of the experience of, and memory for, emotional events operates via strikingly similar cellular mechanisms, as does the cognitive control observed when no strong emotions are involved.[99]

This book emphasizes cooperative interactions between people as well as between neurons, but aggressive and other antisocial behaviours are more prevalent than we would hope. There are two clearly distinct forms of aggression. Reactive impulsive aggression occurs in retaliation to perceived threats. In contrast to that, proactive premeditated aggression is initiated in the pursuit of self-centred personal goals. Although they have distinct genetic, neuronal, and developmental bases, these forms of aggression tend to be correlated. Much is now known about genetic and intracellular mechanisms involved in aggression, allowing us to explore relations between aggressive behaviour and context-sensitive apical function.

Reactive aggression is associated with overactivity of systems that detect threat, such as the amygdala, and underactivity of cortical systems that suppress impulsive reactions, such as regions of the PFC. Some forms of aggressive antisocial behaviour tend to be restricted to the teenage years, but there is also a form that persists throughout life. The lifelong tendency to aggressive antisocial behaviour is associated with a genetic predisposition combined with adverse experiences during childhood. It is also associated with a marked thinning of the frontotemporal cortices. As apical function depends on the length of the apical dendrite, the association of thinner frontotemporal cortices with a tendency for aggression raises the possibility that aggression is associated with apical malfunction. That possibility is also implied by the crucial context-dependence of threat detection and cognitive control. Both will be impaired if there is a malfunction in use of context to disambiguate incoming signals and control ongoing thoughts and actions. Recent advances in our understanding of the genes conferring susceptibility to lifelong aggressive tendencies now suggest that they are related to apical function. The genes most closely associated with those tendencies code for an enzyme that breaks down serotonin, dopamine, and noradrenaline. This also leads to impairments in the function of NMDA receptors, which decreases the ability of the PFC to integrate inputs arriving at different times from a wide variety of sources and impairs its ability to regulate emotional processing.[100] It is likely that impairments to apical function are involved in the control of aggression because these neuromodulators and NMDA receptors all have large effects on apical function. For example, events may be perceived as threats because apical malfunction leads to an emotional state that has a greater effect on the interpretation of sensory signals than the broader context within which they occur. Aggressive reactions to those events are then more likely to occur if cognitive control is also impaired. Further evidence for this is provided by pathologies with known anatomical and physiological impairments of apical function, such as foetal alcohol spectrum disorders, which are well known to strongly increase aggressive tendencies (Chapter 7). Therefore, until evidence proves otherwise, we can assume that some aggressive tendencies and the failure to control them involve apical malfunction.

Given the reality of aggressive antisocial behaviour we must ask how it relates to our emphasis upon cooperation. Firstly, consider aggressive antisocial activities such as those that occur in pursuit of food, mates, territory, or status.

Though they are not common, they are not rare. Nevertheless, the reality of these aggressive interactions within and between species does not provide grounds for doubting that cooperation is far more common than aggression. Twenty-eight experts from a wide range of disciplines, including several anthroplogists, provide strong grounds for supposing that cooperation has a central role in human evolution (Sussman and Cloninger, 2011). In support of Darwin's emphasis upon it, Richerson, Gavrilets and de Waal (2021) argue that it is common across all branches of life and at all levels of organization, from the sub-cellular to the social. Furthermore, they provide ample grounds for supposing that it has a leading role in human evolution.

Now consider use of the word 'control' in the phrase 'cognitive control'. That may greatly overestimate the power that we have over our own mental processes. When discussing cognitive control of our emotions, Ochsner and Gross (2005) review evidence in support of ancient thoughts on this issue by looking at the *Meditations* of Roman Emperor Marcus Aurelius (ruled 161–180 CE). A major Stoic philosopher, Marcus Aurelius noted: 'If you are distressed by anything external, the pain is not due to the thing itself, but to your estimate of it; and this you have the power to revoke at any moment'. Ochsner and Gross summarize evidence in support of this stoical note, but I do not think that their view of it is an accurate description of either our capabilities or of what Marcus Aurelias intended. He intended the note as a reminder of something to be aimed at, rather than as description of what usually happens. Anyone who has attempted to cultivate the ability to control their own thoughts by practicing simple meditative techniques will know that unbidden thoughts tend to come thick and fast, with little heed to our voluntary intentions. Many hours of practice are required for a high degree of cognitive control to be achieved. In context-sensitive cells with two points of integration, the net level of contextual input is computed by summing (integrating) over the diverse set of contextual inputs received. Selective amplification results from an ever-changing combination of contextual inputs from many diverse sources, of which cognitive control from regions of the PFC is but one. Increasing the effectiveness of what cognitive control contributes to the ongoing contextual input requires many hours of rigorous practice.

Nevertheless, despite the lack of full cognitive control over our own mental processes, context-sensitive apical processing does, to some extent, justify holding people responsible for their own actions. By putting the activity of individual context-sensitive cortical cells in the context of neural activity overall, apical amplification engages a large proportion of neocortical cells in a joint enterprise (discussed further in Chapter 10).

5.8 Learning and Long-term Memory

Changes in overt behaviour due to learning depend on using information from past events to guide action in the present. That information must somehow be stored internally, so, as input from internal sources affects neocortical pyramidal cell activity via their distal apical dendrites, they are likely to have an important role in learning. If so, then apical amplification may provide cellular mechanisms for many of the vast body of phenomena revealed by behavioural studies of classical and operant conditioning, reinforcement, discriminative, observational, and other forms of associative learning. Here, we focus specifically on studies of how learning affects the activity of neocortical pyramidal cells.

I have left the discussion of learning and memory until the end of this chapter because they depend on the processes discussed earlier, that is, on whether the events were initially attended, interpreted, thought about, and responded to. A common consequence of how memory of events depends on the way that those events were initially experienced is that different people present at the same event may remember it very differently simply because they each experienced it differently initially. That is, if two people who were present at the same past event insist on contradictory accounts of it, it may be because they experienced the events very differently in the first place— especially if at the time the event had very different emotional implications for each of them.

5.8.1 Cortical Function Depends on Learning

We must learn to live in the world in which we find ourselves. Some events in that world will be highly predictable, such as day length, and others will be highly unpredictable, such as the roll of a die. Most events will be intermediate between those extremes, with probabilities that depend on context and which change over time. Fortunately, as the neocortex is a perpetual building site, it helps us learn about the dependence of regularities on context. Hebb's hypothesis that learning involves modifying the synaptic connections between neurons is now firmly established. Synaptic connection strengths are modified by the flow of neural activity that depends upon and modifies those connection strengths. Thus, learning is analogous to the sculpting of riverbanks by the flow of water that is guided by the banks that the flow helps to create.

The dependence of memory on the way in which events were initially processed and interpreted has wide generality. I assume that it is the consequence of multipurpose learning algorithms that operate across all neocortical regions. I argue that multipurpose learning algorithms are fundamental to an understanding of mind, and so I must first acknowledge that some eminent psychologists are sceptical of general-purpose learning algorithms. They argue that the notion of them makes no more sense than would the notion of a multipurpose sense organ. In contrast, many other experts argue that the evolutionary success of the neocortex arises from the multipurpose learning algorithms by which it can adapt to an indefinitely wide range of ecological niches.[101]

Long-term knowledge acquired by the neocortex includes two distinct kinds of memory: procedural and declarative. Procedural memory is knowledge that is used implicitly in our everyday activities but cannot be explicitly reported. Declarative memory provides information that can be explicitly reported. Procedural forms of LTM include motor skills, habits, and perceptual processes by which we recognize things. The acquisition and use of procedural memories depends on interactions between the neocortex and the subcortical nuclei that guide motor behaviour, such as the basal ganglia and the cerebellum. However, acquisition and use of procedural knowledge does not require input from hippocampal or parahippocampal regions, as indicated by their continued operation following severe damage to those regions. In contrast to procedural memories, the acquisition of new declarative memories does depend on the hippocampal system, as shown by the inability to acquire new declarative memories when that system is severely damaged or prevented from operating. The hippocampal system is not necessary for long-term storage of the information itself, but rather is involved in creating and consolidating declarative memories in the neocortex.

Declarative memory has semantic and episodic forms. Semantic memory can be defined as 'as an organization of relations between memories that compose world knowledge', and represents common properties shared by many different experiences of the same kind of thing. For example, knowledge of a particular place can be acquired by discovering common aspects of the many different experiences that arise from exploring that place. Episodic memory can be defined as 'a representation of relations between events and their context that compose memories for specific experiences', and requires distinguishing between experiences that are similar superficially, as when I try to remember what I had for breakfast on a particular day, rather than what I usually have. For that specific episodic memory, I must remember eating breakfast in a context that identifies that particular day.[102]

The notion of 'context' that is used in definitions of episodic memory is like that used to define cooperative context-sensitivity. For example, one way of testing episodic memory in rodents is by rewarding the choice of one from two or more objects but also making the reward dependent upon the place in which the objects are encountered. As responses to those objects depend on place, learning that contextual dependence is equivalent to making the interpretation of an ambiguous 'O' dependent on the surrounding symbols (Section 5.1). Cooperative context-sensitivity is also implied by successful performance in tasks where a cue or other information held in STM specifies which aspects of a test event are relevant. In auditory fear conditioning paradigms, an initially neutral auditory cue is paired with a mildly aversive stimulus. Success in learning that association is implied by fearful responses that become triggered by the initially neutral cue. Furthermore, the ability to learn that the association occurs only in a particular spatial or other context implies that contextual information is used to modulate response to the cue. Modification of existing knowledge to incorporate new information is known as schema building, which involves interactions between the medial PFC and the hippocampal system during learning. That form of learning facilitates assimilation of the new information into new or improved schema.[103]

5.8.2 Context-Dependent Three-term Learning Has Capabilities That Transcend Two-term Hebbian Learning

From at least Aristotle onwards, mental life has been assumed to involve the association of ideas by similarity, contrast, and contiguity in space and time. The possibility that the neurobiological basis of associative learning and memory involves modifying synaptic connections between cells was debated throughout most of the twentieth century. Donald Hebb (1949) expressed this idea by proposing that when an axon of cell A is near enough to excite B and repeatedly or persistently takes part in firing it, some growth process or metabolic change takes place in one or both cells such that A's efficiency, as one of the cells firing B, is increased. This idea is now summarized within neuroscience by the simple statement that 'Neurons that fire together, wire together'. As this form of learning depends only on presynaptic and postsynaptic events, it is a two-term learning rule. Stated most simply such rules specify how changes in synaptic strength depend on whether there is pre-synaptic activation or not and on whether the cell transmits an action potential or not. When there is both presynaptic activation and cellular firing the synapse is strengthened. There is less consensus on exactly what happens to synaptic strength when there is presynaptic activity without cellular firing, or cellular firing without presynaptic activity, or neither, but it is usually assumed that weakening of synaptic strength occurs in all or some of those cases. As an input to the cell could not take part in assisting it to fire unless the presynaptic input occurs first, the precise temporal order of these events should be crucial. A large body of work on spike-time dependent plasticity (STDP) shows this is often so.

Learning rules that depend only on presynaptic and postsynaptic activity are used in artificial neural networks to discover statistical structure in large multidimensional sets of data. These two-term learning rules are particularly useful in some forms of data mining and in reducing the data as much as possible while preserving all or most of the information that it conveys. They are often referred to as unsupervised forms of learning, although two-term unsupervised learning rules are far from being all-powerful. More discriminating forms of learning are required when the statistical structure that is relevant depends on the context within which the data occurs, whether that is stimulus context, task context, emotional context, or the current state of arousal. Various forms of the three-term learning rule that take context into account have therefore been proposed. Ideally, abstract, mathematically specified forms of learning should specify the goals of learning explicitly, and this has been done for some forms of context-sensitive learning by using information theory (Chapter 8). Here it is sufficient to note that learning in the neocortex involves context-sensitive three-term learning.[104]

5.8.3 Evidence That Learning Involves Apical Amplification

First, synaptic plasticity depends primarily on activities within individual neurons, and they depend on the context-sensitivity of apical dendrites. That makes it possible for learning to be guided towards activity that is globally coherent and relevant to the organism's goals, even though it depends only on local conditions within individual neurons. Second, learning depends on attention and STM, both of which involve apical amplification. Third, learning is affected by emotional prioritization, and in relation to auditory fear learning, connections from the amygdala to apical dendrites have been directly implicated in that learning (Section 5.6). Next, descending input from higher cortical regions has a major role in guiding synaptic plasticity, and much of that input is conveyed by synapses on apical dendrites. Further, there is evidence that calcium currents in the apical trunk have a central role in synaptic plasticity. Finally, inputs that come in brief bursts are far more effective in generating synaptic plasticity than the same number of action potentials spread out more evenly over time, and apical amplification converts a sequence of single action potentials into bursts.[105]

Calcium spikes in the apical dendrites of neocortical pyramidal cells have a key role in synaptic plasticity and depend on current flow through NMDA receptor channels. This plasticity includes modification of synapses that are on the apical branches as well as those that are on the basal dendrites. How this produces all the many phenomena of learning is not yet clear, but we know that, in neurons with two distinct points of integration, it involves the distinct functions of feedforward input to the basal dendrites and of contextual input to the apical dendrites.[106]

5.8.4 Selective Disinhibition of Apical Dendrites Is Involved in Learning

The apical dendrites of pyramidal cells are exquisitely sensitive to inhibition, with major consequences for the synaptic modification on which learning depends.[107] Earlier sections in this chapter discuss its functional implications for the contextual guidance of current processing. Here, we consider its implications for learning, as depicted schematically in Figure 5.8. That shows the dependence of learning on a 'plasticity gate' that directly activates apical dendrites and increases the effects of context by disinhibiting those dendrites. The inhibitory cells shown in Figure 5.8 as being driven by bottom-up sensory input are equivalent to those carried by the class of inhibitory cells that are labelled as PV in Figure 3.8. PV inhibitory cells are those described as basket cells in classifications based on the cell's shape and connectivity. They directly inhibit the soma and its nearby dendrites and have a major role in specifying the cell's feature selectivity (i.e. the input about which the cell transmits information). The bottom-up inhibition tends to make the cell's feature selectivity more precise, while having little effect on the sensory feedforward inputs to which the cell is most sensitive. These bottom-up inhibitory cells are also involved in the generation and precise timing of cortical rhythms. These bottom-up connections are also often referred to as feedforward, although some feedforward signals are not bottom-up (e.g. internally initiated motor commands).

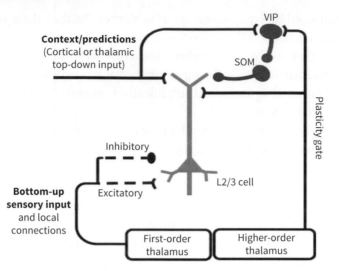

Figure 5.8 The 'plasticity gate' in this figure regulates learning by both directly activating apical dendrites and by disinhibiting them. Connections with a Y-shaped end are excitatory. Connections with a round or oval end are inhibitory. VIP neurons disinhibit apical dendrites by suppressing the SOM, or SST, neurons that inhibit apical dendrites. The inhibitory cells activated by bottom-up sensory input are those classed as PV or 'basket' cells. Some complexities are omitted from this figure, for example, the contrasting sources of input to the two thalamic nuclei, and the dependence of plasticity on cholinergic, adrenergic, and other arousal systems.

Figure from Kahn & Hofer, 2018, as approved by Sonja Hofer, with permission from Elsevier.

The inhibitory cells classified as SOM and as VIP in Figure 5.8 are primarily concerned with regulating activity in apical dendrites. SOM cells (also known as SST cells) predominantly inhibit apical but not basal dendrites. VIP cells disinhibit apical dendrites more than they disinhibit the soma and basal dendrites. Together with direct excitation of apical dendrites this disinhibition has a major role in guiding apical amplification to selected cells. This disinhibition can be thought of as punching holes in the widespread blanket of inhibition that is cast over them by SOM/SST inhibitory cells (Section 3.5).[108]

Studies of many different cortical regions show that the selective disinhibition of selected apical synapses has a major role in learning, including perceptual learning. Synapses conveying information from the sensors to pyramidal cells are modified so that they become sensitive to frequently occurring patterns of input. Different cells learn to detect different patterns such that, across a population of pyramidal cells, they learn to both recognize and discriminate between the patterns of sensory input that they frequently receive. For example, in the rodent primary somatosensory cortex, pyramidal cells in layers

2 and 3 can learn to become selectively sensitive to frequent rhythmic stimulation of their whiskers at a particular frequency. This learning requires the new sensory pattern to be paired with excitatory input to the neocortical pyramidal cells from the higher-order thalamus and involves activating the inhibitory interneurons that disinhibit their apical dendrites.[109]

The disinhibition of apical dendrites also contributes to visual and auditory learning via its role in guiding synaptic modifications in visual and auditory regions of cortex. It also has a major role in the acquisition of motor skills via its role in guiding synaptic modifications in motor cortex. In all these cases, learning depends upon locally specific excitatory input from higher-order thalamic nuclei, and upon diffuse inputs such as those from the cholinergic and adrenergic systems. Learning is also guided by reward signals, such as those from the dopaminergic system.[110]

There are diverse inputs to the apical disinhibitory cells on which learning depends. They are activated by widespread signals of cholinergic arousal and by more locally specific inputs from within the same neocortical region and from other neocortical regions. In the primary somatosensory cortex, for example, locally specific input to the disinhibitory interneurons includes input from the primary motor cortex. In the primary visual cortex it includes input from the cingulate cortex. If the intracortical input to apical disinhibition includes feedback from higher cortical regions, then that feedback can amplify the output of pyramidal cells in locally specific ways, both by direct excitatory input to apical dendrites, and by activating the cells that disinhibit them. Signals that have been learned to have high probability in a specified context carry little information if that is known to be the current context; thus, processing resources would be saved if amplification of those signals by apical dendrites were suppressed in that context. Indeed, there is direct evidence that such signals are suppressed by increased activation of the SOM/SST interneurons. In contrast, signals that contradict those context-dependent predictions will be highly informative, and there is direct evidence that in such cases the signals are indeed amplified by disinhibiting the apical dendrites.[111]

5.8.5 Direct Demonstrations of Learning That Depends on Activating Context-sensitive Apical Dendrites

Evidence from studies of synaptic plasticity that use pioneering physiological techniques confirms the dependence of learning on the activation of apical dendrites. In these studies mice learned that they could obtain sweetened water by licking a tube when a few pyramidal cells in their somatosensory cortex received weak activation from a microscopic electrode. These pioneering studies of learning were thus able to focus on the role of input to layer 1 of the somatosensory cortex from the hippocampal system via the perirhinal cortex. Learning was studied both by observing its effects on the activity of pyramidal cells in the somatosensory cortex, and by observing its effects on overt behaviour, which were in close agreement throughout. Learning to detect the micro-stimulation did not take long, but was prevented by suppressing perirhinal activity, or by inhibiting the apical dendrites in layer 1 to which it projects, or by activating the local interneurons that inhibit those dendrites. Each of these manipulations independently indicated that the learning observed depended on calcium currents in the apical dendrites, which, in this paradigm, were generated by perirhinal input. Learning greatly increased the probability that the cell generated brief bursts of action potentials in response to the micro-stimulation. Learning had far less effect on the total number of spikes generated. Once acquired, retrieval of the learned information did not require perirhinal input and was most effectively retrieved in response to inputs arriving in brief bursts.[112]

Neocortical learning that depends on recurrent connections with the hippocampal system via apical dendrites raises crucial issues concerning relations of that learning to the role of apical dendrites in perception, attention, and working memory. Those ongoing processes involve amplification of the outputs of pyramidal cells when those outputs contribute to the coherence and usefulness of the overall ongoing activity but can still occur in the absence of input from the hippocampus. Therefore, we now need to discover how and why input from the hippocampal system to the apical dendrites of neocortical pyramidal cells has such a large effect on learning. Though the findings outlined in this section also raise many other unresolved issues, they leave little doubt that the amplifying effects of contextual input to the apical dendrites in layer 1 have a major role in some common forms of learning.

Thus, learning depends on at least three kinds of cooperation. First, at the most local level, synaptic inputs to dendritic segments can cooperate to produce a local depolarization that is sufficient to modify those synapses even if there is no action potential. Second, there is cooperation between apical and basal inputs to produce the apical amplification that greatly enhances learning. Finally, there is cooperation between the cell's inputs and outputs.

This raises a rich variety of issues for further exploration. For example, there are some fundamental differences between the plasticity of apical and basal synapses. Inputs to individual basal synapses are not changed if the excitatory inputs that they receive are not soon followed by action potential output. In contrast, apical synapses are weakened if they are not soon followed by an action potential output. Thus, there is a greater need for apical synapses than for basal synapses to be cooperative as apical synapses are less likely to survive unless they cooperate successfully with other synapses. The consequences of this for learning and memory remain to be explored. Another subfield of research awaiting further exploration concerns the dynamic regulation of ion flow through the HCN channels that are especially dense in apical dendrites. They are known to be involved in regulating synaptic plasticity, but exactly how they do so is not yet clear. Another unresolved issue concerns the possibility that reinforcement and other supervisory signals are part of the contextual input to the apical synapses that guide synaptic plasticity.[113] Further issues concerning the role of apical dendrites during the critical periods of early development are discussed in Chapter 6.

5.9 Summary

The class of pyramidal cells described here as cooperative context-sensitive neurons has been implicated in basic cognitive functions. They are common in all neocortical regions. Raw sensory data is typically ambiguous in various ways but is disambiguated by using context at each level of the perceptual hierarchy. This chapter argues that the tendency to create coherent percepts, thoughts, and actions via sensitivity to various forms of context is also central to language, rationality, and other basic aspects of mental life. The tendency of basic cognitive processes to seek coherent internal states can also be seen in the well-known tendencies to reduce mental conflict, including what are known as the many well-established phenomena of 'cognitive dissonance reduction' and 'confirmation bias'. Not all psychological phenomena described as involving context imply cooperative context-sensitivity as defined here, but many do. Evidence indicates that contextual disambiguation in perception involves the capabilities of apical dendrites in context-sensitive neurons, including that from figure–ground segregation, figural synthesis, modulatory interactions between unimodal sensory regions, and object recognition. The chapter posits that the cooperative context-sensitivity that amplifies the outputs of selected cells by directly activating or disinhibiting their apical dendrites operates together with a local form of context-sensitivity that is competitive and attenuates outputs in a way that makes them more informative.

Recent evidence on regional variations suggests that cooperative context-sensitivity may be of even greater importance at higher levels of the cortical hierarchy and in humans than at lower levels of the hierarchy and in other species (see Sections 9.7 and 9.8).

The thalamocortical system provides the stage on which human experience occurs so conceptions of 'consciousness' from the perspective of the cooperative context-sensitive cells that are major players on that stage are examined in depth. Neither that, nor any other perspective, seems likely to disentangle all the many complexities, mysteries, and confusions associated with the nature of conscious experience and its neuronal bases. Nevertheless, it is now clear that the evidence for cooperative neurons offers a new perspective on those issues by identifying a cardinal function of conscious experience as selecting between alternative possible percepts, thoughts, and actions using information from diverse sources concerning the context within which the choice is made. Evidence indicates that cooperative neurons provide a cellular basis for key aspects of each of three prominent theoretical perspectives on consciousness (i.e. recurrent processing theory): the recurrent loops of connectivity includes both loops within the neocortex and loops connecting neocortex with higher-order thalamic nuclei; how global neuronal workspace theory depends on the notion of broadcasting; and Tononi and Koch's integrated information theory. The dependence of conscious experience on fluctuating levels of neuromodulators when awake, such as the cholinergic and adrenergic systems, is then compared with their effects on apical function, which provides further evidence that apical function has a major role in determining both pre-attentive sensory awareness and attended experience.

Evidence relating apical function in context-sensitive neurons to specific cognitive functions that have been inferred from behaviour by psychologists is then examined in depth. These are: selective attention, working memory and imagery, prioritization of emotionally charged events, cognitive control, and learning. It is shown that there are strong empirical and theoretical grounds for supposing that the distinctive capabilities of context-sensitive neurons are implicated in each of those basic cognitive functions. Finally, Section 5.5.16 notes that there is substantial overlap between the perspective advocated here and that advocated by Heeger and colleagues. Their detailed computational model shows explicitly that a combination of divisive normalization and recurrent amplification can account for normalization and contextual disambiguation in perception, selective attention, working memory, and motor planning. The field of cellular psychology would therefore be greatly strengthened by combining their model with the evidence for cooperative context-sensitive cells.

Notes

1. Klink and colleagues (2012) review many examples of the dependence of visual perception on contextual disambiguation.
2. Pally (2005) begins by citing both Hamlet's declaration that 'nothing is either good or bad, but thinking makes it so!', and Nietzsche's declaration that 'there is no such thing as facts, only interpretations'. Pally then uses twentieth-century cognitive neuroscience to argue that these insights are fundamental to our understanding of consciousness, and to her practice as a psychotherapist. Fodor (1983), Firestone and Scholl (2016), and Keane (2018) discuss the limitations on the extent to which higher cognitive processes have been shown to affect perception.
3. Kaaronen (2018) relates cognitive dissonance to current theories of neocortical function.
4. Gennari and colleagues (2007) relate measures of neocortical activity to the disambiguation of word meaning.
5. Grice (1975, 1989) proposed the four maxims of effective communication between humans. Recent advances in Relevance Theory (Sperber & Wilson, 1986) are discussed in a set of papers showing that the context-dependence of human communication has a central role in current research in the philosophy of language, linguistics, and cognitive science (Airenti & Plebe, 2017). Here, the two most crucial of these four maxims imply that neural signals be relevant and true. They must be relevant to the life of the organism, and with adequate objective reality, as shown by the outcome of sensory–motor interactions with the world.
6. Vlaev (2018) provides an extensive and insightful review of evidence that most human judgements and decisions are rational if interpreted within the context within which they were made. Johansson and colleagues (2008) initially reported on the misleading effects of current stimulus cues on memory for our own recent judgements are described as 'choice blindness'.
7. There is a long and rich history of studies showing contextual modulation of the strength with which pyramidal cells respond to their feedforward sensory input (see Lamme, 2004a and Gilbert & Sigman, 2007 for review).
8. Zipser and colleagues (1996) were among the first to show that pyramidal cell output is amplified when it is part of the figure rather than of the ground. Klink and colleagues (2017) show that modulatory amplification of response to a figure in V1 does not occur when micro-stimulation suppresses output from V4. Self and colleagues (2013) show that the response to elements within a figure defined by its texture are amplified by feedback to the most superficial layers and layer 5 of V1. Self and colleagues (2012) show that NMDA receptors for glutamate have a crucial role in figure-ground modulation but not in mediating the cell's response to its driving feedforward input. Though NMDA receptors are distributed widely throughout all the pyramidal cell's dendrites, apical function is particularly dependent on them (Major et al., 2013) as they have a crucial role in coupling dendrites of the apical branches to the cell body (Palmer et al., 2014).
9. Gilbert and Sigman (2007) summarize psychophysical and physiological studies of contour integration. Kovacs and Julesz (1993) first reported greater amplification for closed than for open contours. Li and colleagues (2006) provide direct evidence that in monkeys there is a close correlation between the responses of V1 neurons and the perceptual saliency of contours as measured by their responses in a detection task.

10. Stein and Stanford (2008) provide an influential review of multisensory integration with a focus on cellular activity.

11. Meijer and colleagues (2019) review recent evidence on the inter-regional architecture on which multisensory processing depends. Schuman and colleagues (2021) review evidence convincingly demonstrating that unimodal information transmission is modulated by inputs from other modalities to apical dendrites and to inhibitory interneurons in layer 1 of neocortex.

12. Deneux and colleagues (2019) show that the responses of cells in mouse V1 are amplified when they coincide with a loud sound. Ibrahim and colleagues (2016) show that this amplification sharpens the selectivity of the cell's response to its feedforward sensory input, and that it does so via projections from auditory cortex to layer 1 of visual cortex.

13. Roth and colleagues (2016) show how contextual input from higher-order thalamus to mouse V1 enables it to selectively amplify responses to externally generated changes in the visual image.

14. Using high-resolution fMRI, combined with occlusion of parts of a visual image, Muckli and colleagues (2015) found that contextual information from the surrounding part of a visible scene activates the upper layers of visual cortex. Revina and colleagues (2018) show that these contextual effects generalize across spatial frequency. Revina et al. (2021) report neuroimaging evidence that information from a surrounding context enhances the processing of weak feedforward sensory data. Modelling studies by Morgan and colleagues (2019) show that the information supplied by the context can be described as line drawings. Vetter and colleagues (2014) show that in humans abstract information extracted from auditory input reaches the cortical regions that transmit unimodal visual information. By high-resolution neuroimaging of humans blind from birth, Vetter and colleagues (2020) show that visual imagery is not a prerequisite for the input of auditory information into early visual cortex.

15. Kverga and colleagues (2007) review neuroimaging evidence that orbitofrontal cortex (OFC), provides contextual information that guides visual object recognition in visual cortex.

16. Karnani and colleagues (2014) review evidence that VIP cells specialize in disinhibiting apical dendrites by making small holes in the inhibitory blankets cast over them by SOM/SST cells. Apical disinhibition may be more common than is obvious from the published work on contextual effects in neocortex because most of that work does not distinguish between amplification by direct excitatory input and amplification by disinhibition.

17. Keller and colleagues (2020) show that the effects of surrounding context on the salience with which primary visual cortex of mice transmits sensory information depends on surround suppression mediated by SOM/SST interneurons, and on disinhibition by VIP interneurons that inhibit selected subsets of SOM/SST interneurons.

18. Lee and colleagues (2013) show that apical dendrites of cells receiving sensory information from the whiskers are disinhibited when mice move their whiskers. Xu and colleagues (2012) show that this sensory information is used to estimate the position of objects sensed by moving the whiskers.

19. Pouille and colleagues (2009) show that feedforward inhibition of pyramidal cells via basket cells normalizes input to the soma of pyramidal cells and expands the dynamic range over which neocortical cells operate.

20. Self and colleagues (2013) show that suppression occurs in rodent V1 when stimulation in the surround activates inhibitory interneurons in layers 2/3. Adesnik and colleagues (2012) identify these interneurons with SOM/SST cells, most of which are Martinotti cells that convey inhibitory inputs from other parts of the same region, and which preferentially form inhibitory synapses on the apical branches of nearby pyramidal cells (van Versendaal & Levelt, 2016).

21. Palmer, Schulz, and Larkum (2013) provide an overview of interhemispheric inhibition, and they outline evidence that it inhibits apical dendrites by activating neurogliaform cells in layer 1, thus suppressing the amplifying effects of excitatory input to the apical dendrites.

22. Iurilli and colleagues (2012) show that the net effect of coincident auditory information is to suppress the transmission of potentially distracting visual information by V1.

23. Pyramidal cell activities observed in the neocortex by Kapadia and colleagues (1995) clearly show both surround suppression and the amplifying effects of contour integration.

24. Brosch and Neumann's (2014a) computational model shows how divisive normalizing operations and cooperative context-sensitivity can be combined effectively in neural systems such as the neocortex. Brosch and Neumann (2014b) studied the effects of disinhibiting the apical dendrites in their models.

25. De Meyer and Spratling (2009) is an example of how the divisive aspects of their version of predictive coding can be combined with cooperative context-sensitivity to explain selective attention. Brosch and Neumann (2014a, b) show that normalization operates in a winner-takes-all manner.

26. Harley (2021) provides an exceptionally clear and wide-ranging introduction to the science of consciousness. Reviews of the neurobiology of consciousness that I have found particularly useful include 'Models of Consciousness' by Anil Seth in *Scholarpedia*, and the entry on 'The Neuroscience of Consciousness' in the *Stanford Encyclopedia of Philosophy*. Bjorn Merker (2007), a leading advocate for the view that sub-cortical systems have some kind of 'consciousness', agrees that mature human experience occurs on a thalamocortical stage. His main rationale for locating conscious phenomenal experience in the thalamus, rather than in the neocortex is that those experiences seem to be so definite and fast, whereas neocortical operations seem to be probabilistic and too time-consuming. Therefore, he interprets the evidence as indicating that the decisions that we consciously experience depend on thalamocortical loops. As layer 5 pyramidal neurons have a leading role in those loops that view is largely consistent with the view that context-sensitive cooperative computation in the neocortex has a leading role in human conscious experience.

27. Koch and colleagues (2016) and Lamme (2020) review evidence implicating recurrent connectivity, including feedback, in conscious experience.

28. Larkum (2013) reviews several theories relating consciousness to apical function, such as those of Llinás (1998) and LaBerge (2006). More recent versions include Bachmann and Hudetz (2014), Phillips et al. (2016), Phillips (2017), and Aru et al. (2019, 2020a).

29. Detection of weak whisker stimuli by mice depends on currents in the apical dendrites of pyramidal cells in primary somatosensory cortex that project to sub-cortical sites but not to those that project only to cortical sites (Takahashi et al., 2016, 2020).

30. Van Versendall & Levelt, 2016.

31. Llinás and colleagues (1998) and Halassa and Kastner (2017) show evidence implicating interactions between higher-order thalamus in conscious experience. This evidence has recently been used to formulate the Dendritic Integration Theory of conscious experience

(Aru et al., 2020a; Bachmann et al., 2020). Shepherd and Yamawaki (2021) offer a highly detailed and compelling review of the role of recurrent connections between neocortex and higher-order thalamus.

32. Roth and colleagues (2016) show that input to layer 1 of the neocortex from higher-order thalamus reduces the salience of feedforward visual signals generated by the animals' own movements.

33. Jones, 2001; Collins et al., 2018

34. Blot et al., 2020; Kirchgessner et al., 2021.

35. Komura et al., 2013.

36. Tononi and Koch (2015) provide an overview of the Integrated Information Theory of consciousness. Many experts debate the merits and weaknesses of that theory in Merker et al. (2022), which includes commentaries from many of the leading experts concerned with the neural bases of conscious experience. The wide range of view expressed in that debate is highly disconcerting. It shows unequivocally that there is no consensus on what the word 'consciousness' means, or on whether and how it can be related to its neural bases, either in ways that have already been achieved, or in principle. Statements on these issues should therefore be cautious and accompanied by an attempt to make the meanings of the terms used as clear as possible.

37. Záborszky and colleagues (2018) provide a comprehensive review of the temporal and regional variations in cholinergic activity when awake. Kuchibhotla and colleagues (2017) show that selective amplification of the outputs of a few cells in auditory cortex when performing an active recognition task depends on the cholinergic activation of all three main types of inhibitory interneuron. Williams and Fletcher (2019) show that cholinergic activation increases the electrical excitability of apical dendrites via modulation of calcium channels. Suzuki and Larkum (2020) show that effects of apical activation on the cell's output are prevented by general anaesthetics that either block metabotropic cholinergic receptors or suppress higher-order thalamus.

38. Psychopharmacological experiments in humans directly show the effects of adrenergic activation on perceptual experience (Gelbard-Sagiv et al., 2018). Phillips and colleagues (2016) review findings indicating that adrenergic arousal enhances apical function and that this involves reducing the HCN currents that restrict the effects of apical input. Further demonstrations of that enhancement include studies of the somatosensory cortex of awake mice (Labarrera et al., 2018). Adrenergic activation has often been shown to have a crucial role in attention, working memory, and executive functions of the PFC, implying that those conscious cognitive processes depend upon adrenergic activation (Robbins & Arnsten, 2009; Arnsten et al., 2012).

39. Pal and colleagues (2018) found that activating cholinergic receptors in dorsolateral PFC restored a wakeful state in anesthetized rodents but activating adrenergic receptors did not. Suzuki and Larkum (2020) found that blocking adrenergic receptors on the apical trunk did not affect coupling between the AIZ and the soma, although blocking cholinergic receptors did.

40. Burgess and Peever (2013) conclude that the primary function of adrenergic arousal is to support muscle tone, rather than conscious cognition.

41. Driver (2001) gives a lucid overview of the phenomena and theories of attention as seen from a psychological point of view.

42. Reynolds and Heeger (2009) present an authoritative and highly influential version of the 'biased competition' theory of attention and normalization. They note several possible mechanisms by which the amplification of attended information could be implemented in the neocortex.

43. Spratling & Johnson, 2004, 2006; De Meyer & Spratling, 2009; Spratling, 2008.

44. Other computational models showing how apical function could be involved in attention include those of Brosch and Neumann (2014a, b). Siegel and colleagues (2000) developed a two-layer spiking network built from neurons in which receptive field inputs formed synapses on the basal dendrites, and top-down attentional inputs formed synapses on the apical dendritic tree. The enhancement produced by apical input, specifying what is to be attended in that model, increases burst firing and strengthens the low-frequency components of response (< 20 Hz). Shipp and colleagues (2009) show how input to apical dendrites can amplify transmission of information about properties that did not initially attract attention, as well as about those that did.

45. Jiang and colleagues (2013) show that inputs to some inhibitory interneurons in layer 1 suppress apical activation, whereas inputs to others disinhibit it. They conclude that selective attention amplifies the cell's response to its preferred sensory input and makes that preference more precise.

46. Palmer, Schulz, and Larkum (2013) provide a brief and lucid summary of the work on interhemispheric inhibition.

47. Aru et al., 2019.

48. Zhang and colleagues (2014a) report direct evidence on the role of the cingulate gyrus and its projections to apical dendrites in perceptual regions.

49. Scerra and colleagues (2019) review research on cells in the frontal eye fields and show that they include cells that are primarily sensitive to pre-attentive stimulus salience, rather than to current intentions.

50. Hertag and Sprekeler (2019) review neurobiological evidence on apical inhibition and disinhibition and report extensive computational studies of their role in basic cognitive functions, including selective attention.

51. Zhou et al., 2016; Purushothaman et al., 2012.

52. Sarter and colleagues (2005) review evidence that distinguishes sensory and prefrontal sources of cholinergic activation and relate that to attention.

53. Schmitz & Duncan, 2018.

54. Gazzaley & Nobre, 2011.

55. Liu & Aghajanian, 2008.

56. Berridge and Spencer (2016) review the role of prefrontal noradrenergic activation in the maintenance and switching of attention. Using the effects of an ADHD-related drug, that is, methylphenidate (Ritalin), they suggest that high-threshold adrenergic receptors improve both focused attention and the ability to switch it flexibly as required in the current context.

57. Arnsten, 2015.

58. Oberauer and colleagues (2108) provide a formidable list of phenomena that 16 eminent experts consider to be representative of the evidence on 'working memory'. The evidence that they consider is predominantly psychological, not cellular.

59. For an overview of much of this early work on VSTM, see Phillips (1974, 1983). For a review of subsequent work on VSTM under the title of 'change blindness', see Simons and

Rensink (2005). Norris (2017) presents a strong case for supposing that STM cannot be merely activated LTM.

60. Phillips and Christie (1977) report studies showing that many nonvisual tasks interfere with visual STM. Morey (2018) argues that this indicates that there is no specialized visual STM. It would be more accurate to say that it indicates that there is no specialized visual STM that is independent of a general processing resource of some kind.

61. Phillips, 1983, Fig. 5.

62. Christophel et al., 2017.

63. Velisavljević and Elder (2008) report better STM for coherent than for scrambled scenes.

64. Koch and Crick (1994) suggested that bursting 'turns on' STM. Larkum and colleagues (2001, 2003) discuss long-lasting calcium plateaus in apical dendrites.

65. Xu (2017) argues that visual STM is unlikely to be based on persistent firing in V1.

66. Phillips and Singer (1974) show that there is brief sensory persistence using psychophysical methods, and they also relate it in detail to the activity of cells in LGN.

67. See Guo and colleagues (2020) for studies with implication for the temporal dynamics of recurrent connections between somatosensory cortex and higher-order thalamus. Shepherd and Yamawaki (2021) present an authoritative review of current knowledge relating recurrent loops within the cortex and between cortex and thalamus in fundamental cognitive functions, including consciousness.

68. For evidence of layer-specificity in the effects of attention and working memory on activity in primary visual cortex during mental curve tracing by monkeys, see van Kerkoerle, Self, and Roelfsema (2017).

69. For a review of temporary maintenance of visual information in subregions of the intraparietal sulcus, see Xu (2017).

70. Arnsten and colleagues (2012) and Constantinidis and colleagues (2018) present a robust case for post-stimulus persistence in PFC as a neuronal basis for STM in many simple tasks. Postle (2015) reviews recent fMRI, EEG, and TMS studies of the role of PFC in STM. Bastos and colleagues (2018) also report evidence on persistent activity in the PFC.

71. Merrikhi and colleagues (2017) report direct demonstration of persistent modulatory input from the frontal eye fields of PFC to apical dendrites in perceptual regions.

72. Nakajima and Halassa (2017) and Collins and colleagues (2018) review evidence on the role of recurrent connections between PFC and higher-order thalamus in working memory.

73. Guo and colleagues (2018) report an excitatory thalamocortical loop that generates persistent activity for use in motor planning. Thalamic input to apical dendrites in layer 1 of layer 5B cells are shown to be a key link in that reverberatory loop.

74. Crick and Kock (1998) first proposed the 'no strong corticothalamic loops' hypothesis as part of their search for the neural correlates of consciousness.

75. Wang and colleagues (2004) proposed a microcircuit model of working memory based on physiological and biophysical evidence for a disinhibitory motif. Wang and Yang (2018) review further evidence relating working memory to disinhibition of apical dendrites in the PFC. Sadeh and Clopath (2021) review the stabilization of recurrence by inhibitory interneurons.

76. Wolff and colleagues (2017) report on studies of hidden forms of temporary persistence in perceptual regions.

77. Stokes (2015) and Postle (2015) both review evidence for latent or 'silent' forms of temporary maintenance of selected, but currently unattended, information in the PFC. Lundqvist and colleagues (2018) present a robust defence of temporary maintenance in PFC by dynamic patterns of non-persistent activity as a basis for working memory in complex tasks. Masse and colleagues (2020) review the evidence for such forms of non-persistent STM from a psychological perspective.

78. Mongillo, Barak, and Tsodyks (2008) present a computational model showing how temporary changes in synaptic strength could provide a neuronal basis for working memory.

79. Rose and colleagues (2016) report on the reactivation of latent working memories by TMS. Murphy and colleagues (2016) report the effects of TMS on dendritic calcium currents.

80. For a review of the effects of adrenergic and dopaminergic arousal on STMs and other PFC functions, see Robbins and Arnsten (2009). Dembro and Johnston (2014) review the high sensitivity of activity in PFC to all the main neuromodulators.

81. For evidence on cooperative interactions between dopaminergic and adrenergic modulators in PFC, see Merrikhi et al. (2017) and Lee et al. (2020). For conditions in which they compete, see Robbins and Arnsten (2009).

82. Dembrow and Johnston (2014) outline the effects of cholinergic priming on the responsiveness of PFC pyramidal cells.

83. Adrenergic arousal enhances working memory by activating the low-threshold adrenergic receptors in PFC that block HCN currents that greatly restrict the effects of apical input (Wang et al., 2007; Carr et al., 2007; Barth et al., 2008). Guo and colleagues (2018) directly observed similar effects on HCN currents in premotor regions of frontal cortex during motor planning.

84. Lee and colleagues (2020) find that adrenergic modulation of inhibitory interneurons in the frontal eye-fields of macaque PFC involves specific effects on the interneurons that inhibit apical dendrites.

85. Arnsten and colleagues (2012) review evidence that the adrenergic receptors that respond to high levels of arousal, as when stress is high, impair PFC functions, such as working memories.

86. Unsworth and Robison (2017) review evidence for relations between adrenergic arousal and individual differences in working memory capabilities.

87. Sparing and colleagues (2002) show that imagery reduces the TMS strength required to induce the experience of phosphenes. Spagna and colleagues (2021) show that visual imagery does not depend on primary visual regions.

88. Roldan and Phillips (1980) show that mental rotation does not transform long-term knowledge but uses it to create new descriptions. Phillips (1983) shows that imaging the appearance of handwritten letters greatly interferes with STM for novel patterns.

89. Rollwage and colleagues (2020) provide evidence on the neurobiology of confirmation bias

90. Ma et al., 2014.

91. Halford, Cowan, & Andrews, 2007.

92. On page 13 of supplementary materials for their paper, Heeger and Mackey (2019) note that apical dendrites are a possible biophysical mechanism for recurrent gain. They use the notation a for recurrent gain and b for input gain to indicate a for apical and b for basal.

93. Pessoa, 2017.

94. Smith and Lane (2015) provide a comprehensive review of cortical regions and sub-cortical nuclei involved in emotion. Mather and colleagues (2016) and their many commentators discuss the evidence relating emotional arousal to prioritization and adrenergic arousal. Larkum and Phillips (2016) argue that those interactions are, at least in part, mediated by apical amplification. The effects of adrenergic arousal are complex and not monotonic. Their effects when unusually high may be the opposite of those at more moderate levels. They also depend on cortical region and perhaps on the type of pyramidal cell involved. For example, in contrast to cells in posterior regions, apical dendrites of cells in PFC are disconnected from the soma by unusually high levels of adrenergic arousal.

95. Freese and Amaral (2005) provide detailed information on connections between the amygdala and visual cortex in macaque monkeys.

96. Yang and colleagues (2016) show that auditory fear conditioning in mice depends on direct excitatory connections from the amygdala to apical synapses in layer 1 of auditory cortex.

97. Egner and Hirsch (2005) report selective amplification of perceptual activity by PFC without suppression of irrelevant activity. Other evidence relating cognitive control to context-sensitivity and apical function is reviewed by Phillips (2017).

98. Chiu and Egner (2019) review the evidence for 'context-control learning'.

99. Ochsner and Gross (2005) review the cognitive control of emotion.

100. Kolla and Bortolato (2020) review evidence relating life-long aggressive tendencies to an impaired cellular physiology in PFC that arises from an interaction between genetic susceptibility and an adverse environment during childhood.

101. Phillips and Singer (1997) argued that there are common foundations for cortical computation, including a multipurpose learning rule. Of the 23 expert commentators on our paper, 21 agreed. The other two expressed no opinion on that issue.

102. Eichenbaum (2000) reviews evidence distinguishing declarative from procedural LTM in both human and nonhuman species.

103. Eichenbaum (2017) reviews the role of interactions between PFC and hippocampal regions in episodic memory and schema building.

104. Kusmierz and colleagues (2017) review recent evidence for a third factor guiding synaptic plasticity in the neocortex, but as do many others, they focus on the role of the third factor in learning while neglecting its primary role in guiding current ongoing information processing.

105. Kampa and colleagues (2006) show that calcium spikes in the apical dendrite induce the spike-timing dependent synaptic plasticity (STDP) that underlies learning. They also show that this plasticity is induced by the reception of bursts of two action potentials within 10 ms, but not by single action potentials that are separated by 20 ms or more. These findings have since been confirmed by research from many other labs and extended to show that learning is enhanced by bursting input of the kind that it tends to generate, as in a river carving the banks that guides its flow.

106. Larkum and colleagues (2018) discuss evidence on the functional differentiation of somatic and apical integration zones, and the need for a single coherent theory of apical function, including its role in learning.

107. The selective disinhibition of apical dendrites is outlined in Section 3.5, where it is claimed to have rich functional implications.

108. Tremblay and colleagues (2016) provide an extensive review of the various neocortical inhibitory cells, including the disinhibition of apical dendrites by VIP cells, and relate it to auditory fear learning.

109. The dependence of learning in rodent somatosensory cortex on disinhibition of the apical dendrites in layer 2/3 by higher-order thalamocortical input is reported by Williams and Holtmaat (2019). Letzkus and colleagues (2015) provide a wide-ranging review of the role of disinhibition in learning, including its role in neocortex, hippocampus, and amygdala.

110. Roelfsema and Holtmaat (2018) review current knowledge of synaptic plasticity in the neocortex. They cite many studies showing selective disinhibition of apical dendrites in visual, auditory, somaesthetic, and motor regions. The evidence that they review shows that this synaptic plasticity involves cholinergic and adrenergic arousal, and dopaminergic activation also in the case of the reinforcement learning that depends on reward.

111. Khan and Hofer (2018) review much evidence on the contextual guidance of processing and learning in visual cortex, including input from other cortical regions, such as the anterior cingulate gyrus, and the effects of learning on both apical inhibition and disinhibition. These findings are sometimes interpreted as implying that the learned predictions change what the disinhibited cells code for, that is, what they transmit information about. That change is hypothesized to be such that after learning they transmit information about the difference between what was expected, and the feedforward data received. As I see it these effects of predictability are more accurately described as affecting the salience with which pyramidal cells transmit their signals, however, rather than as changing what the cells 'code' for as discussed further in Chapter 9.

112. These pioneering demonstrations of the role of contextual input to apical dendrites in learning are reported by Doron et al (2020).

113. Williams and Stuart (2002) show that the conditions in which synapses are either strengthened or weakened depends on whether they are located in the apical or in the basal dendritic trees. Sjöström and colleagues (2008) present an extensive review of the distinct roles of apical and basal dendrites in synaptic plasticity. They review ample evidence showing that learning involves cooperative phenomena.

6
Evolution and Development of Cooperative Neurons

Similarities and differences between the mental lives of humans and of other animals raise central and highly contentious issues within the philosophy of mind. Views on these comparisons range from belief in an unbridgeable dichotomy between humans and other species to belief in an essential continuity between all forms of life. French philosopher Rene Descartes (1595–1650) argued that mind–body dualism applied only to humans, and all other organisms were mindless mechanisms. In striking contrast, Scottish philosopher David Hume (1711–1776) emphasized the similarities between humans, primates, and other species and argued for continuities in the evolution of bodies and minds that resonates strongly with the conceptual revolution begun by Darwin and others a century later.

The struggle for survival at the centre of Darwin's view of evolution is often portrayed as the struggle of all against all; this is grossly misleading. Rather, Darwin was concerned (in essence) with the struggle against the ever-present physical forces of noise and disorder and not primarily against other living things. Although he did occasionally use the metaphor of warfare, that is not representative of his perspective in general. Various forms of cooperation within and between species were central to Darwin's thinking, as shown by Gruber's (1974) thorough examination of his books, notes, and letters.

At least three general ways in which cooperation between individual organisms can evolve have been identified: directed reciprocation (i.e. cooperation with individuals who give in return); shared genes (i.e. cooperation between relatives); and by-product benefit (i.e. cooperation as an incidental consequence of selfish actions) (see Sachs et al., 2004). They seem even more likely to apply to cooperation between neurons within a cell because they have the same genes, and because anything that enhances survival of the organism benefits them all; that is, it is a 'common good'. At the level of individual cells the question is not whether cooperation between them has evolved, but rather what forms of cooperation have evolved, and are evolving.

The Cooperative Neuron. William A. Phillips, Oxford University Press. © Oxford University Press 2023. DOI: 10.1093/oso/9780198876984.003.0007

As many ancient species still survive, differences between them provide evidence on the course of evolutionary change. Until recently, differences in gross brain size were widely assumed to be the neuronal complement of differences between the cognitive capabilities of different species. Despite the widespread popularity of that assumption, it is not in accord with either the empirical evidence or our intuitions concerning cognitive capabilities (see Figure 2.2). There is stronger support for the view that cognitive capabilities depend on the total number of neurons and synapses, which is not at all equivalent to sheer volume of the brain because neuronal packing density varies greatly across species, and because miniaturization can have major computational benefits. Using advanced cell staining techniques, Herculano-Houzel (2017) found that the absolute number of neurons in the mammalian cerebral cortex and in the analogous structure in birds correlates better with cognitive capabilities than does either absolute or relative brain size. Humans were found to have about 16 billion neurons, gorillas, and orangutans about 9 billion, chimpanzees about 6–7 billion, African elephants about 5.6 billion, with parrots, corvids, macaques, and giraffes each having between about 1–2 billion.

Though emphasis upon the total number of neurons rather than on gross brain size is a step in the right direction, it is far from adequate, given the evidence reviewed for large differences in the capabilities of different kinds of neurons. Therefore, we can safely assume that it is not only the total number of neurons that evolves, but also their computational capabilities. Until recently those capabilities have been hidden from us by the technical difficulties involved in observing them. However, we can now see that mapping the course of psychocellular evolution is a major scientific task for the coming decades. When we have a better idea of the similarities and differences in the cooperative context-sensitive capabilities of pyramidal cells in the human neocortex as compared with other species, we will be better able to identify ways in which philosophers emphasize continuities (e.g. Hume and others) and discontinuities (e.g. Descartes and others) are valid.

The evolutionary success of the mammalian neocortex is clearly shown by the extent and variety of its evolutionary radiation throughout approximately 6,400 different mammalian species and by the exceptional abilities and achievements of humans. A fundamental goal for the psychological sciences and neurosciences is to discover the special magic of the neocortex from which those successes arise. Given the evidence that some pyramidal cells can operate as context-sensitive two-point processors, we now ask how such cells arose on an evolutionary timescale, and how they develop during the lives of individuals. This requires that we consider similarities and differences in those capabilities between species, as well as between different stages of development.

Section 6.1 outlines evidence that pyramidal cells in ancient three-layer cortex operate as integrate-and-fire point neurons, whereas in the six-layered neocortex, many of them operate as two-point neurons in which apical input provides contextual information that guides the cell's response to the feed-forward (FF) inputs about which they transmit information. This involves the evolution of new ways in which apical function is regulated by inhibitory inter-neurons and by the neuromodulators. The section also reviews the grounds for supposing that these evolutionary modifications involve the prevalence and dynamic regulation of ionic currents through HCN channels in apical dendrites. Section 6.2 outlines differences between species in their context-sensitive cognitive capabilities, and focuses on differences presumably due to evolutionary changes in the deployment and regulation of cooperative neur-onal activity. Section 6.3 reviews evidence for developmental changes in ap-ical function. Section 6.4 then discusses examples of developmental changes in context-sensitive cognitive capabilities that could arise from those devel-opmental changes in apical function. It argues that the evidence on cellular context-sensitive cooperative capabilities provides strong support for the neuroconstructivist perspective on cognitive development, which proposes that highly individual developmental trajectories construct highly diverse cognitive systems that remain (to some extent at least) always open to fur-ther development. Finally, Section 6.5 initiates discussion of the possibility that distinctively human modifications to the capabilities of context-sensitive cooperative neurons provide cellular bases for linguistic and other capabilities that are uniquely human.

I assume that for both the evolution and development of cooperative neurons and their associated microcircuitry the issues and evidence outlined here are merely the tips of giant icebergs, with far more to be questioned and discovered than outlined here.

6.1 Evolution of Cooperative Neurons

6.1.1 The Six-layered Neocortex Evolved from the Three-layered Cortex

Figure 6.1[1] summarizes the similarities and differences between the six-layered neocortex and the three-layered cortex from which it evolved.

Figure 6.1 lists four key differences between the six-layered neocortex and the more ancient three-layered cortex. First, afferent sensory input in the neocortex is predominantly to layer IV in the neocortex, rather than to apical dendrites which receive input from diverse internal sources not shown here. Second, many neocortical pyramidal cells can function as context-sensitive two-point neurons, whereas in the three-layered cortex they all operate as integrate-and-fire point neurons, thus approximating a 'dendritic democracy'.[2] Third, the hierarchies of regions within which successively more abstract things are computed are deeper in the neocortex than in the three-layered cortex. Finally, there is evidence from physiology and neural modelling that learning rules have evolved that are sensitive to the functional

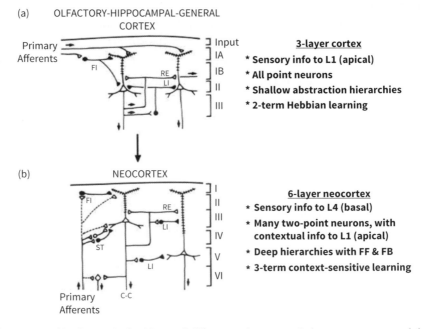

Figure 6.1 This shows similarities and differences between six-layer neocortex and the three-layer cortex from which it evolved. (a) Three-layered cortex. General cortex refers to reptilian cortex, such as that of turtles. Cortical layers are shown on the right of the simplified circuit diagrams. Primary afferents convey information from the sensors to layer I in the three-layer cortex. Inhibitory cells are shown with black cell bodies. There is feedforward inhibition (FI), lateral inhibition (LI), and recurrent excitation (RE), as there is in cortex of both types. (b) Six-layered cortex. Pyramidal cells with cell bodies in layers II, III, and some of those in layer V, transmit their outputs to other cortical regions via cortico-cortical (C-C) fibres. Other layer V cells transmit signals to various sub-cortical sites. Inputs from diverse sources to the apical dendrites in layer 1 of layer II, III, and VI cells are not shown.

Circuit diagrams are from Figure 7 of Gordon Shepherd (2011) and are used with his approval.

differences between apical and basal dendrites, implying that they are 'three-term' learning rules.[3] Output to non-cortical sites is from cells in layer II of the three-layer cortex, but predominantly from cells in layer V of neocortex. Output from layers II and III in the neocortex typically feeds forward to higher cortical regions. In addition to the feedback (FB) information from higher levels that is distinguished from FF input in Figure 6.1, contextual input to layer I also includes input from several other sources.

One way to clarify the evolution of neocortical cooperative neurons and the microcircuits in which they are embedded is to compare them with those in the three-layered hippocampus, to which they have several similarities. Nevertheless, pyramidal cells in the neocortex differ from those in the hippocampus in several ways. First, apical trunk lengths in the neocortex can be up to 800 μm or more, whereas in the hippocampus they are much shorter (they are rarely longer than 400 μm) and have bifurcations closer to the soma. To see the potential significance of this apparently minor difference, note that, in the visual cortex of mice, pyramidal cells with apical trunks shorter than about 480 μm do not have a functionally distinct apical site of integration (Figure 3.7). Second, apical depolarization in the neocortex is opposed by a broad blanket of inhibition cast by several different classes of interneuron, with dynamic selection of a small subset that is released by the activity of disinhibitory interneurons. There seems to be no equivalent inhibitory–disinhibitory circuitry in the hippocampus. Third, the I_h current that reduces the extent of spatiotemporal summation in dendrites, and which is regulated by the neuromodulators, is far larger in neocortical than in hippocampal pyramidal cells and increases more steeply with distance from the soma. Next, in the neocortex, but not the hippocampus, FB from higher to lower levels of abstraction is prominent. Further, input to the apical dendrites in hippocampus is predominantly from a single source (i.e. the dentate gyrus), rather than from many highly diverse sources as in the neocortex. Several other differences between hippocampal and context-sensitive neocortical pyramidal cells may also become clear as this issue is studied in greater depth.

Thus, there is clear evidence that pyramidal cells in the hippocampus tend to operate as point processors, and thus approximate a dendritic democracy in which all inputs, including apical input, have equal opportunities to affect action potential output.[4] In contrast, cooperative neurons in the neocortex typically function as two-point processors in which apical activation greatly increases the probability of action potential bursting in response to weak or moderate basal depolarization with which it coincides. In the three-layer cortex, active dendritic currents in the apical trunk compensate for the distance of apical inputs from the soma. In the cooperative neurons of the neocortex, that distance is greater and not compensated for; instead, it is used as an opportunity to keep the effects of the cell's apical inputs distinct from the effects of its FF basal and peri-somatic inputs. Apical activation can then be used to amplify the transmission of information about FF activation with which it coincides.

However, the contrast between neocortical and hippocampal pyramidal cells is not that simple. Purely apical input from the dentate gyrus can be sufficient to drive the output of pyramidal cells in the hippocampus. Although an analogous effect has not yet been conclusively shown to occur in the neocortex under physiologically realistic conditions, there are grounds for supposing that it does so during dreaming or imagery (see Chapters 4 and 5). If so, that implies that when output from a neocortical pyramidal cell is driven by apical input it involves a reversion to the cell's more ancient mode of operating as a point processor. A more 'primitive' mode of operation seems appropriate for dreaming, but if it provides a cellular basis for imagery and other forms of thought when awake, it therefore must also be combined with mechanisms that prevent imagery being confused with perception. Again, this raises the central issue of how internally generated activity in perceptual systems can operate without corrupting their objectivity.

6.1.2 Evolutionary Changes in Inhibitory Interneurons

Evolutionary changes with fundamental consequences for cognitive capabilities also include changes to the inhibitory–disinhibitory microcircuit upon which apical function depends. For example, there are crucial differences between species in the neocortical disinhibitory motif thought to underlie working memory. For example, the three classes of inhibitory interneuron in this inhibitory–disinhibitory microcircuit are less distinct in mice than in macaques,[5] which suggests that their functions have become more clearly differentiated during mammalian evolution. This may enhance the extent to which the relatively subjective effects of internal variables can be distinguished from the more objective effects of afferent sensory variables.

VIP inhibitory interneurons are at the top of the inhibitory interneuronal pyramid in that they regulate the effects of other inhibitory cells. They disinhibit apical dendrites, and there is a significantly higher proportion of VIP cells in primate than in nonprimate neocortex, whereas the other two main classes, PV and SOM/SST cells, do not show robust evolutionary increases.[6]

Inhibitory interneurons may also be involved in distinctively human aspects of cooperative neuronal function.

6.1.3 Distinctly Human Aspects of Cooperative Neuronal Function

Although the assumption that distinctively human mental capabilities are due to increases in brain size is popular, it does not have general validity. Differences in the total number of neocortical neurons may indeed have major implications for cognition, but evolutionary advances in the capabilities of pyramidal cells and their inhibitory regulation are also involved.

Three key properties of pyramidal neurons and the local microcircuit within which they are embedded contribute to their ability to operate as cooperative neurons. First, there is the apical trunk that segregates the cell's synaptic inputs into two subsets. The longer that trunk, the easier it is for the cell to use inputs to the apical tree to function as a context that guides FF information transmission without imposing itself on that transmission. Second, the contextual guidance of learning and processing is regulated by an inhibitory–disinhibitory microcircuitry whose organization is more differentiated in monkeys and primates than in rodents. Third, the spatiotemporal integration of input to apical dendrites is regulated by HCN currents, I_h, which depend on the levels of arousal that regulate changes of state from slow wave sleep to dreaming to being awake, and which fluctuate over time when awake.

There are good grounds for supposing that there are distinctively human variations in each of these key properties. Each of those variations increases the effectiveness with which apical input can be isolated from the soma except in contexts when its effects are appropriate. Apical input can therefore have larger effects when it is appropriate in the current context. Apical trunks of neocortical pyramidal cells are longer in humans than in rodents, and their apical dendritic branches are larger and have a greater number of synapses. Nevertheless, despite that richer apical input in humans than in rodents, it can be more effectively isolated from the soma (Figure 6.2).[7] Cellular output that is driven by input from internal sources can therefore be more effectively distinguished from that driven by ascending input from external sources, enhancing the objectivity of human perception with far reaching implications for mental life.

The evolutionary alterations just described focus on layer 5 pyramidal cells, but the apical trunks of pyramidal cells in layers 2 and 3 of frontal regions are also longer in monkeys than in rodents (see Figure 3.2). These issues have been explored further by building detailed computational models of pyramidal cells based on data from postmortem human pyramidal cells. The performance of those models has been interpreted as showing enhanced information processing capabilities of the pyramidal cells in the human neocortex, including those in layers 2 and 3. There are some differences between two prominent models of this kind, but both find that the apical and somatic integration sites have distinct functions, with modulatory effects of input depending upon the apical, rather than basal, dendrites.[8]

There is also convergent evidence from cellular morphology, physiology, and patterns of gene expression for a form of apical inhibition in the human neocortex that has never been observed in the neocortex of other species. Extensive investigation provides confidence that this form of apical inhibition is either nonexistent or exceedingly rare in the rodent neocortex. These inhibitory interneurons, or 'rosehip cells', have never been seen in monkey neocortex, so they cannot be common there. Hopefully, using post-mortem tissue or in some other way we will soon determine if they are present in the

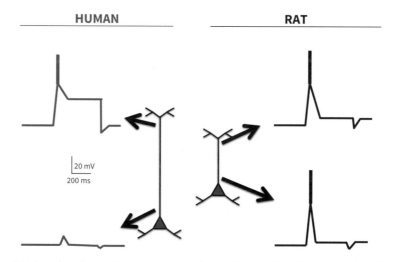

Figure 6.2 Local and somatic responses to depolarizing activation injected to the top of the apical trunk of layer 5 pyramidal cells in human and rat neocortex. The current injected was that sufficient to evoke a calcium spike locally, as shown by the two upper recordings of the local post-synaptic potential near the top of the apical trunk. The two lower recordings show the effect of those local apical injections at the soma. In humans the local calcium spike had little effect at the soma. In contrast to that, in rats it generated three action potentials in such rapid succession that they cannot be distinguished on the timescale shown.

Figure based on the findings of experiments reported by Beaulieu-Laroche et al., 2018.

neocortex of the great apes. This form of interneuron is highly distinctive in that it attenuates the backpropagation of the cell's action potentials into some, but not other, branches of the apical dendritic tree. They can therefore attenuate the contribution of that specific branch to the amplification of the cell's output. The implications of that differential regulation of different components of the context that guides both learning and processing are unknown, but their discovery is likely to greatly advance our understanding of information-processing capabilities that are distinctively human. At the very least, this recent discovery encourages the development of machine learning algorithms that use context to guide both learning and processing and which differentiates the contributions of different sources of information to that context.[9]

The role of I_h in the regulation of neocortical apical functions is greater in humans than in rodents because it has a central role in basic cognitive functions. Gene expression studies show ubiquitous expression of a key HCN channel subunit in the upper layers of the human, but not the rodent, neocortex. Physiological recordings of cellular activity indicate that these differences are greatest near the border between layers 3 and 4 of the neocortex. The greater dependence of human pyramidal cell function on I_h is confirmed by showing that pharmacologically blocking it has more effect in humans than in rodents. In humans, but not rodents, layers 2 and 3 are easily distinguishable, and distinct sublayers can even be distinguished within layer 3. The size of these distinctively human increases in HCN ionic currents increases with depth in the cortical layers such that it is strongest in deep layer 3. In rodents, HCN currents are strong in layer 5 cells, but not in layer 2/3 cells. In humans they are strong in layer 5 and layer 3 cells, thus making human layer 3 cells similar (in this respect) to rodent layer 5 cells. These differences all indicate that human layer 3 pyramidal cells may function more like rodent layer 5 cells than like rodent layer 3 cells.[10] If so, then cognitive evolution in humans involves extending the context-sensitive cooperative capabilities of layer 5 cells to layer 2/3 cells, and as the latter are the predominant source of FF input to higher levels, this implies that information ascending the cortical hierarchy is especially context-sensitive in humans.

The apical dendritic trees of some classes of pyramidal cell are far more extensive than those of others. We can assume that the composition of the context that guides learning, and processing differs across these different classes of pyramidal cell. Some differences in the composition of the contextual input from cell to cell are fixed by the anatomy of the apical tree and cannot change dynamically from moment to moment. In contrast to that, I_h

and local inhibitory and disinhibitory effects can change dynamically from moment to moment. Thus, overall, these differences between species in apical trunk length, local inhibitory microcircuitry, and I_h all suggest that there is an evolutionary trend towards a more differentiated and more dynamically regulated use of the contextual input to layer 1, leading towards forms of context-sensitive apical function that are most clearly differentiated in humans.

A central goal in this field is to discover whether distinctively human cellular processes contribute to the information-processing operations on which human language and rationality depend. We know that those operations include cooperative context-sensitivity and internally generated activity, which depend on apical function (Chapter 5). There is also now rapidly accumulating evidence that there is a greater dependence on cooperative context-sensitivity in higher and later developing cortical regions (see Section 9.8). The role of distinctively human aspects of apical function in the ability of higher cortical regions to imagine things while *knowing* that they are imagined is a key area for future exploration.

6.2 Evolution of Cognitive Capabilities That Depend on Cooperative Context-sensitivity

A vast amount of research has compared the performance of different species in behavioural paradigms designed to assess their cognitive capabilities. Nevertheless, the outline in this section of what has been agreed concerning the role of cross-species differences in apical function to species differences in cognitive capabilities need not be long. Although the cognitive consequences of evolutionary changes in apical function may be extensive, there has so far been little explicit discussion of how that relates to evolutionary changes in cognitive capabilities. My primary aim here is to encourage explicit discussion and empirical exploration of that issue. Instead of thinking of cognitive evolution using concepts like intelligence or the flexibility of processing, it can now be considered in relation to the more precisely defined cognitive capabilities to which apical function has been explicitly implicated in Chapter 5.

It must first be made clear, however, that species without the mammalian thalamocortical system, such as several bird species, can do clever things. Evidence implicating apical function in the cognitive capabilities of mammals does not in any way imply that this is the only mechanism that could possibly support those capabilities. What it implies is that apical function is *one* way evolution has found to be highly effecting in achieving them. In any case, the ability to do things that seem clever to us is not equivalent to having context-sensitive cooperative computational capabilities. So, a major goal for the future is to find out which species do (and do not) have those capabilities.

A major advance in context-sensitive cooperative capabilities may have occurred because of the evolution of sensory systems by which organisms can perceive things that are not nearby. MacIver and Finlay (2022) analysed the computational challenges and opportunities that arise when seeing things on land rather than in the water and suggest that there may have been a major evolutionary transition in cellular context-sensitive cooperative capabilities when life established itself on land about 400 million years ago. Mammals and birds have brains that are at least 10 times larger relative to body size than fish, and they can also see much further. That long-distance perception matters because organisms that can sense things at a greater distance have more time to engage in preparatory planning before action must be taken. Furthermore, the mechanics of life on land led to the evolution of mammalian limbs, together with mobile necks and eyes, which greatly increased the number of motoric variables to be controlled along with the expanded behavioural opportunities thus afforded. Once acquired, by evolution or learning or both, an organism's knowledge of its environment as seen at greater distances enhances its ability to plan behaviour further ahead in time. That planning can involve a form of 'virtual learning' that enables the potential risks and benefits of potential actions to be assessed prior to taking the actions. MacIver and Finlay's analysis of relations between sensory–motor capabilities and neocortical computational style even offers a plausible account of why primate brains evolved new capabilities in savannah-like grasslands.

For comparison with the similarities and differences in apical function across different mammalian species (Section 6.1), the remainder of this section sketches similarities and differences across species in higher cognitive capabilities in which apical function has been implicated, that is, perceptual organization, attention, working memory, and other executive functions.

Some basic aspects of perceptual organization are common to many mammalian species. Segregation of a figure from background has been shown to follow much the same principles of Gestalt organization across a wide range of species. Nevertheless, though these Gestalt organizational processes may remain the same in principle, the sensory modalities and submodalities vary greatly across species, as do the quantitative details of the operation of those Gestalt principles. Nevertheless, close quantitative comparisons of the ability to segregate figure from ground by grouping short line segments to form a continuous contour show there to be few, if any, differences between humans and macaques with respect to those specific perceptual capabilities.[11]

There are also clear differences between species with respect to other effects of context on perception. The effects of a surrounding context can have strong effects on size perception in humans (Figure 6.3). However, that effect of context does not affect size perception in baboons, who are therefore more accurate than humans in conditions where context is misleading. Evidence also shows that, as compared with humans, macaque perception is more biased to a local than to a global style of processing. In contrast, a study of chimpanzees shows that their size perception is affected by the surrounding context in much the same way as in humans. These findings imply that effects of context on perception varies across species and in some cases are greater in humans and chimpanzees than in baboons. However, the effects of context on perception in cases such as that shown in Figure 6.3 also seems to depend on experience because they are much less in cultures where less time is spent looking at pictorial representation of three-dimensional scenes.[12]

There is ample evidence that executive functions are far more effective in humans than in other primates. These executive functions are widely thought to include mental flexibility, voluntary control of attention, working memory and planning, together with suppression of habitual but currently inappropriate responses. In mature chimpanzees these capabilities are broadly comparable to those of preschool children (Völter et al., 2022), but Read and colleagues (2022) show that, in the case of working memory in humans, they continue to improve for many more years. Although we can assume that there are some basic similarities with respect to selective attention and working memory across species, there exist clear grounds for supposing that there are also major differences. First, consider studies of selective attention and short-term memory (STM) in mice. In one recent experiment mice were studied using behavioural paradigms adapted from classic paradigms originally designed to explore selective attention in humans, apes, and monkeys. It was found that, as in those other species, the accuracy and speed of discriminative responses by mice are enhanced by cues that direct attention appropriately and are worsened by cues that misdirect attention. It was also found that mice can learn to actively ignore irrelevant cues.[13] However, there are clear limitations to what can be inferred from that evidence. Firstly, mice do not have a fovea, which is central to the operation of the frontal eye fields (cf. Sections 5.4 and 5.5). Secondly, showing that mice can be trained to use cues to guide attention leaves many issues unresolved. For example, these include what cues they can learn to use, how rapidly and easily they can learn to do so, and how effectively that can be controlled by higher level mechanisms of cognitive control. Upon initial examination, it seems unlikely that those aspects of selective attention

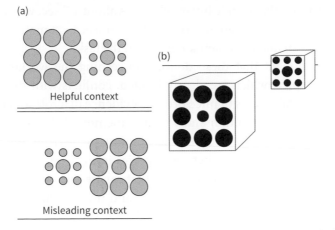

Figure 6.3 This shows effects of context on size perception that vary greatly, both across species and across stages of perceptual development. If you look carefully at the central discs in the two 3 × 3 arrays in the top row of (a) you may be able to see that the one on the right is slightly larger than that on the left. This is not so easy to see when comparing the two central circles in the bottom row of (a), however, even though these two central discs are identical to the two in the top row. This is because the context in the bottom row is misleading. It makes the disc on the left look larger than it is, and the one on the right look smaller than it is. (b) Shows that context can be even more misleading when further cues to pictorial depth are added. Most, but not all, people will see the central circle of the further 3 × 3 array as larger than the nearer one. However, measuring them will confirm that they are the same size.

are the same in mice and humans as the human cortical attention system is greatly expanded when compared to that of mice and even of macaques.

Mice have also been shown to have some form of STM. For example, building on the natural exploratory tendencies of mice and on an analysis of speed–accuracy trade-offs, a recent study found evidence for a higher stage of perceptual processing interpreted as having similarities to visual STM in humans.[14] Nevertheless, there are also basic differences between the STM involved in that study and visual STM in humans. One major difference is that the mouse's STM in that study was for a simple binary decision, so the amount of information stored was only that required to perform one of two highly overlearned responses (i.e. one bit). Despite an extensive search, I have found no reports of evidence for a form of STM in mice that is at all comparable to that found in humans in a paradigm requiring detection of small random changes in complex novel patterns or displays. A second major difference is that the average length of time for which mice can remember the information required to specify that simple binary choice is about 1.7 sec, which contrasts greatly with the ability of humans to visualize a novel 4×4 matrix pattern for as long as they can maintain their attention on the task.

It may be thought that these doubts concerning the working memory capabilities of mice, which are clearly limited, conflicts with the claim that neurophysiological studies of mice provide evidence of a role for cooperative context-sensitivity in attention and working memory. I do not see this as a conflict; on the contrary. I rather see it as pointing to the riches that await discovery concerning differences between species in the extent, differentiation, and voluntary control of the information that can be selectively attended and voluntarily maintained over many seconds and used to guide learning and processing.

The ability of macaques to temporarily maintain information about target location in delayed response tasks is similar, but not identical, to that of humans. Those delayed response tasks do not require information to be stored about complex novel stimuli or displays, however, and so are not comparable to many of the tasks used to study human STM. There is evidence that some monkeys can maintain information that is more complex than the location of a previously presented cue. For example, evidence outlined in Section 6.5 shows that monkeys can perform mental curve tracing in the absence of the stimuli involved. One direct comparison showed that macaque visual STM was qualitatively similar with respect to display size and decay rate to that in humans, but with an information carrying capacity that was at least 50% less.[15]

STM for complex novel displays has been found to be in some ways comparable to that of humans in the case of a chimpanzee who had learned to recognize the digits and to know their order from 1 to 9. The digits were then briefly displayed at randomly chosen locations on a touch screen. Soon after their disappearance from the screen, nine blank squares appeared in those locations and the task was to touch them in the order in which those locations had been numbered from 1 to 9 in the initial brief display. After training the chimpanzees were at least as good at humans at this task.[16] Although this does not show that chimpanzees are strictly comparable to humans in this task had far more training, the results clearly show that they do have an STM for such information that is broadly comparable with that of humans. Thus, as in case of the context-sensitivity of size perception, chimpanzees seem to be more like humans than are macaques or baboons.

As are their cooperative neurons, so are humans exceptional in the amount of information that they can consider when deciding what is relevant to their ongoing decisions. It is therefore possible that the human 'cognitive revolution'

thought to have happened about 60,000–70,000 years ago may involve an enhanced form of apical function. Perhaps that fundamental enhancement lies
not so much in the ability to generate activity from within (i.e. to imagine
things that are not so) but in the clear differentiation between things that are
specified from within and those that are specified from without. Direct evidence for or against this conjecture may be found by comparing the kind of
errors made by different species in tasks in which effects of context can be
strong but misleading. When mice were rewarded for responding only to
trials on which there was a near threshold whisker twitch it was found that
optogenetically activating apical dendrites in primary somatosensory cortex
produced a large increase in false alarm rates (i.e. in responding in the absence of the anticipated stimulation).[17] This shows that activating the apical
dendrites of somatosensory cells (which normally carry information from internal rather than from external sources) was not reliably distinguished from
activating their basal dendrites by external stimulation. Further direct evidence on this issue could be obtained by comparing false alarm rates of different species under comparable conditions, including conditions in which
apical effects are either helpful or misleading and either strengthened or
weakened.

Evidence on these issues could also be sought in various other ways, for
example, by studying species differences in basic cognitive functions and
asking whether they vary with arousal, as they should if they depend on apical function. Another way is by modelling the capabilities of large neural nets
built from reduced compartmental models of cooperative neurons and their
associated inhibitory and disinhibitory microcircuitry. Adding the refinements thought to be distinctively human should enhance the capabilities of
such systems in ways that make them more analogous to those of humans.
Psychopathologies that involve apical malfunction may also help clarify this
issue (see Chapter 7).

Perhaps the human cognitive revolution involved an enhanced ability to
imagine percepts and actions while knowing them to be imaginary. This combination of imagination with objectivity would enhance the ability to use imagination to change the real world. There are strong grounds for supposing
that the human cognitive revolution involves improvements in the cooperative interactions that underlie much of human history. Harari (2011) argues
that if shared by enough people, products of the imagination (e.g. beliefs in
money, religion, country, or a legal system) enabled us to engage in cooperative enterprises that have grown in scale to such an extent that they are now
intrinsic to the globalized world in which we now live.

None of this implies that all consequences of the distinctively human cognitive revolution are fruitful. Only humans make sacrifices to the gods because they fear that, unless they do, the sun may one day fail to rise, and it is only between modern humans that wars wreak such widespread devastation.

The long time-course of human development provides ample opportunity for the culture in which a child is raised to shape what they habitually assume to be relevant, and thus to guide synaptic strengths on which cellular context-sensitivity depends towards those adapted to that culture. Child-rearing practices in all cultures make use of that opportunity. One of many consequences of this may be that East Asian cultures have more context-sensitive styles of reasoning, memory, attention, and perception than Western cultures. Although lower levels of the perceptual hierarchy may be less sensitive to context than higher levels of abstraction, they are present in all cultures; however, the strength of those effects depends greatly on the culture as well as upon the specific context involved. For example, the effects of context on visual size perception shown in Figure 6.3 are much greater in Japan than in the UK. They are also greater for females and those not working in professions associated with high levels of mathematical efficiency, so cellular context-sensitivity presumably varies within as well as between cultures. Furthermore, many of the most cited findings in social psychology are rooted in our intrinsic need to increase peace of mind and reduce cognitive dissonance.[18] Thus, we can hope that a deeper understanding of these differences in context-sensitivity and their cellular bases may help facilitate understanding, and thus cooperation, both within and between cultures.

6.3 Development of Apical Structure and Physiology

A pithy saying relating development to evolution is that 'ontogeny recapitulates phylogeny', that is, the course of individual development from conception to maturity is through a sequence of stages that have much in common with the course of evolution from single cells to complex multicellular organisms. Although an obvious oversimplification, this saying has sufficient validity to make it useful. It broadly applies to similarities between the development of context-sensitive cognitive capabilities in the individual and their evolution on a far longer timescale. By analogy to the course of evolution, we can imagine a course of postnatal development that begins with pyramidal cells operating as point neurons and progresses to a mature stage in which some of them can operate as context-sensitive two-point processors. They may do so with an ever-increasing differentiation in the contexts used to guide learning and processing as development proceeds. Evidence concerning that development is outlined here in the hope of provoking wider interest in relations between cognitive development and the development of cooperative neurons.

The first thing to note is that it is not only the size of the brain that increases during development, but also the size and dendritic complexity of the individual pyramidal cells from which it is composed. Though not showing the full extent of the basal and apical pyramidal cell dendrites, Figure 6.4 correctly reflects the great increase in dendritic complexity during early development. At one month of age, most pyramidal cells do not have an apical trunk that is long enough to reach layer 1, but by six years of age, most of them do. In addition to increases in the length of the apical trunk, there are also changes in the trunk width and other key physiological parameters that fundamentally alter the effect of apical input on the generation of action potentials at the soma. We know that PFC regions are the last to mature, and this prolonged development has recently been linked to an increasing dependence on inhibitory mechanisms that inhibit and disinhibit apical dendrites (see Section 9.8).

The anatomy and physiology of pyramidal cells are not mature in rats until at least the sixth postnatal week, which is analogous to early adulthood in humans. In both species there are fundamental changes in the effects of apical input on cellular output throughout development into early adulthood and beyond. The course of development begins in an initial state in which the apical trunk is short and thin, making the whole neuron electrotonically compact. At this stage of development all pyramidal cells presumably operate as integrate-and-fire point neurons in which apical and basal inputs are summed to generate action potential outputs from the cell. From then until maturity, there are various morphological and physiological changes that increase the electrotonic isolation of apical inputs from the soma and make their effects more dependent on controllable active ionic currents in the apical dendrites and trunk. These changes include increases in the length and thickness of the trunk and increases in apical I_h, that is, the flow of ions through HCN channels, which are most dense in apical dendrites. In contrast to that, basal and somatic I_h change little, if at all, during postnatal development. These developmental changes all increase the default isolation of the apical dendrites in layer 1 from the soma. Apical inputs in adults have little or no effect on the cell's

One Month old   Six Years old

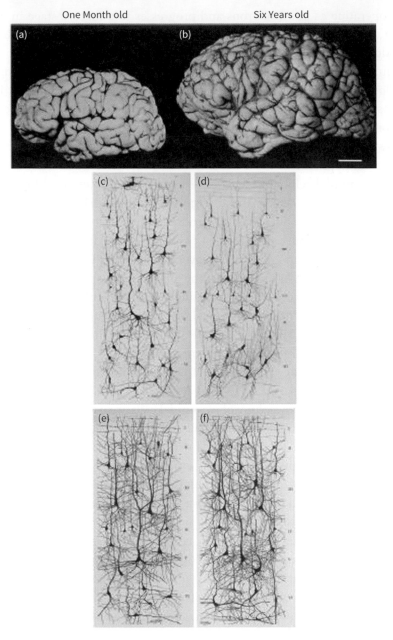

Figure 6.4 This gives an impression of the extent to which the dendritic trees of pyramidal cells in human neocortex become far more extensive during development from one month (a) to six years (b) of age. Drawings (c) and (e) are of cells in prefrontal regions; (d) and (f) are from the orbital gyrus. (c) and (d) are of cells at one-month; (e) and (f) are at six years old.

Adapted from Javier DeFelipe (2011) with his approval.

output unless actively linked to the soma by regenerative calcium potentials in the apical trunk. Only a small amount of apical activation is required to evoke an effect of apical input on cellular output in infants, but that requirement increases during development such that by adulthood the amount of apical activation required to influence output is much greater. The duration of the active calcium currents thus evoked in the apical trunk increases gradually from infancy until well into adulthood. In infants they last only about 15 ms, whereas in adults they last up to at least 60 ms or more.[19] Intuitively, that change may seem to have little or no significance, but it greatly increases the probability that the cells will transmit a brief burst of two to five action potentials, which greatly strengthens the cell's effect on the sites to which it projects. It will also have a large impact on the ability of recurrent circuits to maintain activity in the short term.

Developmental changes in I_h are particularly striking, although they are known only to a small minority of neuroscientists and to a tiny minority of psychologists. However, unlike anatomical features, for example, the length of the cell's apical trunk or the extent of its apical dendrites, these changes are not visible in microscopic images. Furthermore, the anatomical structure of pyramidal cells changes only on long developmental timescales. In contrast to that, I_h is under constant regulatory control such that it can be high when asleep and fluctuate from moment to moment when awake. It has been directly shown that, in rats, HCN channel density in the apical dendrites of layer 5 cells increases greatly from birth to maturity. Thus, L5 pyramidal neurons operate more like compact integrate-and-fire point processors during infancy, but more like context-sensitive two-point processors when mature.[20]

The developmental changes just outlined all concern those observed in rodents, whose whole life span is not much longer than that of infancy in humans. Therefore, we can assume that the developments of apical function in humans involve further elaborations upon those seen in rodents. Given the central role of I_h in isolating the apical tree from the soma, unless it is constrained by arousal systems, and given also that apical input is a mediator of the effects of context on learning and processing, developmental changes in I_h must surely have profound implications for cognitive development that await discovery. Furthermore, these and other discoveries concerning the development of apical function may well have clinical significance, because apical malfunction has been implicated in several neurodevelopmental disorders (see Chapter 7). First, however, Section 6.4 outlines aspects of cognitive development likely to reflect developments of apical function.

6.4 Cooperative Context-sensitivity: A Key Role in Cognitive Development

Neuroconstructivism, a leading theory of cognitive development, has context-dependent cooperation as a core principle (Figure 6.5). The neuroconstructivist perspective on the development of mind and brain emphasizes both competition and cooperation (Quartz & Sejnowski, 1997; Karmiloff-Smith, 1998, 2009). Several key aspects of this perspective on development are as implied by our view of context-sensitive cooperative computation. It is fundamentally dependent on the context within which the development occurs and emphasizes growth in which later stages of development build on earlier stages. The course of development can therefore be highly diverse across individuals. Neuroconstructivism implies that the

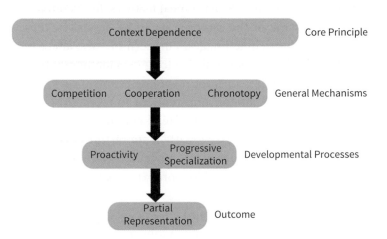

Figure 6.5 This summarizes essential ideas of the perspective on cognitive and neuronal development known as neuroconstructivism. The core idea is that at all levels of organisation, from that of cells to that of whole organisms, mind and brain develop in a way that adapts them to the context within which that development occurs. During development the amount of information used as a context increases and becomes increasingly specific to individual people. This involves progressively increasing levels of functional specialization both within and between neocortical regions. Chronotropy refers to the temporal order in which developments occur, with more abstract concepts being constructed from less-abstract concepts. Proactivity refers to internally generated activity, such as spontaneous actions. The system that is built from these developmental processes is composed of multiple partial representations, each of which is just sufficient to guide behaviour in the specific environmental context to which it is adapted.

This figure, based on Sirois et al., 2008, was supplied by Mike Spratling.

efficiency and effectiveness of 'intelligence' can to some extent rise or fall over time within individuals due to fluctuations in their interactions with the environment (Rinaldi & Karmiloff-Smith, 2017). Neuroconstructivists argue that development constructs many representations, or schema, that are widely distributed across the cortex, and that are 'partial' in the sense that they are sufficient to allow for successful behaviour in each of a particular range of specific contexts. Furthermore, new schema are acquired in the context of the prevailing developmental body state, existing schema, and the current environment.

The neuroconstructive perspective implies that cognitive and neuronal development is a journey without a prespecified destination. The genetic starting points for these journeys have both commonalities and variances across individuals. The strong context dependence of the developmental journey that follows ensures ever-increasing differences between individuals. This echoes a hypothetical proposition that I used to discuss with psychology students: 'every human a species of one'. Here, the term 'species' is not in the sense of taxonomy, of course, but in the sense of amount of difference. It implies that the amount of information needed to adequately describe important differences between any two people is comparable to or greater than that usually needed to describe important differences between any two species.

Neuroconstructivist conceptions of development and conceptions of context-sensitive pyramidal cells as cooperating via their apical dendrites are mutually supportive and complementary. Indeed, neuroconstructivists were among the first to see that input from higher regions to apical dendrites in layer 1 of the neocortex provides cellular foundations for selective attention.[21]

Several aspects of cognitive development may be related to the development of neuronal cooperative context-sensitivity; here I consider only two. The first concerns development of the effects of context on size perception (Figure 6.3. The long time-course over which context-sensitive cooperative computation seems to have evolved is echoed by its long time-course during individual development. Several different and independent studies find that the effect of surrounding context on visual size perception does not reach maturity in humans until about at least seven years of age, or even later.[22]

These maturational processes are so strongly dependent on perceptual experience that people who have grown up in thick jungle with little experience of seeing things at a distance have difficulty believing that things are far larger than they appear to be when seen from far away. Such phenomena may seem strange given that they involve involuntary effects of context on perception. It is hard to believe that preschool children see the world in a way that differs so much from that of adults, but note that the strong effects of context shown in Figure 6.3 involve pictorial cues to depth. Pictures create ambiguities for the visual system, that is, the size and distance of objects on the pictorial surface and their size and distance within the pictured scene. Species or infants who do not see the marks on the observed surface as representing objects at different distances within a pictured scene will be less affected by that ambiguity. I know of no convincing evidence that the late development of these effects of context on size perception are related to the long time-course over which apical function matures, but it is now an obvious possibility that merits exploration. Additionally, for species able to learn to see marks on a two-dimensional surface as also representing things at different distances within a pictured scene, the speed and effectiveness with which they can do so depends upon both the development of context-sensitivity of cells at an appropriate level of abstraction in the visual system and upon the amount of appropriately guided pictorial experience that they have experienced.

Another aspect of cognitive development that may be related to the development of cooperative context-sensitivity concerns intellectual realism in children's drawing of cubes. Figure 6.6A shows examples of ways in which seven-year-old children draw cubes from memory. Although they do not present views of cubes as seen in perspective, their drawings do express intrinsic properties of cubes, such as symmetry, square faces, and right angles. In our study of this phenomenon, 96 children copied simple line drawings of perspective views of cubes and patterns of similar complexity unlikely to be seen as representing three-dimensional objects (Phillips, Hobbs, & Pratt, 1978). The views of cubes were copied much *less* accurately than the unfamiliar and meaningless two-dimensional patterns. The errors made in copying the cubes involved replacing properties specific to the perspective view being copied by properties of the pictured three-dimensional object. They had great difficulty copying the line drawing of a cube correctly even though it remained permanently in view while being copied. The children who were nine years old were far more able to use the simple line drawing being copied than those who were seven years old, but the effects of what they knew about cubes were still clearly present. Indeed, Francis Pratt, a professional artist who played a leading role in these experiments, is convinced by his long experience in teaching advanced drawing and painting skills that subtle effects of internal knowledge on those skills persist throughout life.

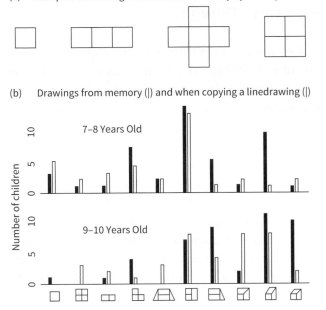

(a) Examples of drawings of cubes from memory by seven year olds

(b) Drawings from memory (|) and when copying a linedrawing (|)

Figure 6.6 Children's drawings of cubes, from memory and when copying a line drawing, are mixtures of what is currently visible and what they know about cubes. The histograms show the number of children producing the kind of drawing shown below. The line drawing copied was that shown on the far right of part B. It was copied correctly by only one out of 48 children who were 7–8 years old, but by ten out of 48 who were 9–10 years old.

Based on Phillips et al., 1978.

When these findings were reported in 1978, it was suggested that they might be due to the computational difficulty of depicting a three-dimensional object on a two-dimensional surface. That may be so, but it must also be explained why the children could not avoid being misled by seeing the simple line drawing being copied as a three-dimensional object. From the present perspective we can now suggest that these findings may reflect development of the ability to select the level of perceptual abstraction that is most appropriate to guide current actions. When copying the line drawing, the higher levels of perceptual abstraction that represent it as a three-dimensional object are not helpful, and so it may be that the older children are more able to select output from the lower levels of abstraction to guide their actions when copying. Whether that is so or not, and, if so, whether it reflects an increasing level and differentiation of apical function in guiding processing to the currently appropriate level of abstraction, remain to be seen.

6.5 Language and Thought

Currently we don't know if linguistic and other capabilities that are distinct-ively human involve the distinctively human refinements of context-sensitive two-point neurons outlined in Section 6.1.3. We discuss it here to provoke broader consideration of this new perspective on the ancient issue of what is distinctively human. In his insightful and wide-ranging (2008) review of 'How the Mind Really Works', Shimon Edelman clearly shows that, although many cognitive capabilities depend on sensitivity to context, it is especially crucial to language. Another simple reason for suspecting that cooperative neurons may be related to language is that humans are the supreme co-operators in the animal world, and language is one of their most effective cooperative con-structions.[23] Another is that language is replete with ambiguities whose reso-lution depends on the use of context (Section 5.1.3). Any attempt to relate the human mind to human neurons must involve the talking and thinking that, when we are awake, are often more continuous than walking, and, if unspoken verbal thoughts are included, almost as continuous as breathing. Finally, there may be a deep analogy between the essential nature of amplification and the semantics of language. Amplifiers strengthen the transmission of informa-tion about something other than themselves. Words transmit information about something other than themselves. A transformation of amplifiers into generators of information may therefore somehow lie at the root of linguistic capabilities.

Linguistic abilities were central to the defence of the classical symbol sys-tems of artificial intelligence provoked by the connectionist neural network perspective that arose in the 1980s. Defenders of classical symbol systems ar-gued that the connectionist neural networks proposed cannot, in principle, account for the flexibility, compositionality, systematicity, and productivity on which human language depends.[24] Compositionality here refers to the ability to select an item without that selection corrupting the meaning of the item selected; systematicity refers to the rules of syntax; and productivity gives us the ability, in principle, to generate and understand an unbounded number of sentences. Those defenders of symbol systems argued that connectionist nets can do no more than learn to associate an input with an output. Furthermore, defenders of classical symbol systems argued that connectionist neural infor-mation processing systems are so massively interconnected that representa-tion is distributed throughout the whole neural network, thus compromising the semantics of its components.

The local neuronal processors used in those connectionist systems are integrate-and-fire point neurons, however. There are at least six grounds for supposing that linguistic capabilities emphasized by the advocates of classical symbol systems can be achieved by neural information processing systems that include context-sensitive two-point processors. First, compositionality is provided at the level of the local processor, which enables context-sensitive selection without corrupting the meaning of the item selected. Second, contextual disambiguation is crucial to language at all levels of organization, from that of the distinctive features that distinguish one phoneme from another to that of conversation (Section 5.1). Cooperative neurons provide a fast and automatic cellular mechanism for much, though not all, of that disambiguation. Furthermore, this clarifies a common misunderstanding of what is and what is not dependent on context. It is the interpretation selected for a given word that is dependent of the context, not the meaning of the internal neural signal selected to convey that interpretation. Third, as cooperative neurons can interact without corrupting the information transmitted by the local elements, localized semantics can be combined with widespread interactions of the kind most emphasized in the early days of the 'connectionism' that critics thought incapable of providing neuronal foundations for linguistic capabilities. Fourth, sensitivity to context enables an increase in coherence and relevance that depends upon what contextual information is used to guide which decisions. Fifth, as the syntactic structures created are in essence sequences, some form of working memory for prior and planned selections is necessary. There are grounds for implicating cooperative neurons in the working memory required (Section 5.5). Finally, the maxims that have been used to describe the pragmatics of human conversation apply with even greater force to communication between neurons. According to those maxims, the signals sent should be clear, concise, true, and relevant. A large body of psycholinguistic research has since been built on these notions, with the need to clarify the notion of relevance being high on the agenda. The evidence for context-sensitive neurons shows that judgements of relevance are so important that they begin at the cellular level.

Thus, context-sensitive two-point neurons, if upgraded in uniquely human ways, might provide a cellular basis for capabilities that are crucial to language, which makes exceptionally great demands on context-sensitivity. That hypothesis points towards a territory that is largely unexplored, but which, in the meantime, could be called 'cellular psycholinguistics'; it raises many new issues. Do uniquely human aspects of apical function help explain uniquely human linguistic capabilities? Do any of the genes associated with linguistic capabilities affect apical function? Does the prolonged developmental time-course of language acquisition depend upon a learning capability that is distinctively linguistic as well as being distinctively human?

Human judgements also have a prolonged developmental trajectory. They can also be seen to be more rational if the context in which they are made is considered (outlined in Subsection 5.1.3). Therefore a major issue for the future is whether and how human language and rationality arise from recently evolved and long-developing forms of apical function.

Notes

1. Based on a figure published by Gordon Shepherd, from Yale, who has been one of the world's leading neurobiologists for many decades.
2. Poirazi and Papoutsi (2020) review evidence that pyramidal cells in the hippocampus function as point neurons, thus providing a basis for 'dendritic democracy' in hippocampus.
3. Sjöström and colleagues (2008) review evidence that changes in synaptic strength due to learning depend on whether the synapses of neocortical pyramidal neurons are apical or basal. Kusmierz and colleagues (2017) review neurobiological evidence for learning rules that depend upon two distinct input variables. Körding and König (2000) study learning with two points of integration in a computational model of pyramidal cell function.
4. Jarsky and colleagues (2005) review evidence on the interaction between the purely apical input to CA1 pyramidal cells from the dentate gyrus and the FF input from CA3. They conclude that either can provide the dominant input, and that they are mutually supportive when weak.
5. Wang and Yang, 2018.
6. Barinka, Magloczky, and Zecevic (2015) argue that VIP cells, identified as those that contain calretinin, are at the top of the inhibitory interneuronal pyramid, and cite articles showing that they are the main class of interneuron involved in evolutionary advance.
7. Beaulieu-Laroche and colleagues (2018) report these revolutionary discoveries concerning the more effective separation in humans of the apical zone in layer 1 from the soma.
8. Eyal et al., 2018; Gidon et al., 2020.
9. Boldog and colleagues (2018) report the discovery of a class of inhibitory interneuron that has never yet been seen in other species. Adeel (2020) and Adeel and colleagues (2022; 2023) present an effective and efficient information-processing algorithm that, inspired by the neurobiology, uses local processors with two points of integration and distinguishes the contribution of different components of the context.
10. Kalmbach and colleagues (2018) show that the effects of ion currents in HCN channels of pyramidal cells in humans differ from those in rodents, as summarized here.
11. Kapadia and colleagues (1995), Kourtzi and colleagues (2003), and Mandon and Kreiter (2005) provide examples of experiments that combine neurophysiological and behavioural methods to demonstrate that Gestalt principles of perceptual organization operate in ways that are very similar in humans and monkeys.

12. Parron and Fagot (2007) show that context does not affect visual size perception by baboons. Parrish and Beran (2014) show that context affects size perception by chimpanzees in much the same way as it does in humans. De Fockert and colleagues (2007) show that these effects of context on size perception are much less in a remote culture where two-dimensional images of three-dimensional scenes are much less common.

13. Wang and Krauzlis (2019) show that mice can selectively attend to relevant stimuli. Patel and colleagues (2015) shows that attention networks in humans are much expanded compared to those in macaques.

14. You & Mysore, 2020.

15. Reinhart and colleagues (2012) show analogous mechanisms of VSTM in macaque and human. Elmore and colleagues (2011) show several aspects of macaque VSTM to be qualitatively, though not quantitatively, similar to those of humans.

16. Inou & Matsuzawa, 2007.

17. Takahashi et al., 2016.

18. For a review of cultural differences in the balance between perception that is highly context-sensitive (i.e. holistic) and perception that is less context-sensitive (i.e. analytic), see Nisbett and Miyamoto (2005). For variations in the effects of context on size perception across cultures, genders, and professions, see Phillips et al. (2004) and Doherty et al. (2008).

19. Zhu (2000) was the first to extensively explore developmental changes in apical function. His focus was on the ease with which apical input can generate action potential output, however, so development of its role in amplifying response to basal input was not explicitly explored.

20. Atkinson & Williams, 2009.

21. Spratling & Johnson, 2004.

22. Weintraub (1979), Kaldy and Kovacs (2003), and Doherty, and colleagues (2010) all find that, for most children, the effect of surrounding context on visual size perception does not reach maturity until about seven years of age.

23. Beecher, 2021.

24. Fodor & Pylyshyn, 1988.

7
Pathologies of Cooperative Neuronal Processing

This chapter discusses neurological and neuropsychiatric disorders in which impairments in the capabilities of context-sensitive cooperative neurons or their use are likely to be involved. It does not attempt to summarize the effects of all the many legal and illegal psychoactive substances that impair or enhance those capabilities. The range of pathologies considered is wide, nevertheless. The chapter discusses five classes of pathology:

1. Epileptic loss or impairment of consciousness, interpreted as a brief temporary loss or severe degradation of all the conscious cognitive capacities in which cooperative neurons are implicated.
2. Schizophrenia spectrum disorders, interpreted as involving impairments of the interactions between information from external and internal sources that do not become acute until late in development.
3. Anti-NMDA autoimmune encephalitis, which has effects similar to the schizophrenia spectrum disorders.
4. Autism spectrum disorders (ASDs), including fragile X syndrome, in which the impairment begins early in development, and causes learning difficulties of various extents.
5. Foetal alcohol spectrum disorders (FASDs), in which context-sensitive cognitive capabilities are due to impaired development of apical dendrites during prenatal development.

All these pathologies involve impairments of basic cognitive functions that are sensitive to context, though which are impaired, when, how, and to what extent varies greatly within and between those disorders. Several other disorders have also been associated with dysfunctions of the apical dendrites that mediate context-sensitivity at the cellular level or of their regulation.[1]

Palmer (2014) reviews evidence indicating that various psychopathologies involve dysfunctions of apical dendrites, or of their regulatory mechanisms (Figure 7.1). Further evidence is included in a more recent review by

The Cooperative Neuron. William A. Phillips, Oxford University Press. © Oxford University Press 2023.
DOI: 10.1093/oso/9780198876984.003.0008

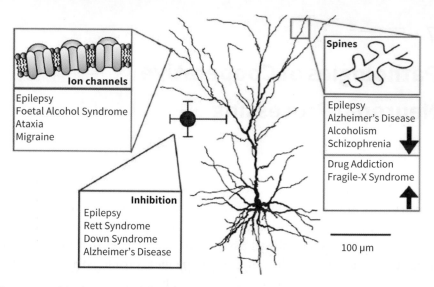

Figure 7.1 This shows some of the disorders that involve dysfunctions of the apical dendrites of neocortical pyramidal cells, or of mechanisms by which their activity is regulated. Some disorders involve modifications of the number or biophysical properties of ion channels that are inserted into the dendritic membrane. Some involve either a decrease or an increase in the density of dendritic spines, and thus of synaptic inputs. A third group involves dysfunctions of the inhibitory input to apical dendrites. Disinhibitory interneurons are not shown. The apical trunks of cooperative neurons are typically much longer than shown here.

Figure from Palmer, 2014, and is copied with her approval, and permission from Elsevier.

Granato and Merighi (2021), who emphasize the role of apical dendrites in guiding learning and processing. Nelson and Bender (2021) present a detailed and compelling account that relates impaired apical function in autism and other neurodevelopmental cognitive disabilities to their genetic roots.

I make no attempt to summarize all that is known about these disorders. Instead, this chapter outlines grounds for supposing that they all involve dysfunctions of the distinctive capabilities of context-sensitive two-point neurons, or of the mechanisms by which they are regulated.

First, it is necessary to distinguish between psychological symptoms, diagnoses, and underlying pathophysiology. As discussed in this chapter, diagnoses based on purely psychological symptoms may be misleading because in the pathologies discussed those symptoms are so various and so distantly related to the underlying pathophysiology, that the psychological diagnoses may be giving a common label to various pathologies that differ in important ways. Furthermore, psychological diagnoses may not adequately differentiate pathologies from nonpathological differences in cognitive style. However, many disorders sharing a common psychological diagnosis may indeed have some things in common. A major advantage of relating them to the underlying pathophysiology is that it can show what different instances of pathology given the same diagnosis have in common, as well as indicating ways in which they can differ. The fragile X form of ASDs, anti-NMDA encephalitis (which has symptoms resembling those of schizophrenia), and foetal alcohol disorders are emphasized here because as their underlying pathophysiology is known we can focus on relating the psychological symptoms to their neuronal bases.

7.1 Epileptic Loss or Impairment of Consciousness

Epileptic disorders are characterized by temporary loss or partial impairment of conscious experience. The temporary loss of consciousness is often accompanied by uncontrolled convulsive shaking. There are diverse forms of these pathologies; some have a genetic aetiology; some are due to various kinds of brain injury; some appear to be spontaneous; others are provoked by an identifiable trigger, such as flickering lights, concussion, low blood sugar levels, or by many other insults to the neocortex. These pathologies have distinct patterns of large slow wave oscillations seen in the electroencephalogram. Absence seizures are characterized by a brief temporary loss of consciousness. They involve large 3–4 Hz rhythms that spread across the cortex and reflect the synchronized activity of an abnormally large subset of pyramidal cells driven by recurrent connections between the cortex and the thalamus.

It is no coincidence that the figure used to show the density and heterogeneity of ion channels in the apical trunk and dendrites (Figure 4.3) is from a paper reviewing their implications for epilepsy. Those ion channels are clearly implicated in diverse forms of epileptic seizure. Furthermore, the studies of anaesthesia discussed in Chapters 4 and 5 demonstrate that loss of consciousness can arise from alterations to the effects of apical input on cellular output. It is therefore no surprise that loss of consciousness during generalized epileptic seizures involves alterations of apical function or of the inhibitory mechanisms that prevent apical dendrites becoming overactivated. In essence, the grounds for associating apical function with epilepsy are simple: apical amplification increases the excitability of pyramidal neurons, and apical drive makes them active. Thus, apical overamplification or apical overdrive are a likely cause of the overactivity that produces epileptic disorders, which are (in general) associated with widespread overactivity.[2]

A study of temporal lobe epilepsy, which is one of the most common forms in adults, observed overactivity that arose from reduced inhibitory input to the apical dendrites specifically, without any reduction of inhibitory input to the soma.[3] Indeed, the inhibitory input to the soma was increased, rather than reduced, which is likely to be a compensatory consequence of the primary pathology, and which, in that form of epilepsy, involves reduced inhibition of apical activation, and thus a loss of conscious experience due to generalized apical overamplification or overdrive. Conscious experience is assumed to reflect the selective amplification of relevant neuronal activities only. If the outputs of all pyramidal cells are amplified, then that selectivity is not possible.

Dysfunctions of I_h in apical dendrites have been strongly implicated in epileptogenesis. As much discussed in previous chapters, the current flow through HCN channels (I_h) is a powerful regulator of pyramidal cell excitability. It is dynamically controlled by several different physiological mechanisms and has exceptionally strong and crucial effects on apical function. Dysfunctions of I_h can arise in various ways, including modifications of the biophysical properties of HCN channels, their dysregulation, or their withdrawal from the dendritic membrane. The net epileptogenic effects of too much or too little I_h are complex and mysterious in several ways, but by relating them in detail to apical overamplification or overdrive, some of that mystery is now being resolved.[4]

Simultaneous recordings from the soma and from the apical integration zone of layer 5 neocortical pyramidal cells have shown that, in rats with genetically induced absence epilepsy, a *reduced* level of I_h contributes to their increased excitability.[5] As the amplifying effects of apical input are specific to the neocortex this explains how we can reconcile apparently conflicting findings concerning the role of I_h in epilepsy. In the neocortex it is a *reduced* level of I_h in the apical dendrites of layer 5 pyramidal neurons that contributes to their increased excitability. In apparent contrast to that, it is an *increased* level of I_h in thalamocortical neurons that impairs their firing pattern in epilepsy. These findings may be reconciled by noting that, in neocortical layer 5 cells, I_h tends to isolate the apical dendrites from the soma, so reduction of I_h produces widespread overamplification and a sudden loss of consciousness. Variations in the level of I_h have different effects in cells that project from the thalamus to the cortex, and which do not have an apical dendritic tree whose communication with the soma is regulated by I_h. Thus, there is no reason to expect that the epileptogenic effects of reduced I_h in neocortex will generalize to subcortical structures.

In a large subset of seizures conscious experience is not completely lost but is altered or impaired to various extents. These are referred to as partial seizures. They typically involve changes in both what is experienced and in the overall state of arousal. Partial seizures originate in specific parts of the cortex, remaining either locally confined or propagating to a few other regions. The temporal lobe is the most common cortical region of origin, although other regions can initiate epileptic overactivity. The contents of any internally generated experiences during an epileptic seizure vary greatly from person to person, but typically have specific emotional and perceptual qualities, as well as expressing information from long-term memory. The amygdala and other limbic structures are also often involved in initiating these internally generated experiences, which helps explain their affective properties. These experiences are often described as dream-like, which, given that they express information from internal sources raises the possibility that they have a basis in apical drive, as do dreams. A further similarity between dreams and experiences during partial epileptic seizures is that both involve altered states of arousal. Neuroimaging evidence indicates that temporal lobe seizures begin with an increase in temporal lobe activation that spreads to the frontoparietal cortex, then to the higher-order thalamus and to the subcortical nuclei of the arousal systems. Whereas abnormal overactivity is associated with a loss of conscious experience, impaired experiences during partial seizures are more like those of dreams. They are associated with underactivity in prefrontal regions and in the higher-order thalamus combined with heightened activity in limbic regions.[6]

These considerations suggest that epileptic seizures involve apical dysfunction. Generalized seizures, in which conscious experience is lost, seem to involve a loss of all those cognitive capabilities in which cooperative neurons are implicated. Partial seizures seem to involve a dream-like state in which internal sources may generate experience by some form of apical drive with similarities to that in dreams. Whether that is so or not is open to further exploration. Nevertheless, there are already grounds for supposing that these explorations may have therapeutic implications. First, advances in our understanding of the cellular bases of overamplification and overdrive must surely have implications for their pharmacological management. Second, transcranial stimulation has already been shown to alleviate some epileptic symptoms, and the predominant effect of that stimulation is to suppress calcium spikes in apical dendrites, thus suppressing apical overamplification.[7]

7.2 Schizophrenia Spectrum Disorders

A diagnosis of schizophrenia-related psychosis is usually given if a person's percepts, thoughts, and actions meet the criteria for a sufficient number of a variety of possible symptoms that have both been present for long enough and that occur together with a decline in everyday functioning. Three broad groups of symptoms are typically distinguished: positive, negative, and disorganized. Positive symptoms include experiences such as intense paranoia, delusional beliefs, and hallucinations. Auditory hallucinations that tell a person to harm themselves or others are not particularly frequent, but, when they do occur, they are ominous because they may be difficult to resist. Negative symptoms include apathy, blunted affect and emotional withdrawal from others, lack of spontaneity, and impoverished speech. Disorganization refers to a cluster of symptoms involving impairment in various cognitive functions, such as those that use context to ensure that percepts, thoughts, and actions are coherent and relevant to current circumstances.

Because the symptoms that occur and their severity both vary so greatly across people and time, schizophrenia is assumed to be a broad group of disorders, rather than a single disorder. Although it is more realistic than the notion of a single monolithic disorder, the notion of a spectrum must be used with caution because psychotic conditions vary within a multidimensional space, rather than being simply variations in severity on a single dimension.

Superficially, these disorders seem to have little in common with epilepsy, but there are commonalities. Both involve dysfunctions of conscious experience. Both wax and wane over time. Both vary greatly across people in the content of the experiences. Furthermore, Hyde and Weinberger (1997) demonstrated an increased rate of epilepsy in people with schizophrenia, and vice versa, and abnormal electroencephalograph (EEG) discharges related to altered neuronal synchrony occur in both disorders (Uhlhaas & Singer, 2006). Finally, both can generate hallucinatory experiences.

In schizophrenia spectrum disorders there are firm psychological and neurobiological grounds for supposing that context-sensitive cooperative computation is impaired. First, if we consider the psychological evidence, it clearly shows that there are impairments of cognitive capabilities that are sensitive to context, including the ability to distinguish imaginary percepts from those inferred from the sensory input. Context-sensitivity in perception, attention, working memory and imagery, emotional prioritization, and cognitive control are all impaired in schizophrenia.

Chapters 4 and 5 argue that feats of the imagination involve generating imaginary percepts via apical synapses whose usual function is to amplify or maintain the transmission of objectively valid percepts. If this occurs when awake the imaginary activity is not usually mistaken for reality but is experienced as a thought of some kind, although information from internal sources is mistaken for reality during dreams. They create imaginary fantasies that are experienced as valid percepts despite their incoherence and absence of sensory detail. This raises the possibility that delusions and hallucinations in schizophrenia spectrum disorders also occur because the ability to distinguish internally generated experiences from those that are externally generated is compromised.

Though less dramatic and less well known than delusions and hallucinations, other more general cognitive impairments are common in schizophrenia disorders and have been clearly demonstrated by many different investigators. Disorders of perceptual organization and interpretation have been studied using rigorous psychophysical techniques for at least fifty years. For example, the role of context-sensitivity in perception has been extensively studied using contour integration tasks. Looking closely at Figure 5.3, you may be able to see an egg-shaped contour around the centre of the display on the left. This shows that elements of a complex scene are more salient when they are coherently related to the local context. These stimuli were used in an experiment relating schizophrenia to perception. Displays containing a contour were presented one at a time, with the task being to decide whether the egg shape outlined by the contour points to the left or the right. The contours were always roughly in the centre of the image, but varied slightly in size, curvature, and location. To assess ability to see the contour, jitter of the orientation of the elements of which it was composed (i.e. its deviation from smoothness) varied from low to high. That ability was clearly impaired in schizophrenia patients, although at first glance, it has little to do with hallucinations or delusions. Furthermore, scalp potentials were recorded while they performed this contour-integration task, and the event-related potentials showed that it was the later stages of processing in both dorsal and ventral visual processing streams that were impaired, not the earlier stages of sensory processing.[8] These impairments could be due to any of a host of underlying causes, for example, refusal to engage in the task, misunderstanding of the instructions, or many other possibilities. However, these impairments of contour integration were much more informative than that: they were specific to perception because they were only present near the perceptual threshold.

Reductions of perceptual context-sensitivity in these disorders have been unequivocally demonstrated using paradigms in which context can be either misleading or helpful. If performance in a task reflects reduced sensitivity to context, then performance should be enhanced, rather than impaired, when context is misleading. This counterintuitive prediction of enhanced performance by patients in those special conditions has been confirmed using the effects of context on size perception (Figure 6.3). Discrimination between things of slightly different sizes is more accurate when context helps (as it usually does), although in some circumstances, such as those in Figure 6.3, context is misleading, thus making size discrimination less accurate. This effect is reduced or absent in schizophrenia disorders, particularly during actively psychotic or highly disorganized states. As these disorders produce size discrimination that is *more accurate* in cases where the context is misleading, as well as being less accurate when it is helpful, it clearly demonstrates reduced sensitivity to context.[9] Behavioural studies provide evidence that schizophrenia also involves disorders of other basic cognitive functions in which cooperative context-sensitive neurons have been implicated, including attention, working memory, emotional prioritization, and cognitive control.[10]

There are also neurobiological grounds for suspecting that cooperative neurons may be involved in schizophrenia spectrum disorders. First, the neocortex is the stage on which psychotic experiences occur, so we can be confident that the activity of neocortical pyramidal cells is modified in some way. Second, the dysfunctions are not confined to any specific cortical region but are widely distributed across many regions of the neocortex. Neuroanatomical investigations, including structural MRI, provide a useful first step towards distinguishing brains associated with psychosis from those associated with other neuropsychological or neurological disorders. To the untutored eye, however, psychosis is not associated with any easily seen anatomical abnormality. A widely distributed dysfunction that cannot easily be seen suggests a more subtle pathology, for example, of pyramidal cells, of the microcircuits that inhibit or disinhibit them, or of the neuromodulators that regulate their excitability, or some combination of all these possibilities. The altered cortical EEG rhythms seen in psychotic disorders provides further evidence for this, and strengthens the grounds for distinguishing positive symptoms, such as hallucinations, from negative symptoms and disorganization.

The main neuropathology underlying schizophrenia has long been thought to involve overactivity of the dopaminergic system. That view was primarily due to two fortuitous discoveries: that drugs that *suppress* dopaminergic activity reduce the probability of hallucinations such as those experienced in schizophrenia, and that drugs that *enhance* dopaminergic activity, such as the amphetamines, increase the probability of such hallucinations. Medications based on this view are still in use today and are helpful for the minority of cases in which positive symptoms predominate. However, in many cases these medications are clearly inadequate, particularly in the frequent cases where it is the negative symptoms and cognitive impairments that are so debilitating. Research on the neuropathology underlying schizophrenia has therefore expanded to include various other possibilities, including an increased emphasis on dysregulation of the NMDA receptors for the main excitatory neurotransmitter in the neocortex, glutamate, and on dysfunctions of inhibitory interneurons.

A simple reason for supposing that underactivity of NMDA receptors may produce symptoms leading to a diagnosis of schizophrenia is that drugs that oppose their activity, such as ketamine and phencyclidine (PCP, or angel dust) produce many of those symptoms. In contrast to that, drugs that produce dopaminergic overactivity mimic only the positive symptoms. This emphasis upon NMDA receptors for glutamate is supported by other evidence that they have a key role in the basic cognitive functions often impaired in schizophrenia. The symptoms produced by NMDA receptor blockade closely resemble those seen in the early phases of these disorders, and more chronic symptoms are interpreted as compensations that become established to deal with the disruptions associated with the acute symptoms.[11] It has therefore been proposed that reduced ion flow though NMDA channels is involved in producing symptoms associated with a diagnosis of schizophrenia. Their voltage-dependence ensures that they have nonlinear effects on the outputs of pyramidal cells, which could impair context-sensitive coordination.[12]

That view faces at least two major difficulties. First, though NMDA receptors are plentiful on pyramidal cell dendrites, they are colocalized with AMPA receptors throughout both the apical and the basal dendritic trees. They are even located on the same dendritic spines. That does provide a mechanism for local nonlinear summing, but it does not provide a mechanism for summing input from a distinct subset of inputs and using that as a context that modulates transmission of information about the cell's receptive field input. Second, a reduction in modulation of response to external input cannot explain positive symptoms, such as hallucinations, because they are not responses to external input.[13]

The evidence for cooperative neurons resolves both difficulties. The well-separated basal and dendritic trees have clearly evolved to receive inputs from different sources. NMDA receptors are more plentiful on apical than on basal dendrites, and the effectiveness of input to the apical tree is more dependent on them than is the effectiveness of the input to the basal tree, which is fed directly into the soma. So, underactivity of NMDA receptors could reduce perceptual context-sensitivity because the contribution of apical input to the cell's output is then reduced, so chronic underactivity of those receptors produces a chronic reduction in sensitivity to context.[14] That does not explain positive symptoms, such as hallucinations, but they may involve some form of apical drive, such as that which occurs in dreams, except that it occurs when awake, though still without the insight that normally distinguishes thoughts from percepts. This implies that the positive symptoms of schizophrenia, such as hallucinations, arise from occasional periods of apical overdrive that occur within longer periods of apical underactivity, and thus of reduced context-sensitivity.

Though this conception of schizophrenia as involving dysregulation of apical function is in its infancy, it is supported by at least four recent advances. The first is from genetic studies of rare neurodevelopmental disorders that indicate that the operation of NMDA receptors is highly intolerant of deviation from the narrow range within which they have evolved to operate (see Section 7.4).

The second recent advance is evidence that hallucinations in schizophrenia involve some form of apical drive. Visual hallucinations occur in various disorders where the feedforward (FF) sensory data is reduced, distorted, or noisy. Hallucinations that occur in schizophrenia are experienced as part of a changed external reality, rather than as a manifestation of internal processes. People who hallucinate in multiple modalities are more likely to describe them as real and distressing and to incorporate them in delusions, such as those of control or thought insertion. The strong emotional tone that is usually associated with hallucinations raises the crucial issue of what it is that serves as 'context', which can vary widely across subjects and mental states. When inputs to the apical dendrites from emotionally loaded memories or from the amygdala make a substantial contribution to generation of a hallucination, the hallucination is more likely to be distressing and is also more likely to be experienced as real because the emotion is real and is highly relevant to self-identity.[15]

The third advance is that we now know that a global systemic reduction in NMDA receptor activity reduces the feedforward transmission of information from the sensors, which increases the dependence of pyramidal cell activity on information from internal sources. In awake and active mice, systemic antagonists of NMDA receptor activity produce a threefold increase in the strength of inputs from the anterior cingulate cortex to the primary visual cortex. The anterior cingulate monitors the effectiveness of behavioural actions and has a major role in emotional prioritization. Additionally, that region includes a class of pyramidal cells, von Economo neurons, which have been found only in species having large cortices and advanced cognitive capabilities (e.g. humans, the great apes, whales). Anatomical tracing clearly shows that the axons from the anterior cingulate to the visual cortex project to inhibitory interneurons in a thin band at the top of layer 1, as well as to apical dendrites. The net effect of a pharmacologically induced global strengthening of inputs from the anterior cingulate to the visual cortex is to lower the spontaneous activity of pyramidal cells in the visual cortex and reduce their response to visual input by about 60%. It reduces the extent to which their outputs are amplified, but without changing the visual input to which they respond most strongly.[16]

Finally, there is now both empirical and modelling evidence that dopaminergic activation reduces the effectiveness of apical inputs by increasing I_h (Mäki-Marttunen and Mäki-Marttunen, 2022), which may help explain much, if not all, of the evidence implicating increases in dopamine in schizophrenic disorders.

If a schizophrenic disorder does involve dysfunctions of ion channels that are particularly dense in the apical dendrites, then it is likely to involve genes specific to those ion channels, and there is already evidence that this is so. Computational modelling of the effects of schizophrenia-associated ion-channel and calcium transporter-encoding genes can indeed alter the sensitivity of the cell's output to apical activation when it is coincident with basal peri-somatic activation.[17]

Translocations of the gene *DISC1* also implicate apical function because they lead to an excessive level of I_h, which reduces the effects of distant apical input on the cell's output. Thus, that can explain why the cognitive impairments of mice with *DISC1* translocation resemble those seen in symptoms associated with schizophrenia.[18]

The *CACNA1I* gene, which encodes a T-type Ca^{2+} channel subunit, has been consistently implicated in schizophrenia risk. These channels are densely expressed in the apical dendrites of layer V pyramidal cells, and a recent computational study indicates that they are necessary to the shunting effects of I_h in layer V pyramidal cells (Mäki-Marttunen and Mäki-Marttunen, 2022). Alterations in the proteins encoded by the *DISC1* and *CACNA1I* genes could thus contribute to psychotic impairments in context-sensitive cooperative computation because that depends on apical currents.

Much more could be learned about the genetic and physiological bases of these disorders from studies of species such as rodents, but disorders in the schizophrenia spectrum are likely to include species-specific aspects, and perhaps some that are distinctively human. Exploration of relations between culturally constructed beliefs and distinctively human cognitive capabilities may therefore provide much-needed insight into the strong cultural influences on diagnosis of these disorders.

7.3 Anti-NMDA Autoimmune Encephalitis

The discovery in 2007 of the rare disorder anti-NMDA encephalitis shows clearly that we can now be confident that NMDA dysfunction can produce many of the symptoms used to diagnose schizophrenia spectrum disorders. Indeed, at an early stage of its development this disorder is often misdiagnosed as a form of schizophrenia. Affected by this disorder, American journalist Susannah Cahalan described it as having a 'brain on fire', and her book documenting her illness was later made into a movie, which is worth watching as it shows the easily observable consequences of this disorder.

Anti-NMDA encephalitis begins with minor sensory and motor symptoms, then rapidly progresses to symptoms that vary widely across patients, but which include some combination of occasional seizures and bizarre behaviour with reduced impulse and emotional control, hallucinations, and paranoid delusions, all of which lead to misdiagnosis as a kind of schizophrenia spectrum disorder. If left undiagnosed, the NMDA impairment soon spreads to more vital physiological functions, leading to an early death. If correctly diagnosed as an autoimmune disorder, however, and treated promptly with steroids and immunotherapy, a full recovery is possible.[19]

Anti-NMDA encephalitis originates at the level of cells and ion channels, and inferences about aberrant ion-channel signalling can now be made via dynamic causal modelling (DCM) of neuroimaging data. These models comprise dynamic equations that describe flow through different classes of ion channel at the synapses of cells in a microcircuit model that is assumed to be variations on a common theme within and across regions. Given that assumption of a common theme, we can calculate the consequences of the ion currents generated by a large population of such circuits for observable variables at the scalp, such as those of EEG and magnetoencephalography (MEG). It is then possible to compute the specific biophysical parameters of the model that are most likely to produce the EEG or MEG spectra observed in any given patient. This biophysical modelling was used to compare resting-state EEGs obtained from three groups of neurological patients: those with anti-NMDA receptor encephalitis, those with other forms of encephalitis, and those without encephalitis of any kind. As expected, when comparing patients with and without anti-NMDA encephalitis, this modelling found group differences only in the model parameters for the NMDA receptors. There was no evidence for differences between the patient groups for other glutamate receptors, nor for inhibitory neurotransmitters. These analyses also implied that it was only the effects of NMDA receptors on excitatory cells that are involved in these group differences, and that, given the model assumptions, NMDA receptor dysfunction tends to produce unstable system dynamics, which would help explain the heterogeneity and volatility of the easily observable psychological symptoms.[20]

Given that EEG data is common and cheap, the possibility that these modelling techniques can be used to provide plausible estimates of ion-channel function and dysfunction in a wide range of neurological and psychiatric conditions is of great clinical and theoretical importance. It will be of even greater importance when the computational modelling used for that analysis advances beyond the point neuron assumption. The evidence for context-sensitive two-point neurons suggests that the canonical model assumed should distinguish between ion flow in basal and apical trees and include the inhibitory interneurons and neuromodulatory mechanisms that have evolved to regulate them specifically. It should also include a major role for the HCN cannels that are so prevalent in apical dendrites, and especially for any modifications to apical function and its regulation that are uniquely human. Finally, these models of NMDA dysfunction would also be more realistic if they included regional variations in the balance between feedforward and contextual effects (see Section 9.8).

7.4 Autism Spectrum Disorders

Symptoms prominently associated with autism spectrum disorders (ASDs) include impairments of social interaction, communication, mind reading, and executive control skills. They also often include a cognitive style that has low sensitivity to context, and thus a local, rather than a holistic, perceptual style. These diverse symptoms can occur in various combinations and with various degrees of severity, so, like schizophrenia, ASD is not a single disorder, but a loosely defined group of disorders. Although the symptoms associated with this group of disorders are clearly not the same as those associated with schizophrenia spectrum disorders, there is sufficient similarity to occasionally make differential diagnosis difficult.

For example, the dynamics of synchronized oscillations in the neocortex are altered in both classes of disorder. There are also several clear similarities between the aberrant oscillatory dynamics observed in schizophrenia and in

ASDs. These oscillatory dynamics have been related to the context-sensitive functions of apical dendrites by a computational model showing how FF sensory processing can be guided by internal top-down information transmitted to the apical dendrites. The model found that adding the top-down guidance altered the frequency spectrum of synchronized oscillations by increasing power in the 0–20 Hz range, while decreasing power in the 20–80 Hz range, but with little effect on the mean overall firing rate. Although this model now needs to be updated (e.g. by including the effects of the dense HCN ion channels that regulate the effects of apical input and by having interneurons that specifically inhibit apical dendrites), it clearly implies that impaired effects of top-down guidance via apical dendrites are likely to alter the power spectrum of synchronized oscillations in the neocortex.[21] A major future task is therefore to relate the evidence on these dynamics and their aberrations to the rapidly growing evidence for the role of context-sensitive apical dendrites in the cognitive functions that are impaired in autism, as well as in schizophrenia and other neuropsychiatric disorders.

As some symptoms occur in both autism and schizophrenia, it is possible that they involve impairment of some of the same underlying mechanisms. However, the dysfunctions usually have a far earlier onset in autism, which impairs the acquisition of the basic knowledge, skills, and shared assumptions that facilitate interactions with the world and with other people. Another major difference between the two groups of syndromes is that the positive symptoms of schizophrenia, such as hallucinations and delusions, are not common in ASD.

7.4.1 Many Psychological Symptoms Used to Diagnose ASDs Arise from Impaired Context-sensitivity

Though many do not, many people diagnosed as being within the autism spectrum have low IQ. In 2013 the criteria for an ASD diagnosis were broadened to include what is described as the Asperger type of ASD, in which several of the symptoms common in the more severe forms of ASD occur, but with little or no intellectual disability; some intellectual skills may even be supranormal. Prominent among the symptoms that comprise criteria for diagnosing the Asperger form of ASD are difficulty with social interactions and with the 'give-and-take' of conversation, a 'desire for sameness', persistent but narrow interests, attention to detail, and hypersensitivity to sensory events, although these symptoms are not all present in every case, However, the more symptoms present, the greater the confidence with which the diagnosis of ASD is made. This diagnosis cannot usually be made on the basis of objective physio-logical or genetic measures, but it can be in the case of Fragile X syndrome, covered later in this section.

Section 7.4.3 explores how many of these symptoms could arise dir-ectly or indirectly from reduced context-sensitivity of cooperative neurons. Some could be a positive benefit in some lifestyles and professions, so an information-processing style can no longer be described as 'impaired' simply because it involves high levels of sensory sensitivity or because it focuses more on locally specifiable details or rigid rules than on broad, holistic, contextual interactions. Even simple tests of context-sensitivity in perception show that there are clear demographic variations in the overall population. For example, the effects of surrounding context on size perception are weaker in males than in females, which may help explain why the majority of those diagnosed as having a kind of autism are male. Furthermore, there are cultural differences, with the effects of context on some aspects of perception being strong in some Asian cultures but weak in some remote African cultures. These differences between cultures may reflect cultural differences in styles of attention or in the time spent looking at three-dimensional scenes represented on two-dimensional surfaces, so there is no need to assume that they reflect either dysfunctions or genetic differences.[22]

The weak sensitivity to context and the bias to local perceptual processing in people diagnosed as being within the autism spectrum have been shown in many ways, including studies of sensory discrimination. Studies of auditory pitch perception provide a simple example of abilities that are often unim-paired or even better than usual. Perfect pitch perception refers to the ability to identify the absolute pitch of a tone without reference to an external standard. It is present in 0.01% of the general population, but in 5% of those diagnosed as being within the autism spectrum. More generally, there is also evidence that, except for those diagnosed as having Asperger's syndrome, people diag-nosed as being within the autism spectrum have an enhanced ability to distin-guish between pure unvarying simple tones.[23]

A bias towards local perceptual processing in those diagnosed with ASD has been shown in various ways, including studies of the perception of faces, words, and impossible objects. Drawing abilities also sometimes show an ex-ceptional eye for detail. Performance reflecting local FF processing of sen-sory detail would then tend to be either preserved or enhanced. They also often find that aspects of performance interpreted as reflecting a global, hol-istic, or context-sensitive processing style are impaired. Even more compel-ling is evidence that where context has misleading effects on size perception

(Figure 6.3), people diagnosed with ASD tend to perceive the sizes *more accurately*. The effects of context are also weak in cases where it needs to be used to disambiguate the local elements or to group them into a larger whole. For example, psychophysical tests of contour integration using stimuli such as those shown in Figure 5.3 find that many, although not all, of those diagnosed with ASD have difficulty detecting the set of elements that form a continuous contour. They are also more likely to have difficulty recognizing objects that are shown as disconnected fragments or in seeing that line drawings (e.g. the devils pitchfork in Figure 5.1) cannot represent a three-dimensional object.[24]

The ability to interpret things in context is also crucial to our use of language (Section 5.1). Many, but not all, people diagnosed with ASD have difficulty using context to disambiguate phonemes, symbols, and word meanings. Interpretation of the body language and actions of others is also highly dependent on context, and many of those diagnosed with ASD have difficulty interpreting such information and in 'mind reading' in general. They also often have executive dysfunctions that are most evident in weakened abilities to adapt to change or novelty, to plan, to change current intentions flexibly, and to suppress habitual responses that are inappropriate in the current circumstances.

7.4.2 Lack of Consensus on the Psychology and Neurobiology of ASDs

At least three theoretical perspectives on ASDs have a substantial amount of empirical support, though that has not yet produced a consensus. One theory proposes that there is 'weak central coherence' and emphasizes a focus on local detail rather than on global context. It implies that difficulties in extracting global form and seeing the 'big picture' can be combined with a preserved or enhanced ability to process local detail. A second theoretical perspective focuses specifically on enhanced local perceptual processes, while acknowledging that some form of global processing is also probably compromised. A third theory suggests that these disorders involve a bias towards 'systemizing' processes that help identify lawful regularities, and which have neurobiological bases that make it more common in males than in females.[25]

It is now widely agreed that local processing is preserved or even enhanced in these ASDs, but there is no consensus concerning *what* it is that is impaired, as made clear by a meta-analysis of research on this issue.[26] It is sometimes assumed that the processing that is impaired can be identified with the 'global' level as specified by paradigms in which subjects are asked to either identify large objects while ignoring the small elements of which they are made, or to identify the smaller elements, while ignoring the larger form composed of them. However, this paradigm has not led to any clear conclusions as it is concerned with difficulties in attending to a specific spatial scale, which is of little relevance to most of the symptoms that characterize ASD.

There is also no consensus concerning the neuronal bases of ASDs, although it is agreed that they involve genetic susceptibility. First-degree family relatives who are not themselves diagnosed as being within the autism spectrum are more likely to have a cognitive style that is locally focused, which may be an advantage in some professions, for example, where sensitivity to local details and well-specified rules is a strength rather than a weakness. The concordance between monozygotic twins is 60%, so we can assume that symptoms of severe forms of ASD arise from genetic susceptibility plus adverse events during prenatal and/or postnatal development. Many different genes are associated with that susceptibility, indicating that there are many ways in which the underlying physiological processes can be impaired.

It is now known that many of the symptoms associated with a diagnosis of ASD can arise from a specific genetic mutation. Studies of the psychological consequences of specific and known genetic mutations offer crucial insights into these disorders. They can help us identify the underlying pathophysiology, and can help us understand precisely why that impairs cognitive function. Fragile X is the most common monogenic cause of symptoms used to give a co-diagnosis of ASD.[27] The aim here is to provide a broad outline of Fragile X and to relate that to the dysfunction of cooperative context-sensitivity. Fragile X affects about 1 in 4,000 males and is less frequent in females. About 5% of cases diagnosed as ASD are found to have a fragile X mutation. People with a Fragile X mutation have a higher probability of epileptic seizures, and of having abnormal shapes of the face, ears, and testes. The gene involved is referred to as *FMR1*. Its mutations vary in severity but typically lead to cognitive, social, and behavioural problems that are common in ASD. In the case of fragile X they arise because the genetic mutation reduces the effectiveness of the FMRP protein, which regulates a wide range of physiological processes, including expression of the *SCN2A* gene implicated in cellular context-sensitivity. In the neocortex, FMRP regulates the excitability of pyramidal cells by its effects on the sodium, potassium, calcium, and HCN channels that are so critical to the operation of pyramidal cells, and especially their apical dendrites. A common conclusion of this research is that neocortical pyramidal neurons become overexcitable when the effectiveness of FMRP is reduced. However, exactly how that explains why so many of the symptoms associated with ASD involve reduced sensitivity to context is not yet clear.

Several ASD symptoms are interpreted as implying an imbalance between excitatory and inhibitory inputs to pyramidal cells. There is substantial evidence for that view, but it would be better able to account for the many symptoms that arise from impaired context-sensitivity if it distinguished between inhibitory inputs to the apical dendrites and inhibitory inputs to other dendrites. For example, there is evidence that some cases of ASD involve a reduction in the number of inhibitory interneurons that target basal/peri-somatic synapses, but not in those that target apical dendrites. This indicates that some forms of ASD may involve changes to the balance between the effects of FF sensory data and the effects of context, as also suggested by computational modelling.[28]

7.4.3 Dysfunctions of Cooperative Context-sensitivity Can Produce Symptoms of ASDs

Given the evidence for cooperative neurons, we can now consider the possibility that many symptoms of ASD involve some form of weak cellular context-sensitivity that varies in severity across subjects and/or across cortical regions and semantic domains. Put simply, this perspective raises the possibility that in ASDs there is less use of context at a cellular level to clarify ambiguous signals and to distinguish between relevant and irrelevant information in all or some domains of knowledge. Disambiguation and selection of the relevant information must therefore occur, if at all, via processes that operate at a higher level of organization, for example, that of selective attention, working memory, and cognitive control. These processes will take more time and will be experienced as being 'difficult' because they compete with other demands on those highly limited cognitive resources. Various performance measures do indeed indicate that people with some form of ASD are more likely to have such difficulties. Furthermore, as those resources depend on apical function, using them to compensate for weak cellular context-sensitivity implies additional demands on reduced resources. Thus, even subtle reductions in the selective effects of apical input could have severe functional consequences.

There are many ways in which the use of apical input as a context to guide learning and processing could be impaired. For example, there could be a greater bias towards net inhibitory input to the apical than to the basal tree, which would weaken the extent to which both processing and learning depend on context at the level of pyramidal cells. The effects of apical input could also be weakened by overactive ion flow, I_h, through the HCN channels that are especially dense in apical dendrites. The effects of apical input could also be weak simply because the apical dendritic tree is less richly branched, thus restricting the range of inputs that can provide contextual information to guide processing and learning.[29] These various impairments of context-sensitivity at a cellular level are not incompatible, so the more of them that apply in any specific case, the more extensive the cognitive consequences. The severity of any impairment can vary across cortical regions and semantic domains because context-sensitivity operates at the level of individual cells, so some can be affected, but not others. As mentioned, context-sensitivity in auditory sensory regions may be preserved in Asperger's syndrome, but not in more severe forms of ASD. However, any weakness of context-sensitivity at the cellular level in autism could not entail complete and persistent loss of all cellular context-sensitivity because that entails a loss of consciousness, as indicated by anaesthesia, epileptic loss-of-consciousness, and slow wave sleep. Nevertheless, the comorbidity between ASD and epileptic disorders does suggest an overlap in their neural bases.

Many symptoms often observed in cases diagnosed as some form of ASD can be understood from this perspective. For example, perfect pitch and better pitch perception imply that the perception of tones is less sensitive to the context in which the tone is heard. From this perspective, it is easier to understand a preference for keeping things the same, as it reduces the amount of context that must be flexibly considered when trying to interpret incoming information (which is often ambiguous), including that from other people. Furthermore, a tendency to 'systemizing' may be increased because it involves dealing with situations in which the context to be considered is highly restricted and well specified.

This perspective on ASD preserves some aspects of the theory of weak central coherence, which emphasizes reduced sensitivity to context. Cellular context-sensitivity amplifies coherent activities by doing so only when both contextual input and FF sense data have net effects that are excitatory. 'Central' processing resources are involved in this cellular context-sensitivity because the prefrontal cortical regions that are concerned with selective attention are a major source of input to the apical dendrites at different levels of perceptual abstraction. The activity of apical dendrites is also highly dependent on neuromodulatory inputs that are largely, though not wholly, shared within and across regions, thus providing what could be described as a widely distributed component of context. Finally, as the effects of context are stronger within sets of stimulus features grouped together and interpreted as being parts of a larger whole, they are, in that sense, 'holistic'.

Although weak cellular context-sensitivity preserves several aspects of the theory of weak central coherence, this new perspective is supported by findings previously interpreted as contradicting the theory of central coherence. For example, studies of linguistically able people with autism are often interpreted as contradicting the hypothesis of weak central coherence. People diagnosed as having the Asperger type of ASD with preserved intellectual and linguistic capabilities have often been shown to disambiguate word meanings by using the local structural context within sentences and/or the broader discourse and environmental context. For example, one study found that people diagnosed as being within the autism spectrum, but with good verbal skills, can easily use contextual cues to disambiguate word meanings in conditions where the choices are clear and simple. Another study found that teenagers diagnosed as being within the Asperger part of the autism spectrum use both structural cues within sentences and the broader discourse context to interpret pronouns such as 'he', 'she', or 'they' correctly.[30] Although the findings of these studies were interpreted as evidence against weak central coherence, there are several ways in which they indicate weak cellular context-sensitivity. First, these studies all confirm that linguistic processes are strongly dependent on the use of context to guide both production and comprehension, which helps explain why language difficulties are so frequent in the autism spectrum. Second, pronouns, which are among the most highly ambiguous of words, are misused more frequently by those diagnosed with autism. Third, those diagnosed with ASD sometimes report difficulties with interpreting pronouns in conversations concerning more than one person, and these studies found that people diagnosed as being within the ASD spectrum took more than the usual amount of time to interpret pronouns. Further, their ability to use context for disambiguation is more dependent on voluntary processing activities such as selective attention and working memory. Also, they have more difficulty using the discourse context to counteract conflicting structural cues from within the sentence. Finally, those diagnosed with ASD are more distracted by information that is irrelevant to what they are trying to do. All of these findings indicate that many of the symptoms associated with a diagnosis of ASD are likely to involve an impairment of the context-sensitivity of cooperative pyramidal cells, even in those diagnosed with less-severe forms of ASD.

There are five further grounds on which reduced cellular context-sensitivity can be shown to be implicated in ASD. The first, and perhaps the most compelling, comes from studies of *SCN2A*, a gene with mutations that are robustly associated with symptoms often seen in ASD. Nelson and Bender (2021) provide an in-depth review of how mutations in this gene leads to changes in pyramidal cell physiology that are strongly associated with a wide range of neurodevelopmental disorders. Their review clearly shows that mutations of *SCN2A* produces symptoms used to diagnose ASD because it codes for the voltage-gated $Na_v1.2$ sodium ion channels that transmit backpropagating action potentials from the soma to the apical integration zone. Until late in infancy, this sodium channel is responsible for axonal action potential transmission. Overactivation of these channels ('gain-of-function') at an early stage of development produces forms of infantile epilepsy with various degrees of severity. At later stages of development and in adult life, however, this subtype of sodium channel is not necessary for the generation of axonal action potentials, but it is necessary for their backpropagation from the soma to the apical integration zone. Physiological studies of these sodium channels show that when they are underactive (loss-of-function), as occurs in some forms of ASD, the backpropagation of signals from the soma to the apical dendrites fails. That greatly weakens the context-sensitive amplifying effects of apical input on action potential generation, and thus on their consequences for synaptic plasticity and learning.

Studies of *SCN2A* mutations in mice suggest that these consequences of their dysfunction depend on sex, which further adds to the grounds for supposing that they are relevant to ASD. The effects of *SCN2A* insufficiency on behavioural flexibility, as measured by reversal learning, seems to be greater in males than in females. Also, there is a trend towards greater effects on sociability in females than in males,[31] which resonates strongly with evidence from Phillips, Chapman, and Berry (2004) that size perception is less context-sensitive in males as measured quantitatively by psychophysical measures of size perception, and who interpreted these differences as arising from sex-linked neurobiological differences of context-sensitivity within the neocortex, and as putting males at greater risk of ASD.

A second source of evidence implicating reduced cellular context-sensitivity in ASD comes from anatomical and neuroimaging studies interpreted as indicating that the disorder involves deficits in the executive capabilities of prefrontal regions. These deficits were seen as arising from an excessive bias towards local rather than to long-range connectivity within those regions, and from a bias against their long-range connections to the posterior regions. That implicates reduced context-sensitivity in these disorders because the consequences of that local bias were described as impairing the ability of frontal regions to integrate information from diverse widespread sources of perceptual, emotional, autonomic, and linguistic information, and to use that rich context to guide processing and learning in lower-level regions.[32]

The third source of evidence comes from anatomical and magnetic resonance imaging studies of mice with the Fragile X mutation, which clearly show that this mutation weakens the effects of long-range inputs to dendrites in layer 1 from other regions and from subcortical nuclei. Studies also show that long-range interactions within the same cortical region are also weakened, whereas interactions between cells that are less than about half a millimetre apart are strengthened. Therefore, these investigations provide direct evidence that the increased fragmentation of processing in Fragile X involves impaired cellular context-sensitivity.[33]

Further compelling evidence comes from intracellular recordings of activity near the top of the apical trunk of pyramidal cells in the somatosensory cortex of mice with a Fragile X mutation. The recordings were combined with calcium imaging of activity in the apical dendrites, with pharmacological effects on awake mice, and with computational modelling, and clearly show that sensitivity to local tactile stimulation is greater in mice with the Fragile X mutation, and that the hypersensitivity is due to reductions in the effectiveness of two classes of ion channel, that is, HCN and BK_{Ca}, that operate as a general restraint on apical amplification. So, when these channels are less effective, the cell responds more actively to sensory input in general, even when it is irrelevant to the broader context.[34]

Finally, the fifth source of evidence implicating apical dysfunctions in cognitive disability come from genetic studies of some rare neurodevelopmental disorders. Those studies found that genes specifically coding for subunits of NMDA receptors are frequently affected, and that the operation of those receptors is highly intolerant of any deviations that either increase or decrease the activity of the NMDA receptors. As the effects of apical dendrites are exceptionally dependent on NMDA receptors, it is their functions that are particularly likely to be impacted by any of these rare mutations.[35]

'Intellectual disability' is a vague cover term that is often used to describe the consequences of neurodevelopmental cognitive disabilities. The evidence for weak cellular context-sensitivity offers a more refined interpretation. It explicitly relates genes and cellular physiology to impairments of the conscious cognitive capacities in which the context-sensitivity of cooperative neurons has been explicitly implicated (Chapter 5). As such disabilities will reduce the likelihood of reproductive success, they have a low probability of being inherited, thus explaining why there is such a high incidence of *de novo* mutations in these genetic variants.

Many unresolved issues are raised by the evidence relating ASD to weakened cellular context-sensitivity, and thus to the function of apical dendrites. Chapter 6 outlines evidence for developmental changes in apical function, and thus in context-sensitivity, but the full implications of those developmental changes for ASD remain unknown. Furthermore, in addition to changes in cellular context-sensitivity across stages of development, species, and cortical regions, there are also differences between types of pyramidal cell within a region. These differences have already between related to the consequences of the Fragile X mutation on activity in the prefrontal cortex (PFC) of mice. That mutation greatly increases the excitability of pyramidal cells with subcortical projections (i.e. pyramidal tract (PT) neurons), but it has little or no effect on those that project only to regions in the neocortex and amygdala (i.e. intra-telencephalic (IT) neurons). The PT neurons are those with by far the largest apical dendritic tree, and they are exceptionally sensitive to local inhibitory and disinhibitory inputs. Furthermore, their increased excitability in mice with Fragile X is due to a reduction in the effective density of the HCN channels carrying the I_h current that so strongly constrains the effect of apical input on cellular output. [36] Therefore we should now explore the possibility that this increased excitability reflects an overamplification that, by being too generalized, reduces the selectivity on which the usefulness of apical amplification depends.

These relations between ASD and I_h also merit much further research, as do relations between ASD and apical dendritic function in general. Nelson and Bender's (2021) comprehensive review of what has been discovered so far about these issues concludes that the cellular mechanisms that support the use of top-down information to guide bottom-up processing have now been convincingly shown to be disrupted in ASD and other forms of intellectual disability. Their review shows in mechanistic detail how these specific cellular impairments can arise from several of the genes known with high confidence to be associated with ASD. Here, we have built on those discoveries by sketching ways in which those cellular impairments can lead to psychological symptoms of ASD via impairments of the cognitive functions that depend on cellular context-sensitivity (Chapter 5).

There is also further evidence implicating apical function in the learning impairments that are common in Fragile X and other forms of ASD. The synaptic plasticity on which learning depends is severely impaired in mice with the Fragile X genetic mutation. That impairment involves reduced calcium signalling in the apical dendrites of pyramidal cells in the PFC and a reduction in their response to excitatory input.[37] That contrasts with the overexcitability of pyramidal cells in sensory regions that is often associated with ASDs. Apical dysfunction is implicated, in both cases, but with decreased effects on apical input in the PFC and increased effects in posterior regions. Although much remains to be clarified concerning the relations of ASD symptoms to apical hypofunction and hyperfunction, a broad outline of mechanistic pathways leading from susceptibility genes for ASD to psychological symptoms now seems to be within reach.

Evidence on the role of apical function in producing symptoms of ASD has even been produced by studies of people without ASD! Snyder (2009) explored the possibility that transcranial magnetic stimulation in healthy volunteers might evoke creative capabilities that are strong in autism. This is relevant to apical function because magnetic stimulation affects apical dendrites in layer 1 more than it affects other dendrites, and the study determined that low-frequency repetitive transcranial stimulation of the left temporal lobe can temporarily induce savant skills such as those sometimes seen in people with ASD.[38] These findings therefore support the view that some skills associated with ASD arise from modified forms of apical function. More importantly, they show a way in which these issues can be studied noninvasively in humans, including those diagnosed with various kinds of ASD.

7.5 Foetal Alcohol Spectrum Disorders

Maternal consumption of alcohol (ethanol) during pregnancy can cause life-long cognitive impairments in the offspring. These disorders are collectively referred to as foetal alcohol spectrum disorders (FASD). They have overlaps with ASDs and attention-deficit-hyperactivity disorder, especially in impairments of cognitive control. FASDs often lead to depression, substance abuse, and criminal activities in adult life. The proportion of people affected is usually underestimated because in less-severe cases, the effects can be subtle and not easily distinguished from those caused by other neurodevelopmental disorders. It has been shown unequivocally that even moderate levels of drinking can cause this enduring brain damage. It is not possible to show that there is a safe lower limit, so Canadian and Scandinavian governments explicitly advise women not to drink alcohol at all when pregnant. This wise advice is now becoming more prominent in the UK, where the National Organisation for FASD estimates its current prevalence to be 1.8–3.6% of all adults (which may well be an underestimate because milder forms are cannot be distinguished from those due to a host of other causes). In the UK, at least 20% of pregnant women drink alcohol, even if only 'moderately', and FASD is therefore one possible cause for many of the symptoms associated with autism, attention deficits, or impaired cognitive control.[39]

Various forms of FASD have been distinguished. The most severe is foetal alcohol syndrome caused by frequent binge drinking when pregnant. This causes distinctive facial abnormalities together with cognitive and behavioural impairments that can be severe, even in the absence of the distinctive facial features. Impairments in language development, attention, and executive control make it difficult to stay alert and focused, to regulate emotions, and to control impulsive behaviour. When less severe, these difficulties may not be apparent until early school days, or later, by when there is no easy way to separate those due to prenatal alcohol from the host of other things that can contribute to such difficulties. Neuroimaging studies have revealed subtle abnormalities of neocortical structure and function in FASD, some being widely spread across cortical regions, others being regionally specific. Several cellular and molecular mechanisms have been implicated, including a reduction in the number of glial cells, which have a key role in guiding neurodevelopmental processes.[40]

Laboratory studies of rodents have directly implicated modifications of apical structure and function in the behavioural and neurobiological effects of prenatal exposure to alcohol. Adult rats that were exposed to alcohol for 12 days before birth via maternal ingestion of alcohol behave more impulsively and show more frequent lapses of attention.[41]

Rigorous investigations of the cellular bases of FASD by the Italian neurologist, Alberto Granato and colleagues, directly demonstrate that prenatal exposure to alcohol produces an enduring reduction in the number of spines on apical dendrites and in the number, duration, and effectiveness of the calcium signals transmitted from the apical integration zone to the soma. Those investigations also show that prenatal alcohol reduces the number of spines on dendrites of the apical dendritic tree of layer 2/3 pyramidal cells, while having little or no effect on the basal dendrites. Further evidence that prenatal exposure to alcohol has effects specifically on apical function is provided by Granato's study of its effects on inhibitory interneurons: it increases the number of interneurons that disinhibit the apical dendrites of pyramidal cells while decreasing the number that inhibit them. In contrast to that, it has no effects on the interneurons that inhibit the soma. As prenatal exposure to alcohol predominantly affects the function of apical dendrites that raises the possibility that its effects on interneurons reflect processes that partially compensate for weakened apical function.[42]

Overall, studies of FASDs indicate that their symptoms arise from dysfunctions of the cellular context-sensitive mechanisms that are now known to provide the cognitive capabilities that are impaired in those disorders (see Chapter 5). As those cellular processes are also implicated in the other disorders discussed in this chapter, the similarities, differences, comorbidities, and interactions between these different disorders provide many new issues to explore.

Considered independently, each of the disorders discussed in this chapter provides strong support for the view that cooperative pyramidal cells amplify response to their FF basal input when it is useful to do so in the current context as indicated by input to their apical dendrites. Considered collectively, they do so even more convincingly.

Notes

1. For example, Down syndrome, Rett syndrome, Alzheimer's disease, and Angelman syndrome.
2. For overviews of ion channel dysfunctions in epilepsy, see Poolos and Johnston (2012) and Child and Benarroch (2014).
3. Cossart et al., 2001.
4. For an overview of the role of HCN ion channels and I_h in epilepsy, see Noam, Bernard, and Baram (2011).
5. Kole, Bräuer, & Stuart, 2007.
6. Cavanna, Rickards, and Ali (2011) outline and assess evidence on partial epileptic seizures.
7. Berenyi and colleagues (2012) show that transcranial electrical stimulation can alleviate epileptic symptoms. Murphy et al (2016) show that this stimulation suppresses calcium spikes in apical dendrites, thus reducing epileptic over-activation.
8. Silverstein and colleagues (2009) found that schizophrenia patients were worse than controls at perceiving contours. That was associated with reduced activation in V2, V3, and V4, although activation in V1 was similar in patients and controls. Butler and colleagues (2013) confirmed the impairment of contour integration abilities in schizophrenia and showed it to involve the later stages of processing in both the ventral and the dorsal visual streams of the human neocortex.
9. The effects of context on perception are much reduced in schizophrenia, and especially during actively psychotic or disorganized acute states (Keane et al., 2013; Silverstein et al., 1996; Uhlhaas et al., 2005; Silverstein et al., 2013).
10. Frith and Johnstone (2003) provide a brief but authoritative outline of schizophrenia.
11. Javitt & Coyle, 2004; Anticevic et al., 2015.
12. Phillips & Silverstein, 2003.
13. Roelfsema and Super (2003) argue that impaired effects of context on perceptual processing cannot explain hallucinations.
14. Major, Larkum, and Schiller (2013) and Palmer and colleagues (2014) review evidence that apical dendrites are especially sensitive to NMDA receptor activation. Phillips and

Silverstein (2013) and Phillips, Clark, and Silverstein (2015) review grounds for relating symptoms of schizophrenia to the function of context-sensitive apical dendrites. Working memory deficits in these disorders have been related to the dysfunction of ion flow through HCN channels (Paspalas, Wang, & Arnsten, 2013).

15. Silverstein (2016) reviews visual processing abnormalities and subjective visual experiences in schizophrenia. Silverstein and Lai (2021) provide a comprehensive review of visual hallucinations in schizophrenia.

16. Ranson and colleagues (2019) studied the effects of NMDA receptor antagonists on the effects of inputs from anterior cingulate cortex to layer 1 of V1.

17. Mäki-Marttunen et al., 2019.

18. Phillips and colleagues (2016) review evidence relating the gene DISC1 to apical function and schizophrenia.

19. Dalmau and colleagues (2011) and Wingfield and colleagues (2011) review anti-NMDA autoimmune encephalitis.

20. Symmonds and colleagues (2018) make these inferences about aberrant ion channel currents using dynamic causal modelling of EEG data.

21. Uhlhaas and Singer (2010; 2012) review evidence showing aberrant high-frequency synchronized oscillations in both schizophrenia and ASD. They find that, although there are some differences between these two groups of disorder, there are also many similarities. The computer model relating both top-down contextual guidance and synchronized oscillations to apical function is by Siegel et al. (2000).

22. Phillips, Chapman, and Berry (2004) show that effects of context on visual size perception are weaker in males than in females. Doherty, Tsuji, and Phillips (2008) show that these effects are strong in east Asian cultures. De Fockert and colleagues (2007) show that they are weak in a remote African culture.

23. Bonnel and colleagues (2010) show that the context-sensitivity of simple auditory pitch perception is preserved or superior in severe cases of autism but not in cases of Asperger's syndrome.

24. For examples of evidence that a diagnosis of autism is associated with a perceptual style that is biased towards local details combined with a reduced emphasis on coherent Gestalt organization and other 'global' or 'holistic' processes, see Happé (1999), Dakin and Frith (2005), Jachim et al. (2015), Booth and Happé (2016), and van der Hallen et al. (2015).

25. Frith (2003) provides an authoritative overview of autism and the theory of weak central coherence. Mottron and colleagues (2006) review evidence for enhanced perceptual function. Baron-Cohen and Lombardo (2017) provide a brief outline of a talent for systemizing in autism and discuss its neural bases.

26. A meta-analysis by van der Hallen and colleagues (2015) of 56 papers reporting studies of 'global' visual processing in autistic disorders found that little could be concluded other than that it is slow in ASD, and not yet adequately defined.

27. For an in-depth review of the genetic and physiological aspects of Fragile X and other neurodevelopmental disorders, see Nelson and Bender (2021).

28. Yizhar and colleagues (2011) review evidence for an imbalance between excitatory and inhibitory inputs to pyramidal cells in autism. Zikopoulis and Barbas (2013) found that in ASD there is a reduction in specifically basal/peri-somatic inhibition in some prefrontal regions, which would decrease the effectiveness of apical input relative to FF input in those regions. Calvin and Redish (2021) present a computational model of how an imbalance

between excitation and inhibition could provide a basis for reduced context-sensitivity in both ASD and schizophrenia.

29. Nelson and Bender (2021) review other ways in which apical function could be impaired, such as those involving metabotropic receptors for the excitatory neurotransmitter glutamate.

30. Hahn, Snedeker, and Rabagliati (2015) find that people with autism and good language skills use sentence context to disambiguate word meanings. Nagano, Zane, and Grossman (2021) review studies of pronoun processing by people with autism and report findings that they interpret as contradicting the theory of weak central coherence.

31. Spratt and colleagues (2019) report key physiological studies of the sodium channels for which the autism-associated gene *SCN2A* codes, and of the consequences of that for apical function. Nelson and Bender (2021) provide a comprehensive review showing that impairments of apical dendritic function have a key role in autism and other neurodevelopmental disorders. They show explicitly how those impairments are made more likely by many genetic mutations known to increase the probability of symptoms used to diagnose autism.

32. Courchesne and Pierce (2005) propose that symptoms of ASD involve local overconnectivity combined with long-range underconnectivity.

33. Haberl and colleagues (2015) provide direct anatomical and physiological evidence for a local overconnectivity and a long-range underconnectivity that is more general than that proposed by Courchesne and Pierce (2005).

34. Zhang et al., 2014b.

35. Vieira, Jeong, and Roche (2021) review the genetic bases of many rare neurodevelopmental disorders and show that NMDA receptor function is highly intolerant of deviation from a narrowly prescribed level of activity.

36. Kalmbach and colleagues (2018) show that the fragile X mutation increases the excitability of prefrontal cells that project to subcortical nuclei, and that it does so by reducing I_h while having little or no effect on prefrontal cells that project only to cortical sites. They note that this is the opposite of what happens in the hippocampus, where pyramidal cells function very differently, in part because the apical trunks in the hippocampus are shorter than the minimum trunk length found to be associated with an amplifying mode of operation in neocortical pyramidal cells (Fletcher & Williams, 2019).

37. Meredith & Mansvelder, 2007.

38. Snyder, 2009.

39. Curtin and Fairchild (2003) and Valenzuela and colleagues (2012) provide useful reviews of the symptoms, epidemiology, and neuronal bases of foetal alcohol spectrum disorders. For an introductory overview of these disorders, see Phillips (2015). In 2022 The National Organization for FASD published *The Time is Now*, which is a report focused on prevention, diagnosis and support, and compiled by people with lived experience of FASD, practitioners, policy makers, and public health experts.

40. Guerri, Bazinet, & Riley, 2009.

41. Wang et al., 2020.

42. For studies of the effects of prenatal alcohol on the function of apical dendrites specifically, see Granato et al. (2003, 2012), Granato (2006), Granato and De Giorgio (2014), De Giorgio and Granato (2015), and Granato (2021).

8

An Information-theoretic View of Context-sensitive Computation

8.1 Distinguishing Abstract Theories from Detailed Models

This chapter outlines a theoretical perspective on context-sensitive computation based on recent advances in the understanding of multivariate mutual information decomposition, which provides a new perspective on neocortical information processing. The computational effectiveness and efficiency of those theories has now been demonstrated by the new machine learning algorithms that they have inspired.

Over the last few decades myriad things have been called 'models' with the result that some fundamental conceptual distinctions have been obscured. The fundamental difference between abstract theories and detailed models is often overlooked, leading to a misunderstanding of what abstract theories can contribute. They are concerned with underlying principles, that is, with what David Marr called computational theory. They are not primarily concerned with algorithms or their implementation. For example, a wing in a wind tunnel is not intended as a model of a bird's wing. Rather, it is made as simply as possible to reveal the essential principles of aerodynamic lift. During the millennia over which we tried to understand how birds fly, those principles were obscured by all the information that people had about birds and their wings, most of it irrelevant to the principles of aerodynamics that were validated when the Wilbur and Orville Wright demonstrated that aerodynamic lift is a way to fly. Thus, theories are improved by discarding all nonessential details that obscure the underlying principles. In complete contrast to that, models are improved by including as many details as possible. They are relevant to abstract theory in that they can be used to explore whether the system modelled operates according to the hypothesized principles.

A related confusion fails to distinguish between realizations and simulations. As a young child I had a toy train driven by a steam engine. Though small and lacking all the complexities of real trains (or any other useful steam-driven

The Cooperative Neuron. William A. Phillips, Oxford University Press. © Oxford University Press 2023.
DOI: 10.1093/oso/9780198876984.003.0009

engine), it was not a model of a steam engine—it *was* a steam engine. It functioned according to the same principles as useful (larger) steam engines. In contrast, weather forecasts are not hot or cold, wet or dry, etc. They are simulations of weather patterns. The abstract neural nets used to explore the capabilities of the style of neuronal computation that we call 'coherent infomax' are realizations of that style of computation—they are not simulations of it. They are analogous to a wind tunnel containing a wing, in which aerodynamic lift is really generated. This chapter summarizes studies of context-sensitive computation using toy examples that have been deliberately simplified to make the essential principles of that style of computation clear. Those studies must then be accompanied by computational studies that explore whether that style of computation can be scaled-up to deal with real-world data to do useful things. Being so abstract, such theories must also be supported by neurobiological, psychophysical, and detailed modelling studies to find out whether the computational principles that they express are used in the biological system studied.

There is a fundamental difference between finding out how the neocortex computes and finding out how birds fly. The ability to fly is easily quantified, but the underlying capabilities of the neocortex are so far from being obvious that there is still no consensus on what they are or on how they can be conceived or quantified. Although Alan Turing famously asked whether machines can 'think', and although computer scientists have since invented algorithms for artificial 'intelligence' and 'big data processing', the notions of 'thought', 'intelligence', and 'big data processing' do not provide adequate definitions of the capabilities to be understood. Machine learning algorithms that pass the Turing test will not thereby resolve this issue until we have adequate criteria for deciding whether those algorithms understand what they say. Chapter 5 avoids reliance on such notions by relating cooperative context-sensitive capabilities of neocortical structures and physiological processes to basic underlying cognitive capabilities inferred from behaviour. This chapter outlines a way of formalizing and quantifying those context-sensitive capabilities using a recent extension to the foundations of information theory.

8.2 Information Theory: A Formal Perspective on Context-sensitive Computation

Information theory, probability, and statistical inference are central to the context-sensitive computation on which the organized complexity of neocortex depends. Probabilistic inference is the most fundamental and general information-processing task that organisms face. Nothing would happen in a completely ordered universe, so there would then be no life, for which some degree of chaotic uncertainty and freedom are necessary. Unpredictability and adequate determinism are inseparable aspects of physical reality. In whatever ecological niche an organism is adapted to live, events occur with a range of predictabilities, from near certainty to complete unpredictability. Organisms discover regularities in their environment by evolution and by learning and embed some of those regularities in their anatomical structure. Reliable order is the foundation of information processing at all levels of organization—from that of neurons to that of societies. However, organisms can discover only some of the regularities that they encounter, so they tend to become highly diverse and with varying abilities to anticipate uncertain but non-random events. As the complexity of organisms increases, so does their ability to anticipate uncertain events. Their diversity therefore tends to increase because different species and different individuals within species discover different regularities to embed within their structure and dynamics.[1]

Claude Shannon defined 'information' transmission as the reduction of uncertainty, which is quantified by the mutual information between an input to a communication channel and its output. That conception of information transmission has been extensively used in neuroscience. It provides a measure of the information that is transmitted by a communication channel about its inputs. That conception of information transmission is adequate for a neuroscience committed to the assumption that all neurons function as integrate-and-fire point processors. To advance beyond that assumption in a way that quantitatively defines the distinct functions of context-sensitivity, we need to extend information theory so that it can decompose the transmitted information in a way that distinguishes the different contributions of different inputs to an output. An extension to information theory that makes this possible has been under development since 2010 (Section 8.4). First, Section 8.3 briefly outlines a theory of the contextual guidance of learning and processing developed by applying the classical definitions of mutual information as defined by Shannon to the case of local processors with two distinct classes of input and one output.

8.3 Coherent Infomax: A Theory of Local Processors with Receptive and Contextual Fields

Coherent infomax is a long-standing theory of processing and learning in neural information processing systems composed of local processors that use their contextual field (CF) inputs to modulate transmission of information about their receptive field (RF) inputs. That style of processing is cooperative in that both its short-term processing dynamics and its long-term learning tend to maximize overall coherence by seeking agreement between the CF and RF inputs. That theory was proposed before we understood the physiological differences between the effects of apical and basal/peri-somatic inputs were known, although now that those differences are better known, there are obvious similarities between apical inputs and CFs and between basal/peri-somatic inputs and RFs.[2]

Endlessly many different architectures can in principle be built from such local processors, but the family of architectures assumed to be most relevant to the neocortex is that of multiple streams of processing that converge and diverge in various ways across a sequence of cortical regions with the information that is dealt with being more abstract at the higher hierarchical levels. In essence, coherent infomax is an abstract idealized theory of cooperative context-sensitive computation, and it is outlined in this chapter to show two main things: that neuronal cooperative context-sensitivity can be rigorously specified and quantified, and that, when applied to physiological data from apical and somatic locations of layer 5 neocortical neurons, the apical input does indeed amplify transmission of information about the more direct somatic input without transmitting information about itself.

The effects of RF and CF inputs within the theory of coherent infomax are intrinsically asymmetric. The long-term objective of the system is assumed to be maximization of the coherence of the activity of the system overall, even though all the RF–CF interactions are strictly local. Those interactions increase the total amount of coherent information transmitted and reduce incoherence. No theoretical limit on the level to which coherence can be increased is assumed, but it is also assumed that if there is life then there is always some incoherence.

This theoretical perspective on context-sensitive cooperative computation was called coherent infomax to both relate it to and distinguish it from Linsker's (1992) prior infomax theory, which showed that the RF selectivity of cells in V1 can be acquired by an activity-dependent learning rule that begins to operate even before visual stimulation occurs at birth, and whose objective is simply to preserve as much as possible of the information that is in the feedforward input from the sensors and concentrate it into far fewer cells. Thus, the objective of Linsker's infomax is to reduce redundancy in the information transmitted. That resonated strongly with the objective of reducing redundancy that Horace Barlow and many others had long seen to be a major principle of sensory information processing in the brain. Maximizing information transmission and reducing redundancy are still long-term goals emphasized by most neuroscientific applications of information theory. Coherent infomax adds a very different objective to that: it maximizes the transmission of information that is coherent and relevant and minimizes transmission of other information. That clearly contrasts with maximizing the transmission of all information received by the local processors whether coherent or incoherent, relevant or irrelevant.

Neurocomputational studies based on simplified toy examples that clearly express the principles of coherent infomax show that sensitivity to context can, in principle, usefully guide both learning and ongoing processing. The information-theoretic objective of coherent infomax was explicitly formulated for local neural processors that receive modulatory CF inputs in addition to the RF inputs about which they transmit information. Learning rules for modifying the strengths of their synaptic connections were then derived analytically from the explicitly defined objective function. Put simply, its goal is to maximize transmission of information in the RF input that is predictably or coherently related to the CF input (Section 8.6). These learning rules can be applied exactly in simple cases and by approximation in more complex cases. They can operate in a supervised mode of learning in that they can discover variables that predict prespecified variables, such as those providing reinforcement. Supervision is not necessary, however, so the learning rules can also be used for data mining. In statistical terms this is a nonlinear form of latent structure analysis such as canonical correlation or principal component analysis. It discovers statistically related variables defined on the input such that those variables and their predictive relationships together describe much of the variance in the input data. It differs from principal component analysis in that it can suppress components of variation that convey much of the variance but are unrelated to other components. The knowledge acquired by learning is embedded in the strengths of the RF and CF connections. When applied to local processors composed of several units receiving inputs from much the same feedforward source, then the coherent infomax learning rules lead to different RFs for the different units. This ensures that (within the limits of their joint channel capacity) they cover the space of input variance effectively. As there will usually be many ways of doing that, there is plenty of room for variation in detailed RF selectivity. Furthermore, these learning rules tend to establish mutual inhibitory connections between units within a local processor, which is analogous to the winner-take-all dynamics of divisive normalization. This implies that the objective of maximizing the coherence of a neural system's overall activities leads to a combination of long-range cooperative context-sensitivity and local competitive context-sensitivity, although we did not describe it in those terms when we first reported these findings in 1998.

Further computational studies of simplified neural nets composed of such context-sensitive local processors extend our knowledge of their information processing capabilities. Such nets can discover and use the coherent and relevant RF variables even if they are not the most informative variables within the distinct streams of processing. They can even do so when there is no information for the existence of those variables within streams, other than the correlation across streams. These abilities are exhibited by a variety of network architectures, including those with multiple streams of RF processing and CF connections across streams. They include network architectures in which CF connections are only between neighbouring streams, nets with multiple RF streams and CF feedback from higher to lower levels, and nets with multiple RF streams that have partial overlap. Phillips and Singer (1997) outline their potential relevance to information processing in the neocortex, where it is also assessed by the commentaries of many different experts.

Coherent infomax as originally formulated depended upon three-way mutual information as defined by Shannon (Kay, 1999), but that does not adequately distinguish the various elementary components of output given two distinct classes of input. Section 8.4 outlines recent developments in the conception of multivariate mutual information decomposition that provide a way of distinguishing those components. Section 8.5 uses it to quantify conceptions of context-sensitivity that are then used to show that many neocortical pyramidal cells are indeed context-sensitive as so defined. Section 8.6 then uses it to express the objectives of context-sensitive learning.

8.4 Decomposition of Transmitted Information

The classical definitions of mutual information have been undergoing revision since 2010 in a field of applied mathematics referred to as partial information decomposition (PID). Surprisingly, it turns out to be far from easy to extend the definitions of mutual information so that they unambiguously distinguish the contributions of two or more classes of input to an output. Williams and Beer (2010) reported techniques for multivariate mutual information decomposition that are still being developed and debated. They have many subtleties and complexities of great interest to applied mathematicians and to those interested in formal mathematical investigations of complex systems.[3] The simplest extension is from systems with one input and one output to systems with two inputs and one output, which is adequate for our purposes because our interest is simply in distinguishing the contributions of contextual and feedforward inputs (e.g. apical and basal/peri-somatic inputs) to the cell's output. Extension to distinguish the contributions of more than a few inputs to an output is unlikely to be needed within neuroscience. That is fortunate because the number of possible components of transmitted information rises more rapidly than exponentially with the number of distinct inputs. Even with only four, there are several thousand possible components of mutual information, so decompositions of neuronal outputs distinguishing ways in which several different subsets of their input contribute to that output are impractical. Naud and Sprekeler's (2018) proposed model shows that pyramidal cell outputs may be able to transmit information specifically about its integrated apical input separately from that about its integrated basal input—a process called multiplexing.

Put simply, partial information decomposition shows that if there are two classes of input, X1 and X2, whose contributions to an output (Y) are to be distinguished then there are five components of transmitted information: first, information transmitted about X1 only (UnqX1); second, information transmitted about X2 only (UnqX2); third, information transmitted about both X1 and X2 because they are correlated, that is, source shared information (ShdS); fourth, information transmitted about both X1 and X2 that is not due to their correlation but to the mechanism by which the output is computed from the inputs, that is, mechanistic shared information (ShdM); and finally, there is synergy, the component of transmitted information that can be obtained from X1 and X2 jointly but not from either separately. Figure 8.1 shows a simple intuitive description of this decomposition. The total amount of information in the output is the information transmitted about the two inputs plus any residual information. That residual information is the information originating from within the system itself, for example, internal 'noise', or from inputs other than the two considered.

Some applications of information decomposition quantify only the sum of the two shared components. They compute that sum of these two shared components without distinguishing between them. It is important to do so when using it, as here, to clarify the operations performed by local neural processors. Components of output that are shared simply because the inputs are correlated have very different implications from those that arise within the local processor itself. Mechanistic shared information is related to synergy. If it is greater than zero, then so is the synergistic component.[4]

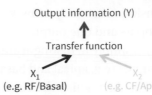

Output information (Y)

↑

Transfer function

X_1
(e.g. RF/Basal)

X_2
(e.g. CF/Apical)

Components of the output information

Unique X_1: Info in X_1 only
Unique X_2: Info in X_2 only
SharedS: Correlated info in X_1 and X_2
SharedM: Uncorrelated info in X_1 and X_2
Synergy: Info that depends on both X_1 and X_2
$H(Y)_{Resid}$: Output info unrelated to X_1 and X_2

Figure 8.1 The components of information transmitted about two distinct inputs by a single output. Each of the two inputs could be an integrated value computed from many different even more elementary variables, such as the thousands of synaptic inputs to the apical and basal dendritic trees. This analysis does not distinguish the separate contributions of those even more elementary variables to the output. It relates components of the output to the two integrated values (e.g. of the integrated apical and basal inputs). It is not assumed that those integrations are linear, nor that they are defined in equivalent ways.

If the two inputs are perfectly correlated, then the shared source component would be the only nonzero component of transmitted information in the output. If the two inputs are completely uncorrelated, then any shared component in the output must be mechanistic shared. Synergistic components cannot be predicted by information in either of the inputs alone. These idealized cases are discussed here only to clarify the distinctive properties of the various components. Typically, for example, as in neuroscientific applications, there will be rich and varied compositions, in which there are few, if any, nonzero components.

These components of transmitted information are related in simple ways to the classical measures of mutual information (I). These relations can be expressed symbolically using a notation in which the inputs whose contributions to an output (Y) are to be quantified are separated from it by a semicolon. If the combined effects of more than one input are to be quantified, then they are separated by commas. If the additional mutual information provided by adding a further input given that the other is already known, then that which is assumed to be known is preceded by a short vertical line. The three-way mutual information is shown by separating all three variables by semicolons.

Using this notation, the components of transmitted information are related to the classical forms of mutual information as follows:

$$I(Y;X1,X2) = UnqX1 + UnqX2 + ShdS + ShdM + Synergy$$
$$I(Y;X1) = UnqX1 + ShdS + ShdM$$
$$I(Y;X2) = UnqX2 + ShdS + ShdM$$
$$I(Y;X1|X2) = UnqX1 + Synergy$$
$$I(Y;X2|X1) = UnqX2 + Synergy$$
$$I(Y;X1;X2) = ShdS + ShdM - Synergy$$
$$I(Y;X1) - I(Y;X2) = UnqX1 - UnqX2$$

So, assuming all components to be non-negative:

$I(Y;X1)$ is an upper bound on UnqX1
$I(Y;X2)$ is an upper bound on UnqX2

It is commonly assumed that information theory has nothing whatever to contribute to our understanding of semantics because it applies to all information, whatever it means. In contrast to that assumption, decomposition of transmitted information into its distinct components shows two ways in which information theory can enhance our understanding of semantics. Firstly, if the information transmitted by a local processor about its RF input contains synergistic components, then the local processor does more than simply pass on the information that it receives. It creates new information from relations between the inputs upon which that synergy depends.[5] Secondly, as Section 8.5 shows in detail, information decomposition can be used to explicitly distinguish between whatever a local processor transmits information about (i.e. the semantics of its output) and whatever amplifies or attenuates transmission of that information. This implies that synergy can arise in two very different ways, with distinct functional implications that could lead to much confusion if not distinguished.

8.5 Transmitted Information Decomposition Quantifies Context-sensitive Computation

Our understanding of context-sensitive computation is being enhanced by the development of these statistical techniques for decomposing information transmission given two classes of input whose contributions to the output are to be distinguished. That development is analogous to the invention of telescopes and microscopes in that it will enable us to see things that could not be seen before. However, use of these new statistical techniques to help us understand neural information processing is in its very early stages, and there is much that needs to be learned if we are to make good use of them. Different techniques for defining the components can produce quantitatively different decompositions, although they are usually qualitatively much the same, so we do not further consider these technical differences here.

Although studies of neuronal information processing using those decompositions have so far been few and fragmentary, those that have been performed clearly indicate that the decompositions observed depend on many things. We can assume that when applied to pyramidal cells they will vary with trunk length, the state of the various neuromodulators, species, region, developmental stage, range of input strengths to which the cell or local processor is exposed, the output variables considered, and their categorizations. Furthermore, these decompositions can be applied to different levels of organization, such as single cells, population codes in microcircuits, cortical regions, and behavioural decisions. The hope that the decompositions observed at different levels of organization will be consistent with each other has been encouraged by comparing the decompositions observed in psychophysical data from humans with those of physiological data from neocortical pyramidal cells.

Here, we outline the use of these decompositions to clarify the theory of coherent infomax. Decompositions of information transmitted by the context-sensitive activation function used in that theory show that CF inputs and RF inputs make fundamentally different contributions to output. RF input specifies the local processor's selective sensitivity (i.e. what it transmits information about). This is shown by a strong component of output information unique to the feedforward RF input. In contrast to that, CF input modulates output strength without transmitting any unique information about itself. It can do so because context-sensitivity contributes to output by affecting only the synergistic and shared (but uncorrelated) components of output.[6]

These distinctive properties of context-sensitive processing have been clarified by contrasting them with the elementary arithmetic operators of addition, subtraction, multiplication, and division. There are many ways in which two inputs can be used to generate output such that they have the distinctive properties of context-sensitive information transmission, but these do not include the pure forms of any of the simple arithmetic operators. Purely additive or subtractive combinations of two inputs produce output decompositions without the intrinsic asymmetry that distinguishes RF inputs from

CF inputs. Instead, they transmit unique components about whichever of the two inputs is strongest. Purely divisive combinations transmit only synergistic components. Purely multiplicative combinations cannot be equivalent to context-sensitive modulation because they have no intrinsic asymmetry. Furthermore, as either term in a multiplicative interaction approaches zero, so does the output, whereas a context-sensitive interaction can generate plenty of output in the absence of any contextual information.[7] Figure 8.2 shows these fundamental differences between the information transmitted by modulatory and simple arithmetic transfer functions.

Many useful things can be inferred by careful examination of the decompositions shown in Figure 8.2. For example, purely additive and purely subtractive interactions produce equivalent decompositions. More importantly, these decompositions clarify the distinctive properties of context-sensitivity. Though modulatory interactions are often assumed to arise from a multiplicative interaction between modulator and modulated these decompositions show that assumption to be mistaken. The decomposition of information transmitted by multiplication (P) is much the same as that transmitted by the modulatory function M2 (r + rc) when the modulated signal (X1) is weak and the modulating input (X2) is moderate or stronger. The consequences of that modulatory activation function are completely different from that of the purely multiplicative activation function when the potentially modulated RF signal is strong, however. All the information unique to the RF input is then transmitted, whereas for a purely multiplicative activation function none is transmitted. Therefore, describing modulation as simply being 'multiplicative' can be seriously misleading, even if it does include multiplicative operations.

Empirical data thought to show context-sensitivity has been obtained from data collected at various levels of organization—from whole organisms to individual neurons. That data can now be examined using information decomposition and compared with the decomposition specified by theoretical forms of context-sensitivity. This has been done in the case of psychophysical data from a much-studied paradigm in which the detectability of a faint line element in a visual display is shown to be affected by flanking line elements. If the effects of the flankers are due to context-sensitivity, then decomposition of the information transmitted by the subject's detection response should have strong components unique to the target to be detected, but weak or absent components unique to the flanking context. It should also have synergistic components iff the target is present but not strong. Decomposition of the stimulus information transmitted by people's responses when performing such a task showed that, for many subjects, the flanker did indeed operate as

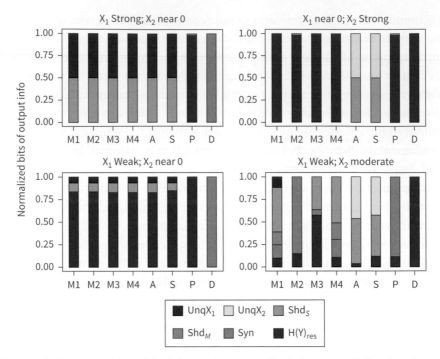

Figure 8.2 Decomposition of the information transmitted about two distinct inputs by four modulatory activation functions (M1 – M4) and by four elementary arithmetic activation functions. This is for the case where the two input variables and the output are binary positive or negative values, where the probability that the output has the positive value is the logistic of the activation, which is a function of r, the receptive field input, where $r = s_1 X_1$ and c, the contextual field input, where $c = s_2 X_2$, and where s1 and s2 are the strengths of the two inputs. As applied to neuronal transmission X_1 and X_2 can be thought of as specifying whether the net input to the somatic and apical integration sites is excitatory or inhibitory; s1 and s2 can be thought of as the depth of excitation or inhibition. The modulatory activation functions are $0.5r(1 + \exp(rc))$ (M1); $r + rc$ (M2); $r(1 + \tanh(rc))$ (M3); and $r2^{rc}$ (M4). The arithmetic activation functions are addition, $r + c$ (A); subtraction, $r - c$ (S); multiplication, rc (P); and division r/c (D). The correlation between X_1 and X_2 in this case was 0.78, which was chosen so that 50% of their entropies is shared. This analysis, and several others, are reported in Kay & Phillips, 2020.

a context that modulated target detection only by its effects on the shared and synergistic components. However, the decompositions were more informative than that, and analysis of the responses provided by individual subjects showed that when the target was near or below detection threshold for a few subjects, the flanker did not operate as a modulatory context but became part of the input about which information was transmitted by their responses.[8]

Schulz and colleagues (2021) and Kay and colleagues (2022) also used three-way mutual information decomposition to decompose the contributions of apical and somatic inputs to the output of pyramidal cells in slices from the primary somatosensory cortex of rats. Figure 8.3 shows the mutual information decompositions typical of apical amplification.

Patch clamp recordings were made either with or without activation of inhibitory receptors in the apical dendrites. In both conditions a substantial amount of information was transmitted uniquely about the current injected into the soma, but very little about the current injected into the apical integration zone, even though it had a large effect on action potential output via synergy. As expected, apical inhibition reduced the synergistic component and increased the amount of information transmitted about the injected somatic current. These two decomposition spectra are comparable to that produced by the modulatory function M1 shown in Figure 8.2 when X1 is weak and X2 is moderate, but not to those produced by any of the simple arithmetic functions. The shared source component is small in this case for the simple reason that the injected apical and somatic inputs were de-correlated by the experimental design (though the binning involved in the analysis may have led to

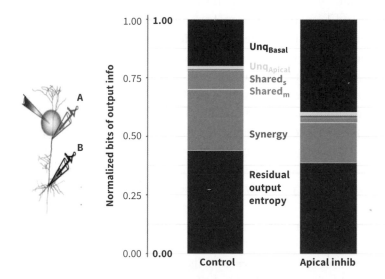

Figure 8.3 The components of information transmitted about physiologically realistic signals directly injected into the apical (A) and somatic (B) integration zones as shown on the left. Patch clamp injections and recordings were made from layer 5B pyramidal cells in 300 mm thick slices of rat primary somatosensory cortex. The components of information transmitted by the cell's action potential outputs are shown for conditions in which, via the other electrode shown in the diagram, inhibitory receptors on the apical dendrites were either activated (Apical inhib.) or not (Control).

The decomposition spectra shown here are from an analysis provided by Jim Kay of data from a pyramidal cell that is representative of those analysed by Schulz et al., 2021, and by Kay et al., 2022.

the tiny source shared component just visible in Figure 8.3). We can therefore predict that the source shared component would be much larger if the two inputs were correlated. The effect of apical amplification was predominantly to increase the probability of the cell firing in bursts of two to four spikes within about 15 ms. It also influenced the total number of spikes produced (i.e. spike rate), but activation of inhibitory receptors in the apical dendrites had a much larger effect on burst probability than on spike rate.[9]

Three-way mutual information decomposition has also been applied to binary output data produced by a highly detailed model of a pyramidal cell. The arguments for distinguishing models from theories do not imply that models are not useful. Indeed, they may be the only way to resolve many fundamental issues. In the highly detailed computational model of a pyramidal cell in layer 5 of neocortex designed by Shai et al (2015) depolarizing input further than 250 µm away from the soma generated brief bursts of action potentials, whereas depolarizing input closer to the soma generated regular trains of single action potentials at a rate dependent on the strength of that depolarization. Output bursts were much more likely to be generated by that model when there was coincident depolarization of both apical and basal trees. This was therefore described as a cellular model of coincidence detection.[10] Decomposition of the information transmitted by that model found that the synergistic and uniquely basal/peri-somatic components are large, whereas the uniquely apical component is small.[11] This is close to the decomposition expected if the apical input amplifies the cell's response to its basal/peri-somatic input. More modelling of this kind is now required, however, because the biophysical parameters used in this specific model may not be representative of all layer 5 cells. For example, the parameters used were based on layer 5 pyramidal cells in mice, and those parameters vary greatly across species, and depend on many other things.

As the notion of context-sensitive processing is a simplifying abstraction it raises important issues that are not easy to see among all the complex phenomena observed at the level of cells and microcircuits. Decomposition of transmitted information helps clarify those issues. One issues concerns relations between gain modulation and context-sensitivity. Leading researchers in biophysics and computational neuroscience have concluded that gain modulation is revealed when one input, the modulatory one, affects the gain or the sensitivity of the neuron to the other input, without modifying its selectivity or receptive field properties.[12] This gain modulation is thought to be ubiquitous throughout the neocortex, and to be crucial to basic cognitive functions such as attention. For several years I assumed that this form of gain modulation is equivalent to the context-sensitivity for which much evidence has been cited here, but things are not that simple. Firstly, the impressive and influential paper from which that definition of gain modulation comes (Salinas & Sejnowsky, 2001) does not mention context, and secondly, it uses coordinate transformation as a paradigmatic example of gain modulation. Coordinate transformation occurs, for example, when information about the location of a stimulus relative to the retina is transformed into location relative to the head or to the body. Thus, gain modulation fundamentally transforms what the cell transmits information about, which clearly contrasts with context-sensitivity, which does not fundamentally change the semantics of the information transmitted. Further, it has been convincingly shown that coordinate transformation can be computed by an approximately multiplicative interaction between the inputs that convey information about location in the primary frame and the inputs that convey information about the relations between the two frames. As they are intrinsically symmetric, purely multiplicative interactions are fundamentally different from context-sensitivity (Figure 8.2). Multiplicative gain modulation, such as that involved in coordinate transformations, is therefore a nonlinear aspect of RF selectivity, which must be clearly distinguished from the context-sensitivity with which it is sometimes confused.

A second issue that arises concerns relations between coincidence detection and context-sensitivity. The only function for coincidence detection mentioned by Shai and colleagues' (2015) detailed cellular model of it was to increase the precision of the cell's RF tuning. However, they did not consider the possibility that apical dendrites amplify transmission of that RF information depending on is relevance and coherence within the broader context of activity elsewhere in the cortex.

A third set of theoretical issues concerns the difference between two fundamentally distinct roles for synergy, that is, synergy that is implicit in RF selectivity and synergy due to context-sensitive amplification or attenuation of response to the RF input. Transmitted information extracted from the RF input would involve synergistic relations between two subsets of input if the information transmitted concerns relations between those two subsets. As the Gestalt psychologists emphasized, most cells in the perceptual cortex detect relations between subsets of their inputs, although those subsets are not usually distinguished by their apical versus their basal/peri-somatic location. Consider that the detector of a vertical brightness edge at some location in the visual field requires there to be a high level of brightness on either the left or the right, but not both, which is logically equivalent to the XOR relation. Information transmitted about such a feature is pure synergy—it transmits no unique information about either of the two inputs.

Schulz and colleagues (2021) and Kay and colleagues (2022) found that decompositions of the effects of apical input on cellular output closely approximated the decompositions expected if apical dendrites were operating as cooperative context-sensitive amplifiers. Nevertheless, it is possible that the synergy observed reflects an interaction that defines the RF about which the cell transmits information. The mere presence of a synergistic component is not proof of context-sensitivity because the two subsets of inputs that interact synergistically may both be part of the RF input about which information is transmitted. However, in cases such as those of the pyramidal cells studied by Schulz and colleagues (2021), we can assume that the synergy observed reflects the amplifying effects of input to the apical dendrites. That is because apical input in the somatosensory cortex is known to come predominantly from the limb opposite to that which specifies the cell's RF, so it is not part of that RF. The question therefore arises as to how we can directly test the assumption that the synergy observed in such cases is due to context-sensitivity, rather than to synergistic contributions to RF selectivity.

Synergy arising from context-sensitivity can be distinguished from synergistic contributions to RF selectivity in at least two ways. First, we can study what happens to synergy as basal excitation increases. Synergy due to synergistic components of RF selectivity increases to a maximum as basal excitation approaches its upper asymptote. Synergy due to context-sensitivity echoes the principle of 'inverse effectiveness' that characterizes the cross-modal interactions (Section 5.2.2). It is at or near zero when RF input is absent or near its upper asymptote. Synergy due to context-sensitivity is greatest when the signal being modulated by context is present but weak. This is also used as a defining property of recurrent amplification in Heeger and Zemlianova's (2020) theory. Figure 8.4 quantitatively shows the stark contrast between synergy due to context-sensitivity and synergy that arises from RF selectivity that is specified by adding the two inputs.

Although decompositions of real or simulated neuronal information processing are few and fragmentary, they already contain key messages. We now know that it is possible for one subset of inputs to amplify the transmission of information about another subset without transmitting any unique information about itself and without compromising the semantics of the information transmitted. This requires the input about which information is transmitted to be present, but not so strong that it drives output

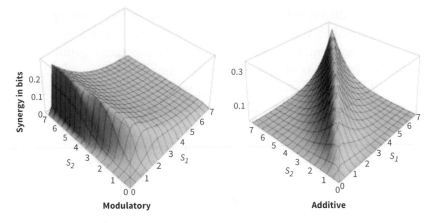

Figure 8.4 The size of the synergistic component, in bits, transmitted by a modulatory and an additive interaction between two binary variables as a function of their strengths. The strength of a binary input X_1 is shown as s_1 and that of a binary input X_2 as s_2. The modulatory function used is that assumed by the theory of coherent infomax (shown as M_1 in Figure 8.2). If X_2 modulates transmission of information about X_1 then synergy at first increases, then decreases, as the strength of X_1 increases from near zero towards maximum. If the activation is additive, then synergy increases monotonically with increases in the strengths of X_1 and X_2 and is higher for balanced than for unbalanced strengths. Kay and colleagues (2017) present such three-dimensional surfaces for all five of the mutual information components given two inputs and one output.

to its upper limit. The few decompositions of empirical physiological data that have been performed so far confirm quantitatively that, in some pyramidal cells in some conditions, apical inputs do amplify transmission of information about their basal/peri-somatic inputs as predicted. Conditions in which input to apical dendrites amplifies response to basal/peri-somatic input by modifying the synergistic component of output are also shown by models of layer 5 pyramidal cells. Decompositions can also be applied to behavioural decisions, and as outlined previously, their application to psychophysical data confirms that people also sometimes use contextual information to amplify their response to the stimuli about which they make the decisions.

The statistician Jim Kay, with whom I have worked since about 1990, explored the decomposition of output information given apical and basal/peri-somatic inputs using data provided by several physiological and modelling studies of layer 5 pyramidal cells. As expected, the decompositions that he observed have been diverse and depended on several things. They do not always conform to those for the modulatory interactions shown in Figures 8.2, 8.3, and 8.4.

We were at first disconcerted by that variability as we were seeking evidence only for a particular version of context-sensitivity. Now we interpret that variability as contributing to the capabilities of cooperative neurons, and as revealing the usefulness of information decomposition as an instrument to explore information processing in neural systems.

Cooperative neurons do not have a single fixed mode of operation determined by their morphology and synaptic strengths, as widely assumed for neurons in general. Apical inputs can operate as amplifiers or drivers, or can be isolated from output generation. The way in which they operate depends on neuromodulatory state, and perhaps many other things, so that vast territory awaits exploration using information decomposition. For example, Chapter 10 discusses the possibility that such explorations may help us understand how the imaginative capabilities of humans can be combined with purposeful objectivity.

8.6 Transmitted Information Decomposition Quantifies Objectives of Context-sensitive Learning

When theories of mental function loosely inspired by neurobiology became prominent in the 1980s under the titles of parallel distributed processing (PDP), or connectionism, they raised doubts in the artificial intelligence (AI) community because of what were thought to be inherent limitations in their ability to learn. The tables are now fully turned by the undeniable success of neurobiologically inspired machine learning algorithms, such as those of deep learning. Many researchers now think that the capabilities of deep learning algorithms may guide us towards a better understanding of learning in the neocortex. Those algorithms do indeed show the impressive learning abilities of systems composed of many local processing elements in networks that are loosely inspired by neurobiology. Being implemented in silicon, however, those algorithms are released from all the biophysical limitations that constrain the operation of the neocortex. The extent to which those algorithms are relevant to learning in the brain is still an open issue, but whether they are or not, neuroscience has other insights to offer the field of machine learning. The possibility of using what is being learned about the contextual guidance of learning and processing in the neocortex to inspire the development of new machine learning algorithms is discussed in Section 8.7. First, here we focus on the use of information theory to specify multipurpose objectives for learning.

To some psychologists, particularly those described as evolutionary psychologists, the notion of a general-purpose learning algorithm makes no more sense than would the notion of a general-purpose sense organ. For example, nonhuman species cannot learn human language, so their learning algorithms cannot be all-purpose. The learning abilities that I have myself are far less all-purpose than I would like them to be. My abilities to learn to think fluently using highly abstract mathematical concepts, for example, are far less than they are in that small minority of people with those skills. Nevertheless, although not all-purpose, my learning abilities are clearly *multi*purpose.

Partial information decomposition provides a general approach to the specification of neural goal functions. Information theory is applicable to information of all kinds, and the objectives of learning can be specified by an objective function that states whether each of the distinct components of transmitted information should be maximized, minimized, or left free to vary.[13] The multipurpose learning objective assumed by coherent infomax is to maximize the amount of coherent information generated by the whole system. It does so by guiding processing and learning at a local level by information from diverse sources in other parts of the system. This learning objective was originally specified using the classical definition of three-way mutual information, that is, given local processors with RFs of strength R and CFs of strength C the objective specified was to maximize the three-way co-information, that is, $I(Y;C;R)$, given that the semantic content of Y is determined by R, not by C and that C amplifies the output, Y, when R and C agree and attenuates it when they disagree. The three-way mutual information $I(Y;C;R) = ShdS + ShdM - Synergy$. In our simplified realizations, ShdM and Synergy tend to be of a similar size and to vary in the same way with the strengths of C and R, particularly when they are not highly correlated. Thus, they will tend to cancel each other out. Maximizing co-information, as specified in the original formulation of the coherent infomax objective function, may therefore be an adequate approximation to maximizing the source-shared information (ShdS), which was assumed to be the basic objective of learning. The theory of coherent infomax specifies learning rules for the local processors in a neural net that were deduced from that objective. They maximize the total amount of mutually predictive, and thus meaningful, information in the system overall. As outlined in Chapter 9, this objective is a special case of the formal objective of a highly influential theory of brain function, that is, the reduction of free energy. Assuming that this is a key objective of learning also expresses the essence of the intuitive notion that dissonance reduction is a major goal for mental life in general, although not the only one.

The viability of coherent infomax as a useful style of computation depends on both the objective of learning and on the requirement that context modifies output without corrupting its semantics. Within those constraints, that learning discovers latent, or hidden, statistical structure in the information upon which it operates. If the latent statistical structure is known, then, from a statistical point of view, it is relatively straightforward to choose actions that maximize reward.[14]

Given the widespread assumption that maximization of information transmission is a general objective of both processing and learning in the brain, I reiterate that maximizing information transmission, that is, infomax, is *not* the objective of coherent infomax. Infomax maximizes $I(Y;C,R)$, that is, the total amount of transmitted information. Coherent infomax maximizes $I(Y;C;R)$, that is, the three-way mutual information, under the condition that C modulates output without corrupting its meaning. Although the difference between these two objectives may seem tiny when expressed in these symbolic terms, the differences in their functional consequences are huge. A key contribution of expressing this difference so simply is that it makes the proposed functional role of context-sensitivity both precise and quantifiable.

The information in neuronal motor outflow is typically far less than that in the sensory inflow. Neural systems do not transmit all the information they receive. A fundamental function of the neocortex is to amplify what matters at that moment, while suppressing the effects of currently irrelevant information, which would otherwise be a nuisance that impedes the discovery of latent statistical structure.[15] Thus, brains acquire and use knowledge of the latent statistical structure of events in their environment, some of which is of their own making. It is therefore necessary to emphasize again that the objective of coherent infomax does not imply that there is some optimum level of coherent information to be reached. On the contrary: it is assumed that it can be increased indefinitely. There is no obvious limit to the organized complexity that may be discovered in the world because much of it is created by living organisms themselves, and especially by humans.

A way of seeing the impossibility of completely optimizing organized complexity is by noticing that organization and complexity are contradictory. Given any set of elements it is impossible that their complexity and their organization can both be at a maximum. Organization reduces the extent to which the elements are free to vary, which necessarily reduces the amount of information needed to specify the overall state of the system, and thus its complexity as implied by standard measures of complexity. A crucial aspect of notions such as that underlying coherent infomax and theories of consciousness such as the integrated information theory (IIT) is that they imply the need to combine the forces of both order and disorder without either being maximized.[16] Both theories emphasize a synthesis that reconciles things that, prima facie, seem to be opposed, which echoes a key aspect of Hegel's proposed dialectical philosophy of history.

To be useful as a conceptual perspective on learning in the neocortex, learning rules must be formulated in a way that is feasible in a net composed of many local processing elements, each of which has many distinct inputs. Large increases in the number of local processing elements poses no problem to the learning rule of coherent infomax because it greatly speeds up learning. That is because a solution to a learning problem found by any one of the local processors spreads rapidly throughout the whole net.[17] Furthermore, the computational load on local processors can be kept manageable when they have many inputs by using Gaussian and nonparametric approximations, which are based on assuming that the RF and CF inputs are each represented by a single integrated continuous variable—what the apical and somatic integration sites presumably provide.[18]

Learning rules for coherent infomax were specified by performing gradient ascent on the objective function relative to the strengths of the RF and CF connections. The learning rules deduced in this way have the same general form for RFs and CFs, but with some small differences. The change in connection strength is proportional to input activity, but it is non-monotonically related to output activity. Connection strengths on active inputs remain unchanged when postsynaptic activity is very low, decrease when it is at intermediate levels, and increase when it is high. The threshold above which connections strengths are increased moves dynamically with the mean level of activity, which ensures that the local processor is neither too active nor too inactive to be of much use as a transmitter of information. Thus, it floats upwards as the local processor's mean level of activity increases towards a maximum, and floats downward as that level decreases towards a minimum. This turns out to be slightly modified version of the computationally powerful BCM learning rule (Bienenstock, Cooper, & Munro, 1982), which is known to be biologically realistic, and to explain much neurophysiological data on synaptic plasticity and learning in the neocortex.[19]

The conceptual framework underlying coherent infomax is in some crucial ways like that underlying neural nets trained by the deep learning algorithms of AI. Indeed, development of coherent infomax in the early 1990s was strongly influenced by what I had learned about 'connectionism' from Geoff Hinton and Jay McClelland when I spent a few weeks with them in Pittsburgh in the late 1980s. The emphasis upon probabilistic inference and information theory was also encouraged by what I learned from Hinton. Coherent infomax and deep learning algorithms are similar in that they both assume that information processing involves adaptive synaptic interactions between many local processors that can be arranged as a sequence of processing layers with increasing amounts of abstraction from layer to layer, as in convolutional neural nets (CNNs), for example. Deep learning has also been extended to nets with recurrent connections that enable them deal with sequential structure, such as that in speech and printed text. The state-of-the art in visual image processing, speech processing, drug discovery, and many other domains of Big Data processing, has been transformed by major advances since 2000 in the available computing power and in the methods for training artificial neural nets, both with and without human supervision.[20]

A key similarity between deep learning algorithms and coherent infomax is that neither of them train the connection strengths to transmit as much input information as possible. On the contrary, local processing elements in each of the internal (or 'hidden') layers of a deep learning net adapt in a way that increases transmission only of the information that is rewarded or shared with a target specified by a 'supervisor' during training. They learn to reduce transmission of irrelevant information in the input data. An analysis of deep learning using classical measures of mutual information confirm that, as learning proceeds, the local processors in the intermediate layers do indeed learn to minimize the transmission of irrelevant input information.[21]

Despite those similarities, nets based on coherent infomax differ from nets trained by standard deep learning algorithms in at least four major ways. First, they use context to guide moment-by-moment processing as well as using it to guide learning. Second, there is no formal difference between supervised and unsupervised learning. Coherent infomax deduces learning rules for modifying connection strengths from a general objective for learning that does not depend on prior knowledge of what is to be learned. Third, in nets composed of context-sensitive two-point local processors the context can come from many different sources, not only by feedback from deeper layers in the net. Finally, output from the net to other sites can come from all layers of the net and can include recurrent feedback from those sites as part of the context that guides learning and processing within the net. Context-sensitive cooperative computation may therefore have much potential as a distinct form of machine learning. Exploration of some of that potential has already begun.

8.7 The Neurobiology of Cooperative Context-sensitive Computation Inspires Effective and Efficient Machine Learning Algorithms

Cooperative interactions between concurrent streams of data processing have many different applications. In one of the earliest demonstrations, Becker and Hinton (1992) showed that stereoscopic depth cues can be discovered in visual images by an algorithm that maximizes the mutual information between the outputs of neural processors receiving their RF inputs from different but neighbouring patches of the image. The underlying rationale for that algorithm is that abstract properties of sensory input that change more slowly than the local details present in the sensory data can be discovered by requiring local processors to devote some of their limited channel capacity to signalling abstract properties shared by separate input streams. Becker and Hinton (1992) exemplified this computational strategy by the unsupervised discovery of stereo depth in visual images. Many other abstract properties could also have been used to exemplify that strategy, including the property of being either a letter or a digit (Section 5.1). This computational strategy has several major advantages. Learning can proceed without requiring any supervisor to specify an expected output because the separate input streams train each other. The abstractions discovered are therefore 'objective' in the sense that they explicitly reveal latent statistical structure implicit in the input data. As a strategy of learning, this shows much promise and is still under active development. The development of such algorithms, for example, in the form of contextually guided convolutional neural nets, has mainly focused on the use context to guide learning only, however, without also using it to guide moment-by-moment processing.[22]

A few applications of machine learning to large amounts of data have used context to guide both learning and processing, so they are of particular interest here. The most recent of which I am aware is that developed in the Subutai Ahmad lab of Numenta, Inc. in California by Grewal and colleagues (2021), in which they use temporal context to learn sequences in a way that greatly reduces the extent to which new learning interferes with previous learning. Ahsan Adeel (2020, 2022, 2023) is developing algorithms for machine learning and Big Data processing that are even more closely inspired by the neuroscience reviewed in this book. Inspired by the discoveries outlined in earlier chapters, Adeel is developing new forms of machine learning that he describes as 'multisensory context-sensitive cooperative computing'. This explicitly extends the sources of contextual input used to include general information about the target domain that has been acquired from prior experience, referred to as the 'universal contextual field'. To explore the capabilities of context-sensitive cooperative computing, it has been applied to the development of hearing aids that use video information from lip movements to selectively amplify speech signals heard in noisy environments. This function is able to remove background noise so well that it can generate speech output in a noisy environment that is as clear as in a noiseless environment. Thus, it is now possible to offer people with impaired hearing intelligent lip-reading hearing aids that greatly enhance their ability to perceive speech.

The capabilities of this form of cooperative computing as applied to audio–visual data processing have been directly compared with those of current deep learning algorithms. Context-sensitive cooperative computing was able to separate the speech from large amounts of noise, whereas deep learning could do so only when there was very little noise. Another major difference is that context-sensitive cooperative computing separates signal from noise using far fewer of the local processing elements. Its operational energy requirements and unwanted heat generation are therefore far less—major advantages in many potential applications. The speed with which the multisensory cooperative computing learns is also greater than that required by current deep learning techniques, thus making training of the algorithms far easier.[23] Thus, although the information-processing capabilities of deep learning algorithms are so great that they have transformed AI and have had a far-reaching impact on our world, context-sensitive cooperative computation may in some ways be even better. It is certainly more closely based on neuroscience and psychology, and thus more likely to reflect the way our minds work.

There are no obvious bounds to the potential capabilities and applications of these and any other context-sensitive cooperative computational techniques. The consequences of releasing that style of information processing from the constraints imposed on it by being implemented in neurons and brains are wholly unpredictable, however. As we, like life in general, cannot avoid those biological constraints, we should surely keep the genie of cooperative context-sensitive computing in its bottle until we have a better understanding of its potential strengths and weaknesses.

Notes

1. Crutchfield (2012) uses information theory to show that the physics of statistical mechanics and deterministic chaos ensure that organisms must evolve and learn to live in a

world that is neither random nor certain. He shows that, as organisms increase in complexity, so does their ability to anticipate uncertain events, but so also does their diversity. Campbell (1982) shows that information theory is ideally suited to describing the linguistic capabilities of 'grammatical man'. In his theory of probability Jaynes (2003) showed that the mathematical equivalence of entropy and information is no accident, and that probability theory and statistical inference are of crucial importance to an understanding of brain function. His arguments for that are summarized and assessed by Phillips (2012).

2. The long-standing statistical theory of coherent infomax and demonstrations of its capabilities in simple systems have been presented in many papers (e.g. Phillips, Kay, & Smyth, 1995; Smyth, Kay, & Phillips, 1996; Kay, 1999; Kay & Phillips, 2011). Kay, Floreano, and Phillips (1998) report on the network in which maximizing coherence led to cooperative context-sensitivity between multivariate (i.e. multicellular) local processors and to competitive interactions within the local processors.

3. Wibral, Lizier, and Priesemann (2015a) provide an authoritative review of mutual information decomposition and discuss its potential relevance to neurobiologically inspired computing. A special issue of *Entropy* presents several papers on partial information decomposition (PID); see Lizier et al. (2018). What is referred to here as 'shared' information is often referred to as 'redundant' information. For further discussion of the distinction between mechanistic shared information and source shared information, see Kay et al. (2017).

4. For rigorous definitions that distinguish all these components see Harder et al. (2013), Wibral et al. (2017), and Kay et al. (2017). Pica and colleagues (2017) provide an enhanced version of these definitions that specifically focuses on the distinction between source-shared and mechanistic-shared components, which they call source redundancy and non-source redundancy. They show that non-source redundancy has some overlap with synergy. If non-source redundancy is greater than zero, then so is synergy, and non-source redundancy is less than or equal to synergy. They focus on applying these measures to issues of coding within neural systems, whereas our perspective on apical amplification uses them to distinguish between information that amplifies selected signals and the information in the selected signals, however coded.

5. Wibral et al., 2017.

6. Kay and colleagues (2017) show that decompositions of transmitted information reveal distinctive properties of contextual modulation. Kay, Schulz, and Phillips (2022) show that several different techniques for performing those decompositions reveal essentially the same distinguishing properties; they are also the first to show directly and explicitly that the effects of apical input to pyramidal cells in slices of rodent cortex meet the criteria for cooperative context-sensitivity.

7. Kay and Phillips, 2020.

8. Kay and colleagues (2017) report this use of information decomposition to analyse psychophysical data obtained from human subjects trying to detect faint line segments. In that experiment the context-sensitivity observed was attenuating, and therefore competitive rather than cooperative.

9. Many basic issues could be investigated using variants of the paradigm reported by Schulz and colleagues (2021) and by Kay and colleagues (2022). For example, it could be used to study whether and how the composition of output signals depends on cell type, cortical region, layers, and developmental stage. It could also be used to test various hypotheses

concerning the information transmitted by different pyramidal cells, including that, in some conditions, they can transmit information uniquely about both apical and basal inputs in a form of multiplexed code (Naud & Sprekeler, 2018).

10. Shai and colleagues (2015) designed this detailed model of a pyramidal cell to study the detection of coincident activations of basal/peri-somatic and apical dendrites. The trunk length beyond which the effect of apical input changes in this model was found to be 250 μm, which is considerably shorter than that observed physiologically by Fletcher and Williams (2019). Amsalem and colleagues (2020) offer freely accessible software for building simplified but functionally realistic models of neurons, including those with distinct basal and apical dendritic trees. This will enable realistic simulations of neural networks composed of various types of excitatory and inhibitory neurons, and with hundreds of thousands of synapses. Although not itself a theory of the function of either the cells or the systems composed of them, these simplified but realistic models of complex intracellular processes provide tools that could be crucial to the computational testing and development of those theories.

11. Kay et al., 2017.

12. Salinas and Sejnowsky (2001) argue that gain modulation is revealed when one subset of inputs modifies sensitivity to the other subset without modifying the cell's selectivity or receptive field properties. They argue that it is widespread and give coordinate transformation as a prominent example.

13. Wibral et al., 2015b.

14. In his *magnum opus* on probability theory, Jaynes (2003) argues that maximizing net reward is relatively straightforward if the underlying statistical structure is known.

15. Jaynes (2003) also makes clear that separating 'relevant' from 'nuisance' variables is one of the most fundamental tasks facing any inferential system operating upon rich real-world data, such as the human brain.

16. Koch et al., 2016.

17. Phillips et al., 1995.

18. Though they have not yet been frequently tested by application to large sets of real-world data, recent advances in machine learning show that the optimization of mutual information measures can be applied to very large sets of data by merging techniques from variational inference and deep learning (Mohamed & Rezende, 2015). Kay and Phillips (2011) outline approximations to the pure coherent infomax learning rules.

19. Intrator and Cooper (1995) review the BCM learning rule, and Sjöström and colleagues (2008) show it to be biologically realistic. Sjöström and Häusser (2006) show that this learning implies cooperativity.

20. LeCun, Bengio, and Hinton (2015) provide an early but authoritative introduction to deep learning as a radically new form of AI, and it has already been cited more than 35,000 times, which is far more citations than most scientists receive in total throughout their lifetime. That paper has been cited so often because the algorithms that it describes successfully perform the information processing tasks for which they were designed, not because they have been shown to be the way that the brain works. I assume that there are both fundamental similarities and fundamental differences between those AI algorithms and information processing in the neocortex.

21. Shwartz-Ziv and Tishby (2017) demonstrate that information transmission in nets trained by deep learning is highly selective. A way to advance beyond this work is therefore to use

context to guide both learning and processing in such nets, and to study their dynamics using multivariate information decomposition.

22. Becker and Hinton's (1992) results have been further developed in various useful ways (e.g. Favorov & Ryder, 2004) and are applicable to both natural and hyperspectral visual images (e.g. Kursun et al., 2021). However, those applications used context to guide learning only, without affecting current processing. That is not biologically plausible and does not capitalize on the possibility of using context to disambiguate ascending data.

23. Adeel (2020; 2022, 2023) proposes that several forms of prior knowledge be included in the contextual inputs to local processors and shows that context-sensitive cooperative computation can be applied to multisensory tasks such as audio–visual processing. His lab is now vigorously exploring the potential of this new form of information processing. It is shown to be both more effective (Adeel et al., 2022) and far more efficient in its energy demands than currently popular machine learning algorithms (Adeel et al., 2023).

9
Difficulties and Unresolved Issues

There is a difficulty that can be overcome only by time. Scientific revolutions are typically described after they have reached maturity (Kuhn, 1962), but the revolution described here is still young and growing rapidly, so it is a revolution in progress. Although that implies that the story this book tells is incomplete, it has the great advantage of inviting further contributions, which is why young people are emphasized on its dedication page.

One of the main issues still to be resolved concerns conceptions of conscious experience and its neuronal bases. The nature and neurobiology of conscious experience is discussed in depth in Chapters 4 and 5, where it is argued that conscious experience involves the use of context to choose between alternative possible percepts, thoughts, and actions and that context-sensitive apical dendrites in layer 1 are a key part of the mechanism by which that is achieved in mammals. However, those arguments do not resolve the issue, and Chapter 4 raises serious doubts concerning the adequacy with which problems related to consciousness are posed, so the problems cannot be resolved until that difficulty is overcome. At that point, we will know and understand the basic similarities and differences between the conscious experiences of humans and chimps, of cats and bats, of fish and octopuses. We are not there yet, but we are on our way.

Another difficulty is that pruning (in which many neurons are eliminated) and competition between those that remain are both common events in the neocortex. That may be seen as showing the emphasis on cooperation to be a subjective quixotic bias rather than an objective assessment of the evidence, but I do not see it that way. The cells that are pruned are those that do not cooperate. The competition produces temporary coalitions of neurons whose activities are mutually supportive.

One more difficulty is that Chapter 8 used an advanced form of information theory to provide a mathematically explicit formulation and quantification of cooperative context-sensitivity, but none of the evidence cited for it in the earlier chapters explicitly used that formulation. In most (if not all) cases, the evidence cited seems to imply that it would meet that formulation if it had been applied, but it wasn't. Even where it was applied to evidence from real

The Cooperative Neuron. William A. Phillips, Oxford University Press. © Oxford University Press 2023.
DOI: 10.1093/oso/9780198876984.003.0010

neurons in Chapter 8, the reduction of synergy as feedforward drive increases (which is a key part of the information-theoretic formalization) was inferred from other data, rather than being an integral part of the specific physiological investigation reported.

Finally, Chapter 3 outlined a specific class of multi-site patch-clamping investigations that are presented as paradigmatic of cooperative context-sensitivity at the cellular level. No specific class of investigations is presented as paradigmatic at the psychological level, however, which may be seen as a weakness, although it would certainly make it easier for psychologists to assess its role in mental life if there were such a paradigm. There are well-established psychophysical paradigms for studying the effects of context on sensory processes in vision, for example, flanker facilitation, contour integration, surround suppression, and size perception. We have in the past used those paradigms as representative of the relevance of context-sensitivity to mental life. Chapter 5 showed that effects of context-sensitivity are seen in many different psychological paradigms, however, and recurrent amplification in the theoretical perspective advocated by Heeger and colleagues is inferred from a wide range of psychological paradigms. Furthermore, many of the unresolved issues noted in this chapter raise the possibility that different kinds of cooperative context-sensitivity may be adapted to different functions. Its relevance to mental life may therefore be more appropriately represented by the absence of any single definitive psychological paradigm, which avoids the mistake of identifying the process being studied with the paradigm used to study it.

This chapter summarizes other difficulties and unresolved issues that arise from the evidence and arguments outlined in earlier chapters.

9.1 Cellular Psychology Is in Its Infancy So Many Issues Are Unresolved

The book's previous chapters raise many difficulties and unresolved issues. At the neurophysiological level far more needs to be done to strengthen the roots of that perspective in the empirical and modelling evidence on the functions of apical dendrites. Abstract computational studies showed long ago that context-sensitive two-point local processors can do useful things.[1] Highly detailed models of layer 5 cells now show that they have some capabilities comparable to those of deep learning algorithms.[2] Although those models did not use context-sensitivity, they do show that layer 5 pyramidal cells are more powerful than integrate-and-fire point processors, with NMDA receptors playing a key role in those enhanced capabilities. Neurocomputational studies of dendritic computation that specifically distinguishes the role of apical dendrites are in progress and indicate that they have a great potential that merits much further exploration.[3]

From a psychological point of view, the links between apical function and cognitive capabilities outlined in Chapters 5 to 7 still need further validation. For example, consider the links between malfunctions at a cellular level and cognitive pathologies outlined in Chapter 7. Genetic, anatomical, physiological, and psychological evidence provides grounds for supposing that context-sensitive cooperative computation at a cellular level is impaired in each of the pathologies considered. Nevertheless, as leading authorities on the psychological malfunctions seen in schizophrenia and autism, Chris and Uta Frith, have said to me those proposed links cannot be conclusively known until a mechanistic cognitive model of symptom formation can be mapped directly on to the anatomy and neurophysiology of cortical microcircuits. As discussed further in Section 9.3, context-sensitive cooperative computation and apical function have not yet been explicitly embedded in a microcircuit model on which there is a widespread scientific consensus.

Another set of issues raised but left unresolved concern relations of context-sensitive cooperative computation to general concepts, knowledge, and beliefs (i.e. semantic memory) and to memories of specific life experiences (i.e. episodic memory). Section 5.1 gave examples of the automatic use of semantic knowledge to disambiguate sentences and visual percepts, and Section 5.2 provided evidence of pyramidal cells that are sensitive to context via their apical dendrites. If those cellular mechanisms are indeed implicated in those psychological phenomena, then semantic memory must be organized such that the information that is used to disambiguate percepts and words is available to the apical dendrites of pyramidal cells whose activities instantiate the relevant concepts. The wide distribution of semantic knowledge throughout the neocortex is compatible with that requirement, but I know of no other evidence that is directly for or against such an organization of semantic memory—and this omission leaves a large gap to be filled.

The rest of this chapter summarizes many other unresolved issues. The first arises because some of the neurobiological evidence cited previously has been interpreted by many researchers as supporting the hypothesis that feedforward signals transmit information in the form of 'prediction error'. This hypothesis is associated with one of the most highly influential neurobiologically based theories of mental function—that based on the principle of free energy reduction. Although the evidence for cooperative context-sensitivity is mostly in accord with that principle, it is not in accord with the associated hypothesis of prediction error coding.

9.2 How Cooperative Context-sensitive Computation Relates to Free Energy Reduction and Predictive Coding

This issue is important for at least two reasons. First, the theory of free energy reduction has much empirical support and is highly influential. The evidence for context-sensitive cooperative neurons provides cellular mechanisms for much of that theory. Second, the notion of prediction error coding, which is emphasized by some implementations of the free energy principle, must be nuanced to be reconciled with the evidence for context-sensitive pyramidal neurons.

9.2.1 Evidence for Cooperative Neurons Mostly Accords with the Principle of Free Energy Reduction

The free energy principle developed by Karl Friston and his many collaborators is currently one of the most influential theories within the behavioural and brain sciences, and no attempt is made to summarize it here. It is presented in many papers of which Friston (2010) is an early representative. Clark (2015) discusses in depth the broad implications of that conceptual framework for philosophy and cognitive neuroscience.

Although developed independently and on distinct empirical grounds, the theories of free energy reduction and of coherent infomax are in essential agreement on many key issues. Both theoretical perspectives assume that a major long-term objective of cortical function is to reduce differences between sensory input and what we predict or intend. Both perspectives are primarily concerned with *how* we know, imagine, or intend, rather than with *what* we know, imagine, or intend. Both perspectives are grounded in the mathematics of information theory and probabilistic inference. Indeed, both Friston and John Hertz (an expert on the application of statistical physics to neural information processing) have independently deduced that the formally specified objective of coherent infomax implies free energy reduction, but I make no attempt to reproduce their proofs here. Another similarity is that both perspectives emphasize the importance of hierarchical sequences of feedforward processing. Recent developments of the free energy principle argue in detail that it can account for the cooperative nature of human social cognition and behaviour, so both perspectives emphasize the importance of cooperation.[4] Coherent infomax and hierarchical formulations of the free energy principle are both concerned with selecting messages that convey precise information relevant to the current context. Finally, both perspectives assume that the local cortical processors of which the neocortex is composed receive information from two classes of input that affect action potential output in different ways, with one being driving and the other being primarily modulatory.

The long-term objective of coherent infomax implies increasing the total amount of information that is correctly predicted at any moment within the neocortex. That sounds as though it must be equivalent to reducing prediction error, as implied by free energy reduction. However, though very similar, these two objectives are not equivalent. Maximizing coherence is not equivalent to minimizing prediction error. Furthermore, the two perspectives differ with respect to the role assumed for prediction error. Another difference between the two theories is that the free energy principle explicitly includes the feedback loop from motor output via the external world and back to sensory input within the formal theory, whereas coherent infomax leaves that interaction with the external world implicit. Free energy theory is therefore more complete in that sense. The perspective advocated here is more complete in that it emphasizes contextual input from a diverse range of sources that extends well beyond feedback from the next region up in the cortical hierarchy to which the cell projects. One further difference between these two theoretical perspectives is that coherent infomax emphasizes cellular processes, whereas conceptions of predictive coding are generally formulated at the level of neuronal population activity of the sort observed by neuroimaging.

9.2.2 Reconciling Conceptions of Predictive Error with Evidence for Context-sensitive Pyramidal Cells

One obvious difference concerns the role of prediction error signals. A much-cited version of the theory of predictive coding emphasizes the forward transmission of errors, and states that the top-down flow of information from a higher to a lower level of perceptual abstraction attempts to predict and fully 'explain away' the forward-flowing sensory signal, leaving only any residual 'prediction errors' to propagate information forward within the system. If so, then there would be no feedforward output from any level when the top-down predictions to it agree with its forward-flowing sensory input. In stark contrast, however, the extensive evidence on context-sensitivity and apical function reviewed in earlier chapters of this book indicates that the feedforward outputs of many pyramidal cells in the neocortex are strengthened when there is agreement between the feedforward and the contextual inputs. Nothing in the evidence cited in support of the hypothesis of prediction error coding casts doubt on the evidence for the amplifying effects of apical activation when it coincides with basal/peri-somatic activation. Proponents of prediction error coding do not claim that it does; in fact, they rarely discuss the issue. Where it has been raised, it has usually been left unresolved.[5]

Although it is unlikely that this issue will be fully resolved easily (or soon), it may be largely resolved by interpreting evidence cited in favour of prediction error coding as showing increases in the salience of unexpected or unpredicted signals, but without changing that for which they code. Context-sensitive cellular and synaptic mechanisms could then provide mechanisms for attention and precision weighting within conceptions of predictive processing and the free energy principle.

Interpreting context as affecting salience—and sometimes precision also (Parr & Friston, 2017, 2019)—rather than coding simplifies conceptions of cortical function in several ways. There is then no need to assume that context is only feedback, nor is there a need to know the context to be able to decode the feedforward signals. Additionally, we need not assume that search is predictive. Search operates as though it were simply saying 'If there is evidence for the thing searched for, then send it loud and clear'. Finally, there is no need to assume that spatial attention predicts what is at the location attended—it simply amplifies the transmission of whatever feedforward information is at the attended location.

Thus, the evidence on context-sensitivity and apical function is in accord with the conception of active inference developed using the free energy principle in a way that does not depend upon the hypothesis that feedforward signals code for errors. It is also in accord with Spratling's (2008) model in which it is inferences, rather than errors, that ascend the perceptual hierarchy.

Thus, findings interpreted as supporting the hypothesis of prediction error coding can now be seen as providing further information on context-sensitivity as described above. Consider, for example, the findings of Keller, Roth, and Scanziani (2020a) and Keller and colleagues (2020b), who contrasted the effects of input to the receptive fields (RFs) of pyramidal cells in the visual cortex of mice with those of inputs to their surrounds. They found that pyramidal cells in layers 2, 3, and 5, but not in layer 4, have two functionally distinct sets of sensory input: inputs from the cell's classical RF and inputs from its broader surround. These two classes of input had very different effects on the cell's output. The effects of stimulating the cell's RF alone were fast with a brief transient burst followed by a lower (but sustained) level of activity. The effects of stimulating the cell's RF surround alone were slower and without a transient burst. The effects of these two inputs when combined could not have been due to any sum of their effects when occurring alone. When both were stimulated, instead of adding to the cell's response, stimulation of the surround attenuated it, thus producing what is known as surround suppression. The role of apical dendrites as a mechanism for this form of contextual modulation was further confirmed by their finding that stimulation of the surround alone generates a response that is too late to affect the cell's initial transient response to its RF input. That also explains why pyramidal cells in layer 4 are unaffected by the context. They do not have apical dendrites in layer 1. Furthermore, because anaesthesia predominantly affects apical function (Chapter 4), we can expect it to predominantly reduce the effects of surrounds. Keller, Roth, and Scanziani (2020a) show that to be so. Finally, they found that the interneurons that selectively inhibit apical dendrites are strongly activated by stimulation of the cell's RF, and by its surround. In contrast to that, interneurons that disinhibit apical dendrites are strongly activated by precisely limited stimulation of the cell's RF and by the figure to which it is sensitive when that figure is presented in figure–ground reversed form. Thus, these findings confirm and provide further information on the apical inhibitory/disinhibitory circuit described in earlier chapters.

So, given these straightforward inferences, we must ask why Keller and colleagues suggest that their findings may support predictive error coding? First, the effects they observed cannot be due to integrate-and-fire neurons but are clearly modulatory, and among the many theories that emphasize modulatory interactions, predictive coding theories are especially prominent. Second, they studied attenuating, or suppressive effects of context. Expected things are not highly informative, so attenuating them may be helpful, but, even if so, making a message less salient because it is not highly informative, or amplifying it because it is, implies that the message conveyed remains the same. Thus, with that interpretation, predictive processing can indeed be seen as making surprising signals more salient, but it does without changing what those signals code for. Third, Keller and colleagues did not study potentially cooperative effects of the surround, so amplification of the unexpected looms large in their findings. A development of their experimental paradigm that includes cooperative effects, as in the case of contour integration, for example, may therefore be highly revealing, particularly if interpreted in the light of theories that combine cooperative with competitive context-sensitivity, as in Heeger and Mackey's (2019) theory, for example.

Thus, overall, the findings of Keller and colleagues (2020a,b) provide further grounds for concluding that, if we are to understand the cellular foundations of mind, we must advance beyond the point neuron assumption—and embrace the cooperative context-sensitive aspects of thalamocortical processing.[6]

9.3 How Cooperative Neurons Are Embedded in Cortical Microcircuits

As already discussed, many different neurobiological investigations have found that the main classes of excitatory and inhibitory cells and the way in which they are interconnected within and between narrow columns of neocortical cells are surprisingly similar across cortical regions and species. This is remarkable because different regions deal with completely different things, such as sensory and perceptual modalities, motor control, and higher cognitive functions, and because different species have such a wide range of different abilities. These findings have therefore led to the assumption that there is a common neocortical microcircuit upon which variations are played within and across regions and species. This pattern of connectivity within a narrow column of the neocortex is called a microcircuit because it contains only a tiny proportion of the cells in the cortex, which is composed of many millions of them. A strategy in which variations are played on common anatomical and physiological themes is common in biology. For example, the shapes, sizes, and properties of the set of bones in hands and feet are variations on a common plan that adapts them to grasping, walking, or other functions, as appropriate to the organism's lifestyle.

Similarly, a microcircuit in the neocortex is composed of a few classes of pyramidal cell that are found in all regions, and which are locally interconnected with each other and with inhibitory interneurons to form a basic cortical microcircuit that is found, with variations, throughout neocortex. If there is an underlying common, or 'canonical', microcircuit then, given its great potential, discovering exactly what that microcircuit is, and why it has such great potential, must be a major goal for neuroscience.

It is now clear that there are three or four main classes of inhibitory cell and three main classes of excitatory cell in the cortical microcircuit. The main classes of inhibitory cell and their interconnections with each other and with excitatory cells are shown in Figures 3.8, 5.9, and 6.1. Three principal classes of excitatory cell are primarily distinguished by whether their outputs go mainly to other neocortical cells, that is, intra-telencephalic (IT) cells, or to the thalamus, that is, corticothalamic (CT) cells, or to thalamic and subcortical sites via the pyramidal tract (PT) cells. Various patterns of interaction between these subtypes of excitatory cell within the cortical microcircuit have been inferred from the anatomical and physiological evidence. Although there is not yet a settled consensus on the nature of any such common microcircuit, some inferences do seem to be reliable. For example, excitatory cells in layer 4 receive feedforward input from the sensors, their output goes to IT cells in layers 2 and 3, whose output then goes to IT and PT cells in layer 5.[7] Some other long-standing inferences concerning connectivity between excitatory cells within a microcircuit are now looking more doubtful, however, such as the presumed prevalence of recurrent connections between excitatory cells in different layers within a microcircuit.[8]

A major task for neuroscience in this decade is therefore to discover whether or not there is a common microcircuit that uses connections to the apical dendrites of some pyramidal cells as a context that guides both learning and processing. That requires anatomical and physiological studies of connectivity within the local microcircuits that adequately distinguishes between apical and basal/peri-somatic connections of pyramidal cells. There is as yet no consensus on any such microcircuit. Nevertheless, there have been important steps in the development of computational microcircuit models that do clearly distinguish these two distinct classes of excitatory input. One is that developed by David Heeger and colleagues as discussed in several previous chapters. Another studies the consequences of regulating these two classes of excitatory input by distinct classes of inhibitory interneuron. It shows that, via a pattern of connections between inhibitory interneurons (Figure 3.8), transient inputs can persistently switch the microcircuit between a state in which apical input affects the cell's output and a state in which it does not. Analysis of that model also concludes that each of these classes of inhibitory interneuron acts cooperatively as a population rather than as a set of independent individuals.[9] Given models of this high quality, I predict that there will soon be a consensus on the essentials of the neocortical microcircuit.

Many more detailed issues arise concerning the architectures and dynamics of the microcircuits in which context-sensitive cells are embedded but here only three groups of issues are noted. First, there are major issues concerning subtypes of context. What are the main subtypes? Do they include differences between stimulus contexts, task contexts, short-term memory contexts, and emotional contexts? Do different types of context project to different parts of the apical tree, and is that relevant to their functionality?

A second group of issues concerns regulation of the extent to which apical input affects the cell's output. At one extreme there is apical isolation. At the other there is apical drive in which apical input alone is sufficient to generate salient bursts of output. The intermediate mode of operation is apical amplification in which apical input amplifies response to feedforward input. These different modes of operation have huge implications for mental state and cognitive capabilities. There is much evidence that the mode of apical function is itself modulated by a variety of mechanisms. These seem to include mechanisms that increase basal inhibition when apical dendrites are disinhibited, thus decreasing the effectiveness of basal inputs when apical input is made more effective, so that offers a large territory to be explored.

Finally, there is a group of issues concerning energy demands that mainly involves the signals transmitted by excitatory cells because connections to and from inhibitory cells are mostly confined to the local microcircuit and its near neighbours. There is now growing evidence that excitatory cells communicate via sparse burst firing, which is both fast and highly energy efficient. Therefore, it may be no accident that apical input primarily amplifies its response to basal input by converting the response from a single spike to a brief burst. Even more importantly from the viewpoint of energy efficiency, the primary function of apical amplification is to amplify transmission only of the information that is currently relevant, implying a large reduction in energy demand.

9.4   How Cooperative Neurons Are Regulated by the Neuromodulators

Changes in mental state from deep sleep, to dreaming, to quiet wakefulness, to active wakefulness, and to stressful emergencies are regulated by the neuromodulators and are reflected by distinctive changes in electroencephalograph (EEG) signals that can be recorded on the scalp. These changes in the EEG predominantly reflect changes in the operation of pyramidal cells. In part this is because EEG signals are generated in the neocortex, and about 80% of neocortical neurons are pyramidal cells. More importantly, EEG signals are almost entirely determined by the electrical field dipoles across the axis linking the apical branches to the soma of pyramidal neurons. So, the changes in mental state that are reflected by the EEG involve changes in the apical dendritic currents on which context-sensitivity depends. This is also implied by evidence that the neuromodulatory systems that regulate mental state have particularly large effects on the relative effectiveness of apical and basal dendrites, thus regulating the extent to which pyramidal cell activity is affected by internally stored information.

Chapter 4 explained how mental state is regulated by orexinergic inputs to the neocortex from the hypothalamus, by cholinergic input from the basal forebrain, and by adrenergic input from the locus coeruleus. These neuromodulators operate in concert with more locally specific inputs to the cortex from the higher-order thalamus. As a result of these neuromodulatory and thalamic inputs, apical dendrites amplify or drive the activities of highly selected subsets of pyramidal cells far more effectively when awake or dreaming. The subset of pyramidal cells whose activities are currently relevant changes rapidly from moment to moment and from location to location in the cortex. As a result, the frequency and heterogeneity of EEG signals increases with arousal, while their power decreases, thus producing changes that are easily observed via EEG.[10]

All cortical regions receive input from the subcortical neuromodulatory systems that regulate arousal. In addition to their recurrent connections with the thalamus, some cortical regions also have recurrent interactions with the subcortical neuromodulatory nuclei, thus giving the neocortex some say in the regulation of its own state of arousal. The moment-by-moment pattern of cortical activity that results from this is complex with some regularities that are now becoming clear, but with many issues that remain unresolved.

First, consider the effects of the arousing neuromodulator orexin (hypocretin), which is a neuropeptide synthesized in a hypothalamic nucleus and transported to sites that are widely distributed throughout subcortical nuclei and cortical regions. It affects the cortex indirectly by orchestrating other neuromodulators that directly regulate the mode of neuronal activity in the cortex, but it also directly affects the neocortex itself. Thus, orexin orchestrates the activities of subcortical arousal systems in preparation for motivated actions of various kinds. Some of those actions express internal drives, for example, search for food or mates, but many of them are responses to external opportunities or threats. In preparation for the motivated actions, orexin increases the depth of breathing by modulating the respiratory rhythm generator in the brainstem. Subtle variations in mental and cortical states are coupled to these respiratory rhythms of breathing. This is in part because of the effects of orexin on adrenergic arousal. Some malfunctions of this system lead to sleep apnoea, which involves inadequate breathing when asleep. Other malfunctions lead to narcolepsy, which is a rare but serious and chronic neurological disorder in which people suddenly fall asleep because of a malfunction in the subcortical systems that regulate sleep–wake cycles. Narcolepsy is often confused with more complex disorders, but when appropriately diagnosed it can to some extent be managed by using stimulants that compensate for the malfunctions.

Orexin also contributes both directly and indirectly to the orchestration of neocortical activities and affects various cognitive functions, especially attention and some forms of learning. This is achieved via direct projections to medial prefrontal cortex (PFC), and indirectly by its effects on cholinergic and adrenergic arousal. To be able to selectively enhance just those actions that are most appropriate in the current situation, for example, in approach–avoidance dilemmas, orexinergic arousal must somehow be embedded in a system of functional connectivity that is sufficiently heterogeneous to produce such a diverse range of behaviours. There is some locally specific heterogeneity in the subcortical population of orexinergic cells, their inputs, and their outputs, but that heterogeneity by itself is insufficient to produce the diversity of motivated behaviours. It is therefore likely that orexin operates in a qualitatively similar manner across different cortical regions, but in interaction with a system that does have the local specificity required. How that is achieved is currently unknown.[11]

One way in which orexin could have locally specific effects is by increasing cholinergic and adrenergic arousal, which would increase the effectiveness of contextual input to pyramidal cells, and thus leverage the high degree of local specificity of that contextual input (Chapters 4 and 5). It is also possible that orexin could enhance the effectiveness of apical input directly by reducing current flow through HCN channels, which, as noted in several previous chapters, will greatly increase the effectiveness of apical input.[12] A way in which the heterogeneity of orexinergic arousal might contribute to deciding what to do is by being part of the emotional prioritization discussed in Section 5.6. Finally, heterogeneity of the effects of orexinergic arousal might arise from its especially large effects on cells in the lower levels of layer 6 in the cortex. These cells are sensitive to the activity in the specific column of which they are a part, and project to higher-order thalamic nuclei, which in turn regulate the excitability of neocortical cells in a way that depends on their locally specific apical inputs in ways that remain to be clarified.[13]

We can be confident that a better understanding of the effects of orexinergic arousal on the function of apical dendrites will have clinical utility. Orexinergic arousal decreases greatly when animals are subject to aversive stressors from which there is no escape. The reduction in motivated behaviours that results has many similarities to some forms of depression in humans. So, the advice to 'cheer up' may sometimes be asking for something of which we are not directly capable. We may be able to do so indirectly, however, for example, by focusing on wholesome things, by avoiding inescapable stressors, or by cultivating a mindset in which inescapable stressors are perceived in a way that makes them less stressful. These issues therefore merit far deeper investigation.

In cholinergic arousal, the ascending cholinergic projections from the brainstem induce large changes in mental state. When directly stimulated, cholinergic cells in the basal forebrain produce powerful changes in the state of the neocortex as seen in the EEG. They increase high frequency rhythms, such as gamma, and reduce slow wave rhythms. When we are awake, smaller fluctuations in the level of cholinergic arousal also occur with major implications for mental function (Chapters 4 and 5). Cholinergic arousal has particularly large and distinctive effects on apical function, for example, the activation of muscarinic cholinergic receptors selectively boosts the excitability of apical dendrites of layer V pyramidal cells via facilitation of the flow of calcium ions into the cell.[14] There are also several other ways in which cholinergic arousal modulates context-sensitivity in the cerebral cortex, but explorations of these possibilities and its relevance to context-sensitive cognitive functions still have far to go.

Finally, adrenergic arousal occurs when the locus coeruleus releases noradrenaline (NA) widely throughout the brain, including all neocortical regions. Earlier chapters discuss research on its role in context-sensitivity and conscious experience, although that is only a tiny fraction of the experimental evidence available, so we do not yet have an adequate understanding of its role in mental life. Adrenergic arousal has long been thought of as a global brainwide influence that is either on or off, but it is now clear that adrenergic arousal is more heterogeneous, both across time and across different locations in the brain. Adrenergic levels can fluctuate rapidly on a timescale of seconds or less and may vary across different locations within the cortex. Though the locus coeruleus is small relative to the whole brain, in rodents the adrenergic cells within it receive inputs from up to 111 distinct brain regions. There are about 50,000 of these adrenergic cells in the human brain, and they project widely to all cortical regions and to most subcortical nuclei. There is direct anatomical evidence that different adrenergic neurons preferentially target one cortical region, even though they also innervate other regions to some extent.

As discussed in earlier chapters, adrenergic arousal further enhances responses to salient events while further attenuating responses to less salient events. Local release of NA in specific cortical regions enhances their usual functions. The normal dependence of those functions on adrenergic arousal is confirmed by showing that blocking the effects of adrenergic arousal can worsen those functions. For example, local release of NA in sensory or perceptual regions enhances their selective sensitivity. Similarly, local release in the anterior cingulate region of the PFC enhances sustained attention and decision making. In rodents, local release in prelimbic or infralimbic regions (which are part of their version of the PFC) improves their ability to learn new associations. Thus, whereas adrenergic arousal was long assumed to exert a global uniform influence on its many targets in subcortical nuclei and neocortical regions, it is now thought to have more heterogeneous effects across time and across the diverse brain locations that it effects, but that further clarification is still needed.

Two theories have long been dominant concerning the function of adrenergic arousal: the theory of adaptive gain-modulation and the theory of network reset. The theory of gain-modulation proposes that adrenergic activity optimizes the trade-off between exploiting knowledge already acquired and acquiring new knowledge by exploration and learning. It proposes that exploitation is produced by phasic (i.e. brief) adrenergic bursts, and that exploration is produced by tonic (i.e. sustained) adrenergic activity. Network reset theories emphasize a role for adrenergic arousal in suppressing the use of prior knowledge and maximizing the use of sensory signals to acquire new knowledge. Neither of these views alone gives an adequate conception of the functions and mechanisms of adrenergic arousal, but there has been little progress in either refining or unifying them over the past 15 years. They are not mutually exclusive, however, so some theory that combines the best of each of them might be possible.[15] The evidence for the contextual guidance of learning and processing supports aspects of both theories and provides cellular mechanisms for them. Therefore, it raises the possibility that the strengths of these two theories can be combined by explicitly relating them to that evidence. That has not been attempted yet, but it soon may be as research on apical function becomes more prominent.

The effects of adrenergic arousal on apical function depend on many things including neocortical region, species, and level of arousal. As noted in previous chapters, the effects of arousal on cellular and cognitive function are not monotonic. Increases from moderate to high can have effects that are the opposite of those caused by increases from low to moderate. The focus of those earlier chapters was on the increased role of cooperative context-sensitivity as arousal increases from very low, as in slow wave sleep, to moderate levels of arousal during quiet and active wakefulness. However, it has been observed that when adrenergic arousal increases even further, as in emergencies or other highly stressful situations, input to apical synapses was disconnected from the soma via a class of adrenergic receptor with a high threshold. The effects of thoughtful deliberation may then be reduced, with fast stereotyped responses mediated by the basal dendrites alone being facilitated, although these observations were from studies of the hippocampus. Hippocampal pyramidal cells differ in many ways from those in the neocortex, resulting in our need to explore the effects of high levels of adrenergic arousal on apical function across cortical regions, species, and developmental stages.[16]

9.5 How Cooperative Neurons Relate to the Speed of Thought

There is ample evidence that mental processes that are fast and automatic can be distinguished from those that are slow and voluntary,[17] but how is that related to the evidence for context-sensitivity? It is unlikely that the slow processes can be identified with those that are context-sensitive because the effects of stimulus contexts on perception can be fast, as shown in several of the demonstrations given in Chapter 5. A more plausible possibility considers the effects of context that are not direct but conveyed by intermediaries. If cell A receives direct contextual input from cell B, and cell B from cell C, etc., then cell A can, given enough processing time, be indirectly influenced by contextual input from cell C, and by reiteration of that to a much wider set of cells than that to which it is directly connected. This mediated contextual guidance depends upon the intermediaries being active, however. So, it is possible that slower processes of thought involve activating potential intermediaries in search of coherence between a wider population of cells than those that are directly connected via apical dendrites. This possibility remains to be explored.

9.6 How Cooperative Neurons Relate to Hobson's and Freud's Views on Dreams

Chapter 4 provides evidence for three distinct modes of apical function, and thus of mental state. It indicates that when we are in a deep dreamless slow wave sleep, the effects of apical dendrites are at a minimum, and when we are awake, apical amplification provides cellular mechanisms for perceptual awareness. Similarly, apical drive provides a cellular mechanism for our dreams when we are asleep, but the cortex is active with its sensory inputs and motor outputs being blocked.[18] There is now much evidence for these claims, but we are only starting to explore their implications. To start, I first briefly relate context-sensitive cellular mechanisms to J. Allan Hobson's theory that sees dreaming as occupying a particular region within a three-dimensional view of mental state. I then connect evidence on apical function to the unconscious mind of Freudian psychoanalysis.

Hobson, emeritus professor of psychiatry at Harvard, was a leading international authority on the neurophysiological bases of the differences between waking, dreaming, and dreamless sleep. He concluded that mental states vary within a space specified by the levels of three variables: activation (A), input–output gating (I), and modulation (M). (A) is the overall level of neuronal activity and energy consumption, which is at a minimum during dreamless sleep and at a maximum during active wakefulness. It can be increased by either external or internal events. (I) facilitates or suppresses interaction of the cortex with the outside world via sensory input and motor commands. It is high when awake, but low during both dreaming and dreamless sleep. (M) is high when aminergic arousal, such as that due to NA, is higher than cholinergic arousal and low when it is the other way round. It is at a minimum during dreaming, which occurs when adrenergic arousal is at a minimum but cholinergic arousal is at a maximum. All modulatory systems slow down during dreamless sleep, but they do not shut off completely. According to Hobson's AIM theory, aminergic activation, which includes adrenergic activation, is at a minimum when dreaming.[19]

There are obvious similarities between Hobson's AIM theory of mental state and the modes of apical function described in this book. Both imply that dreams are a direct expression of the contextual information that is used to guide perception and learning when awake. States where (A) is low are analogous to apical isolation. Dream states are dominated by apical drive, and waking states are characterized by open (I) and adrenergic arousal in Hobson's AIM theory, which is analogous to the state in which apical activation occurs. However, these analogies require much closer examination.

There are also some contrasts between the perspective advocated here and Hobson's three-dimensional state space theory. Hobson (2009) proposes that waking consciousness, with its impressive secondary features (i.e. self-awareness, language, and volition) might be present only in humans. In contrast, the direct evidence for context-sensitive cellular mechanisms comes mainly from rodents. So, what Hobson refers to as primary conscious awareness (which he ascribes to all or most mammals) may also include ancient versions of cognitive capabilities that he claims are distinctively human. Another contrast is that Hobson assumes that the activation that generates dream content is random, so he argues that there is no point in trying to interpret dreams. However, the input to apical dendrites that guides perception and learning when awake is far from random. Thus, as long argued by many psychoanalysts, it is possible that dream content does have some meaning.

One simple way in which this evidence resonates with Freudian psychoanalysis is that both emphasize fundamental differences between dreaming and states of conscious wakefulness. Freud argued that dreams reflect mental processes of which we are usually not aware, which resonates with the objectively established differences between dreaming and wakeful awareness (Chapter 4). This view also resonates with the evidence indicating that dreams are a direct expression of synaptic connections that primarily operate as amplifiers of response to feedforward signals when awake. We usually have little or no direct knowledge of those context-sensitive operations because, ideally, they operate behind the scenes of conscious experience. If dreams are the direct expression of contextual interactions that guide learning and processing when awake, then they may tell us something about those interactions. Although this is more plausible than some other aspects of Freudian theory, I know of no previous discussion of it, though that is surely worthwhile. For example, do dreams reflect properties of components of the apical input that still operate when adrenergic arousal is low? If so, that is likely to be those components of apical synaptic input that are especially strong or arrive at synapses close to the apical integration zone. Do such components include inputs to apical dendrites from the amygdala, and, if so, does that explain why dreams are usually emotionally charged? Does the anomalous incoherence of dreams reflect a loss of the modulatory processes that operate to enhance coherence when awake? I assume that some valid insights concerning the dynamics of unconscious processes have accrued over more than a century of psychoanalytic observation and thought. Can any of them be related to evidence on the different modes of apical function or to evidence on stratification of contextual input to apical dendrites?

9.7 Are There Distinctively Human Forms of Cooperative Context-sensitive Computation?

There are distinctively human cognitive capabilities, including language. However, there is no consensus on either precisely what those specific capabilities are, or about their neurobiological bases. Even if either absolute/relative brain size or number of neurons were consistently associated with those capabilities, why do these specific quantitative changes result in specific cognitive consequences, and how do these cognitive changes relate to changes in lifestyle?

About 40,000 years ago *Homo sapiens* became the only surviving species in the genus, and via conceptual and technological revolutions transformed their lifestyle at an increasing rate, leading to unprecedented growth in the number of people on the planet.[20] Although each revolution occurred as a result of a cultural accumulation of conceptual and technological innovations combined with increasing population density and favourable climatic and other environmental conditions, I see no firm grounds for ascribing any of those historical revolutions to changes in the underlying cognitive capabilities of humans. This suggests that the cognitive capabilities on which cumulative technological culture depends evolved more than 40,000 years ago.

First, about two to three million years ago, several species in the genus Homo separated from other primates. Their spread from East Africa throughout Africa and Eurasia during a sequence of ice ages and interglacial periods shows that those early hominoids had the ability to adapt rapidly to a wide variety of prevailing conditions. Nevertheless, their cognitive capabilities were not equivalent to ours, and their technologies advanced little, if at all, for thousands of years. Then, between about three and four hundred thousand years ago rapid technological advances included the building of shelters, and the use of fire for multiple purposes, including cooking. Individuals were able to voluntarily control body temperature using clothing, and with adapted teeth and digestive systems they became opportunistic omnivores. The information processing capabilities on which such adaptations depend require high energy input to the neocortex, which was provided by the energy-rich diet that those capabilities made available.[21] *Homo sapiens* remains the only species that, in addition to all our modern luxuries, has lifestyles that usually depend on cooking, clothing, and extensive technologies for cooperative hunting, gathering, and sharing. Given the great benefits of those technologies and lifestyles, is there a reason for their restriction to a single species? We do not yet know whether there is or not, but we do known that around sixty to seventy thousand years ago, the rate of technological advance greatly increased, resulting in major developments in pictorial art, language, and the use of an even wider range of tools.

With this in mind, the cognitive foundations on which human cumulative technological culture depends may well be multifactorial (see Chapter 6) for at least three different aspects of cooperative neuronal function that may be distinctively human. These include changes in the length of the apical trunk, in inhibitory interneurons that target apical dendrites, and in I_h (current flow through HCN ion channels).

Current attempts to identify the cognitive and neuronal foundations for advances in human lifestyles focus on debates concerning the extent to which they involve social cognition, non-social cognition, language, imitation, and teaching.[22] These issues have not yet been related to enhancements of cognitive capabilities in which cooperative neuronal function have been implicated. It is likely that such enhancements are involved because tool use, social cognition, and language are all highly context-sensitive. Language and thought are especially dependent on the use of context to disambiguate the meaning of items within dynamically created syntactic and semantic structures— something not easily explained by networks of integrate-and-fire neurons.[23]

While working for Google on the role of attention in natural language processing, Vaswani and colleagues (2017) developed a neural network algorithm for machine translation that outperforms prior algorithms to such an extent that their paper has now been cited more than 46,000 times! It is based on processes of normalization and selective attention that resemble those outlined in Chapter 5, where they are shown to involve the operations of cooperative context-sensitive neurons. In a personal communication Peter König, a cognitive neuroscientist in the University of Osnabrück, has told me that he sees a way of implementing that algorithm using a plausible cortical microcircuit that could provide a mechanism for cooperative context-sensitive computation. If so, and if what is distinctively human about that microcircuit can be identified, then that would be a truly historic advance.

It is commonly assumed that the ancient enhancements in hominid cognitive capabilities can be explained by increases in either brain size or number of neurons. However, those types of evolutionary change are common and do not easily explain cognitive capabilities that evolved over more than three billion years, and then only in humans.[24]

It is now possible to relate cognitive evolution to neuronal capabilities that transcend those of integrate-and-fire point neurons. Chapter 6 discusses evidence for properties of human cooperative neurons not yet seen in the neocortex of either rodents or nonhuman primates and Section 6.3.1 outlines discoveries showing that apical dendrites of layer 5 pyramidal cells can be more effectively isolated from the soma in humans than in rodents. Apical dendrites are longer, thicker, and more complexly branched in humans than in other species, so, we can be confident that they have major functional implications for human cognition. Chapter 5 shows that in perceptual regions those functions include using information from internal sources to amplify the information transmitted about sensory input when appropriate. If apical inputs are more effectively isolated from the soma when inappropriate, this will produce a closer approximation to the use of apical input as a pure amplifier and will more effectively distinguish the objective sensory information to be transmitted from subjective decisions concerning the interpretation or importance of that information. In short, some of the intracellular changes leading towards human cognitive capabilities may enable perception to be both more objectively realistic and thought to be more subjectively selective. We now need to discover whether or not this is so.

Thus, in addition to a role in making perception both more objective and more relevant to current intentions, apical dendrites of human neocortical pyramidal cells might also provide a basis for other cognitive capabilities. For example, Gidon and colleagues (2020) reported that a distinctive capability of apical dendrites of layer 2/3 pyramidal cells excised from the temporal lobe of humans can generate output from the cell by themselves, but with that capability reducing as apical input strength increases. They suggest that this may enable layer 2/3 cells compute the XOR relation between two different components of the apical input, that is, either one component of input, or the other, but not both.[25] Of even more importance may be the evidence implicating apical drive in dreaming (Chapter 4) and in imagery when awake (Chapter 5). I know of no research focused on the possibility that distinctively human cognitive capabilities depend on evolutionary advances in apical function, but it is surely a tantalizing prospect for future research.

We may clarify these issues by studying how specifically human intellectual abilities typically develop and the ways in which those abilities are enhanced or impaired by specific psychoactive substances. We can do this via methods such as transcranial magnetic stimulation or direct current stimulation, or by studying genetic mutations shown to affect both cooperative neuronal function and higher cognitive functions (Chapter 7). Indeed, a review being compiled by Albert Granato, Mototaka Suzuki, Jan Schulz and myself of the pathophysiology of neurodevelopmental learning disabilities shows that unbroken paths from the cellular dysfunctions to the psychological symptoms can now be sketched.

9.8 Are There Regional and Developmental Variations in Cooperative Context-sensitivity?

Grounds for supposing that there are regional and developmental variations in cooperative context-sensitivity are provided by Anderson and colleagues' (2020) review of regional variations in the densities of parvalbumin (PV) and somatostatin positive (SOM/SST) inhibitory interneurons using genetic, transcriptional, and neuroimaging methods. They finds that variations in these densities are strongly linked to both development and pathology. PV densities decrease along a gradient from posterior sensorimotor to higher more abstract prefrontal regions, whereas SOM/SST densities do the opposite; therefore, they are anticorrelated. These differential densities first emerge in the final prenatal month or two and continue to change until early maturity. This is so in vivo in both human and nonhuman primates and, in a simpler form, in rodents. In humans these densities are strongly correlated with heritable individual differences in large-scale BOLD neuroimaging measures of resting state signal amplitudes and with risk genes for schizophrenia and other disorders such as major depression.[26]

We can assume that these findings are relevant to the functions of apical dendrites because PV inhibitory interneurons mostly target basal/perisomatic locations, whereas SOM/SST inhibitory interneurons mostly target apical locations. Anderson and colleagues (2020) also implicate PV inhibitory interneurons in gamma band dynamics and synchronization. They implicate SOM/SST inhibitory interneurons in slower dynamics and in filtering out irrelevant activities while increasing the salience of relevant activities.

Almeida (2022) relates these findings to the function of apical dendrites at two levels of conscious awareness. One level is graded and associated with awareness of a richly detailed sensory field. It is predominantly associated with regions that are low in the cortical hierarchy, and thus close to the sensory–motor interface. The other is associated with regions that are higher in the neocortical hierarchy. It is discontinuous because it must pass a high, context-sensitive, threshold set by the inhibition of apical dendrites. Signals emerge into higher-order awareness when direct excitation or disinhibition of those dendrites are sufficient to exceed that threshold. The complexity of these higher-order processes may increase with hierarchical level, and thus distance from the sensory–motor surface, but without necessarily diminishing the importance of direct contact with the external world in mental life. The increasing role of cooperative context-sensitivity with distance from the sensorimotor periphery may even be visible in the exceptionally exuberant apical branches of the lateral prefrontal cortical cells of monkeys (see Figure 3.2).

Increased dependence on SOM/SST inhibitory interneurons in higher cortical regions seems to resonate well with our view of apical dendrites as a mechanism for cooperative context-sensitivity in a large class of neocortical pyramidal cells. Thus, the need to clarify the implications of these discoveries for variations in the capabilities and vulnerabilities of apical function across regions, developmental stages, and pathologies may provide happy hunting grounds for cognitive neuroscientists and others for many years to come. Furthermore, as inhibition increases I_h, which tends to suppress the effects of apical input and which also depends on neuromodulatory state, relating these interdependencies to regional variations in the relative amounts of somatic and apical inhibition raises many issues for future research.

An increasing role for cooperative context-sensitivity in higher and later developing cortical regions is implicit in Sydnor and colleagues' (2021) wide-ranging review of the hierarchy of neocortical regions, whose 14 authors come from departments or institutes of brain and mind, psychology, psychiatry, neurology, bioengineering, electrical and systems engineering, physics and astronomy, paediatrics, biomedical imaging, and neuromodulation, developmental neurogenomics, and biomedical image computing and analytics. Comprehensible themes, such as cooperative context-sensitivity, may underlie the discoveries of those multidisciplinary collaborations, and Sydnor and colleagues (2021) show that processing is more dependent on stimulus and task contexts at higher levels of the neocortical hierarchy. One way in which this increased flexibility is revealed is by the increasing heterogeneity of a region's inputs and outputs. A region's pattern of connections tends to be more local and stereotypical across individuals at lower hierarchical level and more long-range and variable across individuals at higher levels. This echoes our emphasis upon the heterogeneity and adaptability of apical inputs. Higher regions process their inputs on a longer timescale, have more abstract multimodal semantics, develop for much longer before becoming mature, have evolved in mammals over several hundred million years, and confer uniquely human risks of pathology. Much of the variation across this hierarchy seen in macroscopic neuroimaging data is shown to reflect microscale variations in cellular and molecular properties. Thus, increased dependence on intracellular capabilities, including cooperative context-sensitivity, may be a key marker of a region's place in the cortical hierarchy. These anatomical, functional, evolutionary, and developmental variations of cooperative context-sensitive apical function with position in the neocortical hierarchy resonate so strongly with the perspective advocated in this book that they must surely point to the future of cellular psychology.

9.9 Technological Potential of Cooperative Context-sensitive Computation

Inspired by the discoveries outlined in this book, a new kind of context-sensitive information processing (called multisensory cooperative computing) is being developed. The sources of contextual input used by those algorithms include general knowledge about the target domain acquired from prior experience—the 'universal contextual field'. To explore the capabilities of this style of context-sensitive cooperative computing, it has been applied to the development of hearing aids that use video information from lip movements to selectively amplify speech signals heard in noisy environments (Section 8.7).[27] The consequences of releasing the cooperative context-sensitive style of information processing from the constraints imposed on it by being implemented in living cells are unpredictable, however, so use of its potential should proceed with great caution.

Notes

1. Phillips, Kay, & Smyth, 1995; Körding & König, 2000.
2. Beniaguev, Segev, & London, 2020.
3. Poirazi & Papoutsi, 2020.
4. Veissière et al., 2020.
5. Phillips, Clark, and Silverstein (2015) and Phillips (2017) raise, but do not resolve, the issue of reconciling findings interpreted as evidence for prediction error coding with evidence for apical amplification. Karl Friston has suggested to me (pers. comm.) that 'Mathematically, the resolution is likely to be found in the notion of precision weighted prediction errors'. In other words, the prediction errors fed forward in hierarchal predictive coding are afforded a gain or weighting in proportion to their precision (Parr et al., 2018; Limanowski, 2021) Precision here is just the inverse variability or reliability ascribed to a prediction error. This means that there are two determinants of precision-weighted prediction error: the prediction error per se and the precision of the prediction error that can often be associated empirically (Kok, Jehee, & de Lange, 2012; Kok et al., 2012). As precision is thought to be closely related to salience, this suggests that processing under the free energy principle is more concerned with the salience and precision of the information selected for enhanced processing rather than with coding and the feedforward transmission of errors. If so, then, this nuancing of the free energy principle may not only be a step in the right direction, but also compatible with other broad views of thalamocortical function, including that of coherent infomax.
6. Although Keller and colleagues' (2020a, b) results are interpreted here as contributing to our knowledge of context-sensitive cells with two points of integration, we cannot be confident of that for at least four reasons. First, the distinct effects of input to apical and somatic

integrating zones integration zones within pyramidal cells were not studied directly. Second, the cells studied were not shown to be in that part of visual cortex where pyramidal cells with two points of integration have been shown to occur in mice. Third, many of their findings were from cells whose soma are in layers 2 or 3, rather than in layer 5, where those most typical of context-sensitivity lie. Fourth, they did not explicitly study bursting, which is the output variable most affected by context.

7. Harris & Shepherd, 2015.

8. Thomson, 2021.

9. Hertag & Sprekeler, 2019.

10. Tantirigama and colleagues (2020) review the multiple pathways by which neuromodulators regulate cortical dynamics and mental state. They include clear accounts of their relation to basic physiological processes such as breathing, and of their relations to the higher cognitive functions of neocortex.

11. Mahler and colleagues (2014) provide a fascinating account of orexin as a general orchestrator of the states of arousal on which motivated behaviour depends.

12. Li and colleagues (2010) report anatomical and physiological studies indicating that orexin has large effects on currents that flow through HCN ionic channels in mouse prelimbic cortex, which is part of its version of the PFC.

13. The review by Tantirigama and colleagues (2020) contains an extensive section on the special properties of pyramidal neurons whose cell bodies are deep in layer 6, and whose functions remain unclear.

14. Williams & Fletcher, 2019.

15. Breton-Provencher, Drummond, and Sur (2021) provide a detailed review of the many anatomical inputs to and outputs from the adrenergic cells in the locus coeruleus. They also discuss theories concerning its function, but do not consider the evidence relating adrenergic arousal to apical function and context-sensitivity.

16. Abdallah and colleagues (2016) discuss several of the complexities underlying the effects of adrenergic arousal. Pedarzani and Storm (1995) and Storm and colleagues (2000) observed effects of an adrenergic receptor with a high opening threshold.

17. Kahneman, 2011.

18. Marvan and colleagues (2021) review the evidence indicating that apical amplification provides a cellular mechanism for perceptual awareness. Aru and colleagues (2020b) review evidence indicating that apical drive provides a cellular mechanism for dreams.

19. Hobson, 2009.

20. Harari (2011) gives an enthralling account of these revolutions in the evolution of *Homo sapiens*.

21. Bentsen (2020) provides a highly accessible review of the evolution of the use of fire, including cooking. This shows that there is clear evidence of its habitual use from about three to four hundred thousand years ago, but we have no evidence for its use much earlier than that.

22. Commentaries in Osiurak and Reynaud (2020) show a wide variety of views on cumulative technological culture and its evolution, although none consider the possibility that changes in cellular information processing capabilities may be involved. For a review of the role of teaching in cumulative culture, see Caldwell, Renner, and Atkinson (2018).

23. Fodor and Pylyshyn (1988) present a highly influential critique of connectionist theories based on integrate-and-and fire point neurons, with an emphasis on their inability to represent combinatorial syntactic and semantic linguistic structure (Section 6.5).

24. For an impressive attempt to explain distinctively human cognitive capabilities by relating them to the total number of neurons, see Herculano-Houzel (2017).

25. Gidon and colleagues (2020) report extensive investigations of pyramidal cells from layer 2/3 of human neocortex and suggest that such neurons may provide a cellular mechanism for the computation of RF properties that cannot be computed by single integrate-and-fire point neurons.

26. Kim and colleagues (2017) review regional variations in the densities of different inhibitory interneurons.

27. Adeel et al., 2022; Adeel et al., 2023.

10

Mind's Place in Nature

The research summarized in this book offers a new perspective on deep, enduring, and unresolved philosophical issues of central importance to human mental life, independently of any knowledge of, or theories about, neuronal function. These questions concern knowledge and doubt, self-identity, and purpose in life. Though they are not centre stage moment-by-moment, they run implicitly throughout our daily lives. Shakespeare's plays dramatize these issues exceptionally well, as shown be their enduring appeal to different cultures throughout the world. Shakespeare was strongly influenced by sceptical humanist philosopher Michel de Montaigne, as shown by Colin McGinn (2006), who argues that these three issues are central to Shakespeare's philosophy.

10.1 Knowledge and Doubt

In human minds, Nature has some knowledge of itself. In 1862 the American poet Emily Dickinson wrote

> The Brain—is wider than the Sky— For—put them side by side
> The one the other will contain With ease—and you beside.

Without knowing it, mindless forms of life changed the earth's climate a few billion years ago by greatly increasing the amount of oxygen in the atmosphere. Now, by an explosive rate of reproduction, humans are changing the climate, but only *we* know it. Any adequate management of global warming requires global cooperation, but as the computational capabilities of potential collaborators increases then so does the difficulty of overcoming the obstacles to their collaboration. As their cognitive capabilities increase, they become more able to see ways of increasing short-term benefits for themselves. We must therefore hope that our understanding of the long-term benefits of global cooperation will soon be sufficient to adequately counteract the attractions of short-term selfish benefits.

The Cooperative Neuron. William A. Phillips, Oxford University Press. © Oxford University Press 2023.
DOI: 10.1093/oso/9780198876984.003.0011

However, presumed knowledge comes with doubt, which applies just as much to our daily lives as to global issues. Therefore, how confident can we be in whatever we think we know, and to what extent is scepticism justified? We can take it for granted that perceptual systems are usually trustworthy in that they are well suited to the organism's needs and ecological niche. The multi-disciplinary investigations summarized in this book show how that object-ivity can be flexibly modified to suit the current situation and goals without compromising the validity of the information abstracted from the current sensory data. The delight that we take in direct sensuous experience of the external world is a clear reflection of that objectivity, and of the limitations of imagination. There would be no point in looking at a red sky at night, or in attending to familiar works of art or music, if we could recreate the same sensory experience from within.

Our phenomenal awareness of sensory data is usually reliable (Section 5.3), and includes sensitivity to an amount of sensory information that is far greater than we can imagine or briefly keep in mind (as shown by the evidence for sensory storage; see Section 5.5). We now know that context-sensitivity can in principle guide both learning and processing without compromising the objectivity of the information transmitted (Chapter 8). If subjective context is mediated by apical dendrites then the ability to distinguish it from objective reality may be exceptionally well developed in humans, because their apical dendrites can be more effectively isolated from the soma than in other species (Subsection 6.1.3; Section 9.7).

One way in which context-sensitive cooperative computation makes a major contribution to our insight into objective reality is via its enhance-ment of supramodal abstractions that are 'closer' to external realities than the modality-specific information that we receive from them. Consensus between information arising from highly disparate sources witnesses more than the sum of each alone. The intuitive understanding of this simple observation gives rise to the ancient notion of the *sensus communis* in which the different sensory modalities are combined to reach a common sense decision. Context sensitivity at a cellular level contributes to that by cross-modal amplification of unimodal information (Section 5.2 and Figure 5.4).

Thus, scientific evidence supports the everyday assumption of objectivity that we take for granted in our everyday lives. Nevertheless, and more im-portantly, I draw from the evidence for cooperative neurons that personal subjective contributions to our direct experience of external events are un-avoidable. Earlier chapters show how there is some subjectivity in all realism— as Nietzsche put it (somewhat over-dramatically), 'There are no such things as facts, only interpretations'. We are personally involved in our perception of the external world. We can attend and respond to only a small selected fraction of the sensory information available at any moment and we interpret that from our own point of view. There are many involuntary effects of stimulus context on how we perceive sensory data. For example, humans and chimpanzees both perceive the size of a portion of food as being, in part, relative to the size of the plate. Putting it on a smaller plate makes it appear larger, which is a version of the contextual guidance of size perception (Figure 6.3).[1] Another subjective contribution to our experience of the external world concerns the emotional context within which it occurs, for, as Hamlet said, 'there is nothing either good or bad but thinking makes it so' (2.2.247–248). The anatomical and physiological evidence clearly indicates that emotional evaluation, perception, and learning are all closely intertwined at the level of cooperative neurons (Section 5.6).

We can therefore be confident that, because perception and learning are so highly context sensitive, different people experience and remember the same events from their own perspectives, which can be very different. It may be that they experienced that event in very different ways initially, which is particularly likely to be the case if the event had very different emotional implications for them.

Objectivity of our direct experience of the external world is also strictly limited to the information transmitted—although it may be the 'truth', it cannot be the 'whole truth'. As is often said 'absence of evidence is not evidence of absence'. Twentieth-century atomic and particle physics shows us that the *reality* of physical things is very different from our *experience* of them. Having initially started university as a physics student, I still expect theories to reveal aspects of things that differ greatly from our own direct experience of them. Therefore, I feel reassured, rather than discomforted, by theories of the cellular foundations of mental life that sometimes differ in basic ways from my own direct experience and intuitive expectations.

Given the crucial role of imagination in human mental life, it is necessary to consider its relation to the objective aspects of perception and to the function of apical dendrites. The evidence indicates three distinct modes of apical function: apical amplification, apical drive, and apical isolation (Chapter 4). Though we rarely confuse waking states with dreaming, dreaming is typically confused with the waking state, and has been interpreted here as a paradigmatic example of experiences created from within in a way that involves apical drive. Hobson, Hong, and Friston (2014) show this interpretation to be compatible with the free energy theory principle, which is reassuring, as there is plenty of other empirical support for that principle, if not for the hypothesis of prediction error coding.

Thus, the evidence for cooperative context-sensitive cells indicates that imagination is the creation from within of experiences that have much in common with the perception of external reality. However, there is one crucial way in which that evidence contradicts a common assumption about internally generated experience. It is widely claimed that imagined experiences, whether they occur when awake or asleep, are as vivid as direct perceptual experience. However, the difference between the vast amount of information that is briefly stored within the primary sensory systems and the small amount that can be kept in working memory contradicts those claims. Furthermore, my own study of the ratings by psychology students of the vividness of their images showed them to have little objective validity (Section 4.6). It also showed those ratings to be easily modified. When presented with demonstrations that cast doubt on the notion of vivid images, most students changed the rating of the vividness of their own images accordingly.

These considerations imply that creative imagination when awake involves generating perceptual experiences at abstract levels of representation. Many mysteries as to how that is achieved are left unresolved, but if this does involve apical drive that occurs when adrenergic arousal is high, then we are closer to uncovering some answers. It implies that thinking of the creative imagination as daydreaming has some empirical validity.

Distinguishing between knowledge and imagination is most important, and most difficult, when the presumed knowledge concerns other minds. The physical world never tries to deceive us, but other minds sometimes do. Our knowledge of other minds can (in some ways) be more valid than our knowledge of any other external thing because other human minds are surely the closest thing in the universe to our own minds. However, our attempts to read other minds also result in the ever-present dangers of deliberate deception and of over-confidence in our own interpretation of another person's mind. There is always the danger of a substantial mismatch between the mental events that *did* generate a person's overt behaviour and the mental events that an observer *supposes* to have generated them. That danger is particularly great when the events are complex or heavily laden with emotion. Deliberate deception, though not common, may do great harm when it does occur. According to McGinn, many of Shakespeare's greatest plays present deliberate deception as one of the most serious of all human vices in that it undermines the interpersonal trust on which the essentially cooperative nature of human life depends. So, given the importance and difficulty of knowing other minds, it is no surprise that this is a central aspect of cognitive development (Chapter 6) and of neuropsychiatric disorders (Chapter 7).

Finally, consensus between people helps us to distinguish things in which we can be confident from those that we should doubt (Section 5.5.14). Science is a cooperative enterprise in which consensus is sought on the interpretation of observations that are as diverse and as objective as we can make them.[2]

10.2 Self-identity

To what extent is self-identity fixed, and to what extent adaptable? A person's genome is fixed, but a genome is not a person. We do have some enduring traits, abilities, and disabilities, but they are far from being the only things that influence the course of our lives. Fortune, both good and bad, is also a major influence. Furthermore, conceptions of neuroconstructivism within developmental psychology, with which the evidence for context-sensitive cooperative neurons is highly compatible, implies that self-development is a journey, not a destination (Section 6.4).

At both psychological and cellular levels, those aspects of our self-identity that are expressed at any moment are strongly dependent on context. We play different roles in different circumstances in the sense that we tend to act as we think we *should* act in those circumstances. This is often described as implying an essentially theatrical notion of self-identity, which entails a lack of authenticity only if those actions conflict with how the person *believes* they should act in those circumstances, but chooses not to. The contexts that guide processing and learning at the level of neocortical pyramidal cells are a heterogeneous mixture of impersonal external influences and personal internal influences. Although not intuitively obvious, only some of those internal influences are under voluntary control. Internal and external contextual influences are intertwined at a level of processing within pyramidal cells to which we have no direct conscious access. The importance and heterogeneity of those contextual influences have only recently started to become clear to neuroscience.[3] Semantic and episodic memories presumably contribute to that contextual input, so the context that amplifies selected signals varies from person to person, and moment to moment. At the cellular level, it is also locally specific in space and time.

Some psychiatrists suggest that a normal sense of self arises in part from the consistency with which internal knowledge is used as a context that guides the processing of sensory input. Psychoses, such as schizophrenia, are then interpreted as involving disruption in that sense of self.[4] Self-identity is thus seen as an enduring viewpoint from which the world is experienced. However, I see no evidence for a single enduring 'self' in the context that guides processing and learning at a cellular level, even though it may be that some of its components are long lasting and common to many of the locally specific contexts.

Another key inference is that, as perfect coherence between all that we know, believe, intend, and hope is impossible, we must expect (and learn to live with) cognitive dissonance. The context-sensitive cellular mechanisms do indeed cooperate in a way that tends to increase coherence and reduce incoherence, but those effects are strictly local in space and time. They do not (and cannot) take everything that might be relevant into account. The devil's pitchfork (Figure 5.1) provides a simple example. The locally coherent pictorial cues to a three-dimensional shape keep operating, even though they are not coherent overall. Furthermore, you know that this is not a three-dimensional shape but simply a two-dimensional set of lines contrived to look like an impossible three-dimensional object. That knowledge, however, does not prevent the persistent attempts of your perceptual system to make sense of the whole as a three-dimensional structure, given the local coherence.

Limitations on the extent to which we can expect perfect coherence in our mental lives does not imply that mental processes are necessarily irrational. On the contrary; they suggest that they can be seen to be more rational if viewed as bounded by the local contexts within which they occur (Section 5.1).

We can also infer that the mental lives of different people will be highly diverse because perception, thought, and action are all open to such a wide range of contextual influences. Different people live in different circumstances, have different options, and make different compromises between incompatible beliefs and between conflicting goals. The unique history of each person's life is replete with the effects of chance and marginal decisions that could easily have been otherwise, but that, once taken, could not be reversed. The context-sensitive cooperative computational capabilities that expand the diversity to which this leads helps us create, adapt, and pursue our own personal goals. A simple implication of the evidence for these fundamental differences between people is that we should expect, respect, and—indeed—revel in them.

A related set of unresolved but unavoidable problems concerns relations between personal freedom, social organization, and the allocation of responsibility. Are we free to choose between alternative possible percepts, thoughts, and actions? Of all the problems that philosophers have considered, the problem of 'free will' is one of the most challenging. Many theological debates, wars, and other conflicts have, to a significant extent, centred around free will.

There is no consensus on how it is best resolved, and no final resolution is proposed here. Nevertheless, the perspective advocated here suggests some working assumptions. First, though much of perception given a particular pattern of sensory input is not open to our voluntary control, we do have a substantial amount of voluntary control over the sensory input to which we expose ourselves. Second, as regards freedom of thought, there is a sense in which the evidence for context-sensitive cooperative computation can be seen as supporting Sartre's startling claim that 'Man is condemned to be free'. From the viewpoint of context-sensitive neuronal activity, voluntary decisions can provisionally be considered to involve selective amplification of subsets of context-sensitive activities that maximize their mutual agreement and minimize their disagreement. The integrated contextual inputs to apical dendrites and the integrated feedforward inputs to basal dendrites are each a nonlinear sum of many separate input signals. In apical dendrites, these inputs come from many highly diverse sources that, to a large extent, can vary independently. There are recurrent nonlinear interactions between the different cells such that the contextual input to each can be indirectly influenced by a large fraction of the other cells, if they are active (Section 9.5). All this implies that, whether deterministic or not, the outcome of all those processes is not reliably predictable and depends not on any one cell alone but on many of them operating in a coordinated way. Thus, if we think of ourselves as being that which generated the mental activity and behaviours that occurred, we are no more slaves to our cooperative neurons than we are to our genes. As the banks of a river guide the flow that modifies the banks, so context-sensitive cooperative interactions guide the flow of neuronal activity that modifies those interactions. Thus, widespread thalamocortical activity is involved in what we choose to think and do, and what we choose has major consequences for who we become.

Bob Doyle clearly describes the dilemmas underlying the common-sense notion of free will (https://informationphilosopher.com/books/Free_Will_2 016.pdf), and shows errors in arguments against it. They include the argument that if determinism is true then there is no freedom and that if determinism is false then events are due to chance, so cannot be willed. Doyle shows how that dilemma can be resolved, and personal responsibility preserved, by combining limited indeterminism in the choices that are available with adequate determinism in choosing between those alternatives. This leads to a two-stage, free-then-will notion of voluntary decision making which he sees as building on prior views of philosophers such as Aristotle, William James, and Daniel Dennett.

In essence, that two-stage free-then-will resolution resonates strongly with the neurobiological and psychological evidence reviewed in this book. The two stages have much in common with the pre- and post-attentive processing stages in vision (Figure 5.5). Furthermore, there is evidence that pre-attentive processing is predominant at lower levels of the neocortical hierarchy and attentive processing becomes of increasing importance as that hierarchy is ascended. Thus, on that interpretation, the adequately determined willed choices are more concerned with the higher, more abstract levels of processing than with the lower, more detailed sensorimotor levels of processing. That conclusion is compatible with common sense. Thus, research on cooperative context-sensitive neural computation offers philosophers a new and promising perspective from which to consider free will.

Philosopher Daniel Dennett (2004) argues that people's freedoms depend on cooperative social organization. Individuals have more choices in well-organized societies. Thus, from that point of view, it is not freedom *from* social organization that is to be cherished, but freedom *through* social organization. So, does the evidence for cooperative neurons bear on this issue, and if so, how? This could in part be investigated by relating cooperative neurons to the theory of morality as cooperation. We can also ask whether context sensitivity in any sense increases the 'freedom' with which cooperative cells operate. Perhaps it does—at least in the sense that sensitivity to a rich and unpredictably varying context reduces the extent to which the cell's output is rigidly determined by its basal input.

It may seem that political theory and social policy should be founded on the sovereignty of the individual, with that view being justified by interpreting evidence from evolutionary biology as implying the 'survival of the fittest in a competition between individuals'. In apparent contrast to that view evolutionary biologists, ethologists, and geneticists are all well aware that cooperation is common throughout all levels of biological organization, from genes to societies. Though he is most famous for his emphasis upon selfishness, Richard Dawkins is well-aware that genes must be cooperative. He says that the title of his book *The Selfish Gene* could equally well have been *The Cooperative Gene*, because genes operate as cartels of mutually compatible cooperating genes.[5] However, the title of this book could not have been *The Selfish Neuron*. Life, brain, and mind are marvels of cooperation, not triumphs of selfishness. At the level of genes and neurons the notion of cooperation is meaningful, but the notion of 'selfishness' is not. If organisms inherit tendencies to avoid enhancing short-term individual gain at the expense of the long-term benefit of the species, then that will improve the long-term prospects of the species. This is particularly important in species (e.g. humans) with cognitive abilities that enable them to see many ways of enhancing short-term individual gain. The negative connotations of the word 'selfishness' can then be seen as referring to actions that deny our inherited tendencies to be cooperative. These connotations of 'selfishness' do not apply to either cells or genes.

The individual cells of a single organism are necessarily team players for the simple reason that they share identical genes, so cooperation between them is an example of 'kin selection' par excellence. Nevertheless, a form of cooperation in which cells know about and cooperate with others while maintaining rich and individual identities that transcend anything known to their genes is very different from cooperation that is imposed by obedience to a totalitarian authority. The emphasis on cooperative interactions in which individuals develop and enhance their individuality through cooperation echoes long-lasting and widespread intuitions concerning the importance of mutually beneficial social interactions. In the African philosophy of Ubuntu this is expressed by saying 'I am because we are', which contrasts neatly with the individualism expressed by Descartes's starting point of 'I think, therefore I am'.

This emphasis on deep-rooted tendencies towards cooperation resonates with a recent conception of morality as cooperation, which sees our tendency to be biased towards cooperation with others as biological and cultural ways of reaping the benefits of cooperation at a social level. Although still in the early stages of development, that conception has been shown to have firm grounds in evolutionary biology, game theory, genetics, ethology, and anthropology.[6] Examples of cooperative interactions commonly seen in humans and some other species are identified as allocation of resources to kin, coordination to mutual advantage, reciprocal social exchanges, non-destructive conflict resolution, fair division of resources, and property rights. As those cooperative interactions must surely involve decisions made by the neocortex, we can now ask whether and how these cooperative interactions between individuals involve cooperation between the neocortical pyramidal cells that have a key role in generating their behaviour.

These considerations suggest that it is important to distinguish between voluntary cooperation and cooperation that does not involve freedom of choice. As cognitive capabilities evolve, so will the opportunities for individuals to cooperate in novel ways to meet novel circumstances; but so will the ability of individuals to see opportunities for private profit. The evidence for morality as cooperation may therefore reflect the evolution of mechanisms that to some extent bias voluntary social interactions towards cooperation when it conflicts with opportunities for private selfish profit.[7] If so, we need to discover what specifies the extent of that bias, how it operates, and whether it involves the mechanisms by which the activity of selected neocortical pyramidal cells is amplified when in harmony with the context of neural activity elsewhere, including the sensory and perceptual mechanisms by which they receive information about other minds.

To see how context sensitivity may have implications for responsibility consider issues that arise if our mental lives must tolerate some degree of incoherence. Some impulsive acts occur before there is time to think about them, so they may be regretted in retrospect. Where does responsibility for those acts lie? From a legal point of view, it could be argued that, on the condition that they have adequate cognitive capabilities, adults should have acquired the ability to suppress impulses known to be illegal or immoral. Those cognitive capabilities surely involve the neocortex, so is the whole neocortex responsible for the decisions taken, or only parts of it? The possibility of mediated contextual interactions suggests (what seems to me) a plausible attitude towards this question. No cell can receive direct inputs from more than a tiny proportion of other neocortical cells. Nevertheless, individual pyramidal cells can be indirectly influenced by a much larger proportion via contextual effects that are mediated by active intermediaries (Chapter 9). Thus, given time to think about it, a large part of what the neocortex knows, believes, and intends can be brought to bear on the activity of all or many of the neocortical cells involved in the decision taken. As they operate in a way that seeks coherence, their activities can be considered as constituting a joint enterprise. Thus, this is compatible with holding the whole person responsible for their actions.

However, adequate cognitive capabilities are a key part of the prevailing conditions, and they are clearly constrained by various psychopathologies in which context sensitivity and apical function are impaired. For example, impulse control is weak in several pathologies, such as foetal alcohol spectrum disorders (Chapter 7). Presumably, some of the responsibility in such cases lies with maternal drinking, but, more importantly, it also lies with societal practices that encourage that drinking.

In contrast to societal practices that are harmful to mental life, there are also many that are wholesome, including practices that promote calm equanimity and the reduction of mental stress. Various meditative traditions teach ways of cultivating states of mind that increase coherence while reducing mental conflict and suffering. Both cortical and subcortical contributions to mental state are involved in these practices. The neocortex is involved because it is the main stage upon which conscious experience is played. Subcortical contributions are also involved because they regulate the relative effectiveness of information from internal and external sources in the generation of that conscious experience. Although some of the benefits of these practices require many years of training, some can be reaped from shorter investments of time and effort. For example, I have learned the simple lesson that, as minds are highly sensitive to stimulus contexts as well as to internal contexts, the ability to focus on difficult internally specified tasks (such as reading complex scientific or philosophical papers) can be greatly increased by the simple expedient of avoiding as many potential distractions as possible (such as background music or other salient stimulus events). These long-established practices indicate that a healthy mental life does not require the preservation of a fixed self-image. As teachers of those meditative practices sometimes say, 'no self, no problem'. From that perspective, individual freedom can be conceived of as a freedom from habit and coercion that evolves in interaction with the environment on both short and long timescales, but with responsibility for the way in which its exercise affects other lives.

10.3 Life's Purposes

Issues concerning purpose in life are the most insoluble of all. No more is attempted here than to note some perspectives on these issues that are encouraged by the research outlined in this book—a patchwork quilt of arguments and evidence drawn from many different disciplines and sewn together in a way that seamlessly connects what psychology tells us about minds to what neuroscience tells us about brains. Much of that territory connecting brains and minds has not yet been explored in detail, but some possible paths through it are now visible.

One obvious conclusion drawn from this patchwork quilt is that different purposes are seen in life if considered from different perspectives. From the viewpoint of evolutionary biology and genetics, preservation of the germ line and its ever-expanding distribution may seem to be an ultimate purpose. Others are suggested by the viewpoint advocated here. They include reducing mental suffering and cognitive dissonance, developing a coherent understanding of events, and advancing towards goals that are coherent and meaningful, both personally and socially.

Personal purposes are obviously highly dependent on the current context, and particularly on the current state of mind, so they can vary greatly over time and circumstance. It is perhaps partly because of this that all human cultures inform personal purposes by conceptions of purposes that extend beyond self-interest. One way of looking for purpose that extends beyond self-interest is by asking whether any purpose can be discerned in the long-term history of life. This can be rephrased as one of the most vexed questions in all of biology: is evolution progressive? In relation to the aspects of mental life discussed here this question can be given concrete form: has the effectiveness of apical function evolved? If so, in what way does that imply progress? Does it involve progress toward an objectivity that is more objective, toward a subjectivity that is more effectively creative, or toward an increase in individual freedom because more complex organisms have more options from which to select? If any or all of these are so, as implied by earlier chapters, it strengthens belief in progressive aspects of the evolution of life on earth. Darwin assumed that there were while insisting that his theory did not imply that progress is either ubiquitous or inevitable.[8] If it is neither, as Darwin also assumed, then its occurrence here on earth and its progressive enhancements are of even greater value. Furthermore, though the evidence clearly shows that there have been progressive aspects to the history of life on Earth, it also shows that history to be a journey without any signs of having a destination.

Another way of looking for purposes that extend beyond short-term self-interest is by considering the analogy between the importance of an appropriate balance between order and disorder in society and between order and disorder in the brain. The difficulty of finding and securing that balance within society is made manifest in the variations that range across time and place from beliefs based on order imposed by some ruler or government to beliefs in a laissez-faire individualistic market economy. Carried to their extremes, both conceptions of society have bad outcomes, but there is endless debate about where and how the balance should be drawn (Williams, 1961). One thing that seems clear is that neither extreme can be justified. Too much order leads towards the stability and sterility of a crystal, and too much disorder leads towards the decay and eventual collapse of the marvels of organization by which life has arisen and flourished (despite the ever-present forces of noise and disorder). The abstract issue underlying these debates is that of how complex living systems composed of many diverse individuals can be organized in the interests of one and all. That abstract issue is relevant to the evidence for context-sensitive cooperative neurons and the theory of coherent infomax because they imply that, by blind evolutionary search through a vast space of possibilities, nature has slowly found a way of reconciling order and disorder in the neocortex. Whether we can find a way of reconciling them within a society of cooperative individuals by imaginative design grown from some understanding of the deep issues involved will be known, if at all, only in the unforeseeable future.

The view of mental life presented here implies that it seeks to reduce mental conflict and to increase the coherence between its many highly differentiated activities. Coherent infomax made that abstract objective precise by expressing it as maximizing the three-way mutual information between the context, the information transmitted, and the output of the local processors of which neocortex is composed (Section 8.3). This explicitly defined objective is sufficiently abstract to encompass many of our own personal goals as well as broader conceptions of human flourishing. That resonates with the widespread supposition that happiness depends on inner harmony and relational connectedness to others (Fave et al., 2016). Put simply, that objective maintains and enhances organized complexity (i.e. life), so what merit is there in that? Although the intrinsic value of life is taken for granted by most people, we are also often encouraged to suppose that life is common throughout the universe. The most special thing about life on Earth, it is that it exists. Life is so highly improbable that we have still not found out how it began. Whatever the events were by which life began on earth, however, they seem highly improbable because they have happened once and once only throughout the whole of Earth's long history. Furthermore, life depends on a molecule with unique properties, H_2O, and on that being in a liquid state that it becomes only within a narrow window of temperatures and pressures. Even that apparently simple requirement for life is not easily met! The requirements of life beyond that simple starting point are even harder to meet, so there are good grounds for supposing that, though many forms of life have evolved on Earth, life as we know it may be rare (or even absent) elsewhere in the galaxy.[9]

Mental life with the epistemological and creative capabilities that are manifest in humans is even more improbable. It took more than four billion years to evolve on earth even given those favourable conditions. As eminent physicist Enrico Fermi asked, if intelligent life is common in the galaxy, where is everybody?[10] Life is rare in the universe—especially mental life. We can safely assume that the prospects for our part of the cosmos are known only to us, so therefore only we can take any responsibility for them.

None of these abstract considerations usurp our own purposes in life, of course. They must be personal and pursued within our own specific circumstances. For me, writing this book became a central and challenging purpose—pursued as part of a broad cooperative effort. In addition to the host of people involved in acquiring the empirical data and in developing concepts central to the view presented, many of them provided helpful comments on various sections of the book as they were being drafted. Thus, this book itself is an example of the organized complexity that can be produced by the cooperative enterprise that it extols.

Notes

1. Parrish and Beran (2014) show that humans and chimpanzees eat less if it is on a smaller plate.
2. Harari (2011) shows that consensus on some 'imagined' things, such as the value of money and national identity, can be seen as underlying much of human history.
3. Schuman et al., 2021.
4. Helmsley, 1998.
5. Dawkins, 2016, pp. 346–347.
6. A view of morality as cooperation is proposed by Curry et al., 2019. Rigorous and extensive reviews of the evolution of cooperation lead to similar conclusions (Sussman and Cloninger, 2011; Richerson and colleagues, 2021).
7. Ridley (1996) presents grounds for supposing that the origins of human virtue and morality involve inherited and acquired tendencies to cooperate. Rilling and colleagues (2002) identify specific cortical regions that are associated with reciprocal altruism, such as that involved in food sharing in humans.
8. Gruber, 1974, p. 371.
9. Conway Morris, 2003.
10. https://www.space.com/25325-fermi-paradox.html.

List of Abbreviations

5-HT	serotonin
ACh	acetylcholine
AI	artificial intelligence
BAC	backpropagation-activated calcium spike
bAP	back-propagated action potential
BOLD	blood oxygen-level-dependent
Ca	calcium
CF	contextual field
CT	cortico-thalamic
DA	dopamine
EEG	electroencephalograph
FASD	foetal alcohol spectrum disorder
FB	feedback
FF	feedforward
GABA	gamma amino butyric acid
HA	histamine
HCN	hyperpolarization-activated cyclic nucleotide-gated
I_h	deactivating electric current flow (I) through HCN ion channels
IT	intra-telencephalic
K	potassium
LFP	local field potential
MEG	Magnetoencephalography
MT	visual motion area
NA	noradrenaline (aka NE)
Na	sodium
NE	norepinephrine (aka NA)
NGF	neurogliaform
NMDA	N-methyl-D-aspartate
OFC	orbitofrontal cortex
PCP	phencyclidine
PFC	prefrontal cortex
PID	partial information decomposition
PT	pyramidal tract
PV	parvalbumin
RAS	reticular activating system
REM	rapid eye movement
RF	receptive field

SOM	somatostatin positive (aka SST)
SST	somatostatin positive (aka SOM)
STDP	spike-time dependent plasticity
SWS	slow-wave sleep
TMS	transcranial magnetic stimulation
VIP	vasoactive intestinal peptide positive
VSSP	visuospatial sketchpad

Bibliography

Abdallah, C. G., Averill, L. A., Krystal, J. H., Southwick, S. M., & Arnsten, A. F. (2016). Glutamate and norepinephrine interaction: Relevance to higher cognitive operations and psychopathology. *The Behavioral and Brain Sciences*, *39*, e201.

Adeel, A. (2020). Conscious multisensory integration: Introducing a universal contextual field in biological and deep artificial neural networks. *Frontiers in Computational Neuroscience*, *14*, 15. https://doi.org/10.3389/fncom.2020.00015

Adeel, A., Raza, M. Franco, M., & Ahmed K. (2022). Context-sensitivity transforms the effectiveness and efficiency of neural information processing. *Arxiv* [preprint], 15 July. https://arxiv.org/abs/2211.01950

Adeel, A., Adetomi, A., Ahmed, K., Hussain, A., Arslan, T., & Phillips, W. A. (2023). Unlocking the potential of two-point cells for energy-efficient and resilient training of deep nets. *IEEE Transactions on Emerging Topics in Computational Intelligence* (in press).

Adesnik, H., Bruns, W., Taniguchi, H., Huang, Z. J., & Scanziani, M. (2012). A neural circuit for spatial summation in visual cortex. *Nature*, *490*, 226–231.

Airenti, G., & Plebe A. (2017). Editorial: Context in communication: A cognitive view. *Frontiers in Psychology*, *8*, 115. https://doi.org/10.3389/fpsyg.2017.00115

Almeida, V. N. (2022). The neural hierarchy of consciousness: A theoretical model and review on neurophysiology and NCCs. *Neuropsychologia*, *169*, 108202.

Amsalem, O., Eyal, G., Rogozinski, N., Gevaert, M., Pramod, P., Schürmann, F., & Segev, I. (2020). An efficient analytical reduction of detailed nonlinear neuron models. *Nature Communications*, *11*, 1–13. https://doi.org/10.1038/s41467-019-13932-6

Amunts, K., & Zilles, K. (2015). Architectonic mapping of the human brain beyond Brodmann. *Neuron*, *88*, 1086–1107. dx.doi.org/10.1016/j.neuron.2015.12.001

Anderson, K. M., Collins, M. A., Chin, R., Ge, T., Rosenberg, M. D., & Holmes, A. J. (2020). Transcriptional and imaging-genetic association of cortical interneurons, brain function, and schizophrenia risk. *Nature Communications*, *11*(1), 1–15.

Anticevic, A, Corlett, P. R., Cole, M. W., Savic, A., Gancsos, M., Tang, Y., Repovs, G., Murray, J. D., Driesen, N. R., Morgan, P. T., Xu, K., Wang, F., & Krystal, J. H. (2015). N-methyl-D-aspartate receptor antagonist effects on prefrontal cortical connectivity better model early than chronic schizophrenia. *Biological Psychiatry*, *77*(6), 569–580. https://doi.org/10.1016/j.biopsych.2014.07.022

Arbib, M. A., & Erdi, P. (2000). Precis of neural organization: Structure, function, and dynamics. *Behavioral and Brain Sciences*, *23*, 513–571.

Arnsten, A. F. T. (2009). Stress signaling pathways that impair prefrontal cortex structure and function. *Nature Reviews Neuroscience*, *10*(6), 410–422. https://doi.org/10.1038/nrn2648

Arnsten, A. F. T. (2015). Stress weakens prefrontal networks: Molecular insults to higher cognition. *Nature Neuroscience*, *18*, 1376–1385. https://doi.org/10.1038/nn.4087

Arnsten, A. F., Wang, M. J., & Paspalas, C. D. (2012). Neuromodulation of thought: Flexibilities and vulnerabilities in prefrontal cortical network synapses. *Neuron*, *76*(1), 223–239.

Aru, J., Suzuki, M., Rutiku, R., Larkum, M. E., & Bachmann, T. (2019). Coupling the state and contents of consciousness. *Frontiers in Systems Neuroscience*, *13*, 43.

Aru, J., Suzuki, M., & Larkum, M. E. (2020a). Cellular mechanisms of conscious processing? *Trends in Cognitive Sciences, 24,* 814–825.

Aru, J., Siclari, F., Phillips, W. A., & Storm, J. (2020b). Apical drive: A cellular mechanism of dreaming? *Neuroscience and Biobehavioral Reviews, 119,* 440–455. doi.org/10.1016/j.neubiorev.2020.09.018

Aston-Jones, G., & Cohen, J. D. (2005). An integrative theory of locus coeruleus norepinephrine function: Adaptive gain and optimal performance. *Annual Review of Neuroscience, 28,* 403–450.

Atkinson, S. E., & Williams, S. R. (2009). Postnatal development of dendritic synaptic integration in rat neocortical pyramidal neurons. *Journal of Neurophysiology, 102,* 735–751.

Baddeley, A. (2012). Working memory: Theories, models, and controversies. *Annual Review of Psychology, 63,* 1–29. http://dx.doi.org/10.1146/ annurev-psych-120710-100422

Bachmann, T. (2015). How a (sub)cellular coincidence detection mechanism featuring layer 5 pyramidal cells may help produce various visual phenomena. *Frontiers in Psychology* [online], 6, Article 1947. https://doi.org/10.3389/fpsyg.2015.01947

Bachmann, T., & Hudetz, A. G. (2014). It is time to combine the two main traditions in the research on the neural correlates of consciousness: C = L × D. *Frontiers in Psychology* [online], 5, 940. https://doi.org/10.3389/fpsyg.2014.00940

Bachmann, T., Suzuki, M., & Aru, J. (2020). Dendritic integration theory: A thalamocortical theory of state and content of consciousness. *Philosophy and the Mind Sciences, 1*(II), 2. https://doi.org/10.33735/phimisci.2020.II.52

Baker, A., Kalmbach, B., Morishima, M., Kim, J., Juavinett, A., Li, N., & Dembrow, N. (2018). Specialized subpopulations of deep-layer pyramidal neurons in the neocortex: Bridging cellular properties to functional consequences. *Journal of Neuroscience, 38,* 5441–5455.

Barendregt, H., & Raffone, A. (2013). Conscious cognition as a discrete, deterministic, and universal Turing Machine process. In B. Cooper & J. van Leeuwen (Eds.), *Alan Turing: His work and impact* (pp. 92–97). Elsevier.

Barendregt, H., & Raffone, A. (2022). Axiomatizing consciousness with applications. In N. Jansen, M. Stoelinga, & P. van den Bos (Eds.), *A journey from process algebra via timed automata to model learning: Essays dedicated to Frits Vaandrager on the occasion of his 60th Birthday* (pp. 46–62). Springer.

Barinka, F., Magloczky, Z., & Zecevic, N. (2015). Editorial: At the top of the interneuronal pyramid-calretinin expressing cortical interneurons. *Frontiers in Neuroanatomy, 9,* 108.

Baron-Cohen, S., & Lombardo, M. V. (2017). Autism and talent: The cognitive and neural basis of systemizing. *Dialogues in Clinical Neuroscience, 19,* 345.

Barth, A. M., Vizi, E. S., Zelles, T., & Lendvai, B. (2008). α2-Adrenergic receptors modify dendritic spike generation via HCN channels in the prefrontal cortex. *Journal of Neurophysiology, 99*(1), 394–401.

Bastos, A. M., Loonis, R., Kornblith, S., Lundqvist, M., & Miller, E. K. (2018). Laminar recordings in frontal cortex suggest distinct layers for maintenance and control of working memory. *Proceedings of the National Academy of Sciences of the United States of America, 115,* 1117–1122.

Beaulieu-Laroche, L., Toloza1, E. H. S., van der Goes, M.-S., Lafourcade, M., Barnagian, D., Eskandar, E. N., Frosch, M. P., Cash, S. S., & Harnett, M. T. (2018). Enhanced dendritic compartmentalization in human cortical neurons. *Cell, 175,* 643–651. doi.org/10.1016/j.cell.2018.08.045

Becker, S., & Hinton, G. E. (1992). Self-organizing neural network that discovers surfaces in random-dot stereograms. *Nature, 355,* 161–163.

Beecher, M. D. (2021). Why are no animal communication systems simple languages? *Frontiers in Psychology*, *12*, 602635. https://doi.org/10.3389/fpsyg.2021.602635

Beniaguev, D., Segev, I., & London, M. (2020). Single cortical neurons as deep artificial neural networks. *bioRxiv* [preprint]. doi.org/10.1101/613141

Bentsen, S. (2020). Fire use. In M. Aldenderfer (EIC), *Oxford research encyclopedia of anthropology* [online], 27 October. doi.org/10.1093/acrefore/9780190854584.013.52

Berényi, A., Belluscio, M., Mao, D., & Buzsáki, G. (2012). Closed-loop control of epilepsy by transcranial electrical stimulation. *Science*, *337*, 735–737. https://doi.org/10.1126/science.1223154

Berger, T., Larkum, M. E., & Lüscher, H. R. (2001). High I(h) channel density in the apical dendrite of layer V pyramidal cells increases bidirectional attenuation of EPSPs. *Journal of Neurophysiology*, *85*, 855–868.

Berger, T., & Lüscher, H. R. (2003). Timing and precision of spike initiation in layer V pyramidal cells of the rat somatosensory cortex. *Cerebral Cortex*, *13*(3), 274–281. https://doi.org/10.1016/j.brainres.2015.11.024

Berger, T., Senn, W., & Lüscher, H. R. (2003). Hyperpolarization-activated current I_h disconnects somatic and dendritic spike initiation zones in layer V pyramidal neurons. *Journal of Neurophysiology*, *90*(4), 2428–2437.

Berridge, C. W., & Spencer, R. C. (2016). Differential cognitive actions of norepinephrine α2 and α1 receptor signaling in the prefrontal cortex. *Brain Research Reviews*, *1641*(Pt B), 189–196. https://doi.org/10.1016/j.brainres.2015.11.024

Biel, M., Wahl-Schott, C., Michalakis, S., & Zong, X. (2009). Hyperpolarization-activated cation channels: From genes to function. *Physiological Reviews*, *89*(3), 847–885.

Bienenstock, E. L., Cooper, L. N., & Munro, P. W. (1982). Theory for the development of neuron selectivity: Orientation specificity and binocular interaction in visual cortex. *Journal of Neuroscience*, *2*(1), 32–48.

Binzegger, T., Douglas, R., & Martin, K. (2004). A quantitative map of the circuit of cat primary visual cortex. *Journal of Neuroscience*, *24*(39), 8441–8453.

Blot, A., Roth, M. M., Gasler, I. T., Javadzadeh, M., Imhof, F., & Hofer, S. B. (2020). Visual intracortical and transthalamic pathways carry distinct information to cortical areas. *BioRxiv* [preprint]. https://doi.org/10.1101/2020.07.06.189902

Boldog, E., Bakken, T. E., Hodge, R. D., Novotny, M., Aevermann, B. D., Baka, J., Bordé, S., Close, J. L., Diez-Fuertes, F., Ding, S.-L., Faragó, N., Kocsis, Á. K., Kovács, B., Maltzer, Z., McCorrison, J. M., Miller, J. A., Molnár, G., Oláh, G., Ozsvár, A., … Tamás, G. (2018). Transcriptomic and morphophysiological evidence for a specialized human cortical GABAergic cell type. *Nature Neuroscience*, *21*, 1185–1195. https://doi.org/10.1038/s41593-018-0205-2

Bonnel, A., McAdams, S., Smith, B., Berthiaume, C., Bertone, A., Ciocca, V., Burack, J. A., & Mottron, L. (2010). Enhanced pure-tone pitch discrimination among persons with autism but not Asperger syndrome. *Neuropsychologia*, *48*(9), 2465–2475. https://doi.org/10.1016/j.neuropsychologia.2010.04.020

Booth, R. and Happé, F. G. E. (2016). Evidence of reduced global processing in autism spectrum disorder. *Journal of Autism and Developmental Disorders*, *48*(4), 1397–1408. https://doi.org/10.1007/s10803-016-2724-6

Boudewijns, Z. S. R. M., Groen, R. M., Lodder, B., Minni, T. B., McMaster, M. T. B., Kalogreades, L., de Haan, R., Narayanan, R. T., Meredith, R. M., Mansvelder, H. D., & de Kock, C. P. J. (2013). Layer-specific high-frequency action potential spiking in the prefrontal cortex of awake rats. *Frontiers in Cellular Neuroscience*, *7*, 99. http://dx.doi.org/10.3389/fncel.2013.00099

Breton-Provencher, V., Drummond, G. T., & Sur, M. (2021). Locus coeruleus norepinephrine in learned behavior: Anatomical modularity and spatiotemporal integration in targets. *Frontiers in Neural Circuits*, *15*, 638007. https://doi.org/10.3389/fncir.2021.638007

Brombas, A., Fletcher, L. N., & Williams, S. R. (2014). Activity-dependent modulation of layer 1 inhibitory neocortical circuits by acetylcholine. *Journal of Neuroscience*, *34*(5), 1932–1941.

Brosch, T., & Neumann, H. (2014a). Computing with a canonical neural circuits model with pool normalization and modulating feedback. *Neural Computation*, *26*, 2735–2789. doi.org/10.1162/NECO_a_00675

Brosch, T., & Neumann, H. (2014b). Interaction of feedforward and feedback streams in visual cortex in a firing-rate model of columnar computations. *Neural Networks*, *54*, 11–16. doi.org/10.1016/j.neunet.2014.02.005

Brown, R. E., Basheer, R., McKenna, J. T., Strecker, R. E., & McCarley, R. W. (2012). Control of sleep and wakefulness. *Physiological Reviews*, *92*, 1087–1187. doi:10.1152/physrev.00032.2011

Burgess, C. R., & Peever, J. H. (2013). A noradrenergic mechanism functions to couple motor behavior with arousal state. *Current Biology*, *23*, 1719–1725. doi.org/10.1016/j.cub.2013.07.014

Butler, P. D., Abeles, I. Y., Silverstein, S. M., Dias, E. C., Weiskopf, N. G., Calderone, D. J., & Sehatpour, P. (2013). An event-related potential examination of contour integration deficits in schizophrenia. *Frontiers in Psychology*, *4*, 132. https://doi.org/10.3389/fpsyg.2013.00132

Byrne, A., & Hilbert, D. R. (2003). Color realism and color science. *Behavioral and Brain Sciences*, *26*, 3–64.

Caldwell, C. A., Renner, E., & Atkinson, M. (2018). Human teaching and cumulative cultural evolution. *Review of Philosophy and Psychology*, *9*(4), 751–770. https://doi.org/10.1007/s13164-017-0346-3.

Calvin, O. L., & Redish, A. D. (2021). Global disruption in excitation-inhibition balance can cause localized network dysfunction and schizophrenia-like context-integration deficits. *PLoS Computational Biology*, *17*(5), e1008985. doi.org/10.1371/journal.pcbi.1008985

Campbell, J. (1982). *Grammatical man: Information, entropy, language, and life*. Simon and Schuster.

Carandini, M., & Heeger, D. J. (2012). Normalization as a canonical neural computation. *Nature Reviews Neuroscience*, *13*, 51–62.

Carhart-Harris, R. L., Leech, R., Hellyer, P. J., Shanahan M., Feilding, A., Tagliazucchi, A., Chialvo, D. R., & Nutt. D. (2014). The entropic brain: A theory of conscious states informed by neuroimaging research with psychedelic drugs. *Frontiers in Human Neuroscience*, *8*(20), 1–22. https://doi.org/10.3389/fnhum.2014.00020

Carr, D. B., Andrews, G. D., Glen, W. B., & Lavin, A. (2007). Alpha2-noradrenergic receptors activation enhances excitability and synaptic integration in rat prefrontal cortex pyramidal neurons via inhibition of HCN currents. *Journal of Physiology*, *584*, 437–450.

Cauller, L. (1995) Layer I of primary sensory neocortex: Where top-down converges upon bottom-up. *Behavioral Brain Research*, *71*, 163–170.

Cauller, L. J., & Connors, B. W. (1994). Synaptic physiology of horizontal afferents to layer I in slices of rat SI neocortex. *Journal of Neuroscience*, *14*(2), 751–762.

Cavanna, A. E., Rickards, H., & Ali, F. (2011). What makes a simple partial seizure complex? *Epilepsy and Behavior*, *22*, 651–658.

Celada, P., Puig, M. V., & Artigas, F. (2013). Serotonin modulation of cortical neurons and networks. *Frontiers in Integrative Neuroscience*, *7*, 2.

Child, N. D., & Benarroch, E. E. (2014). Differential distribution of voltage-gated ion channels in cortical neurons. Implications for epilepsy. *Neurology*, *82*, 989–999. https://doi.org/10.1212/WNL.0000000000000228

Chiu, Y.-C., & Egner, T. (2019). Cortical and subcortical contributions to context-control learning. *Neuroscience and Biobehavioral Reviews, 99*, 33–41.

Christophel, T. B., Klink, P. C., Spitzer, B., Roelfsema, P. R., & Haynes, J. D. (2017) The distributed nature of working memory. Trends in Cognitive Sciences, *21*, 111–124.

Clark, A. (2015). *Surfing uncertainty: Prediction, action, and the embodied mind.* Oxford University Press.

Collins, D. P., Anastasiades, P. G., Marlin, J. J., & Carter, A. G. (2018). Reciprocal circuits linking the prefrontal cortex with dorsal and ventral thalamic nuclei. *Neuron, 98*, 366–379.

Constantinidis, C., Funahashi, S., Lee, D., Murray, J. D., Qi, X. L., Wang, M., & Arnsten, A. F. T. (2018). Persistent spiking activity underlies working memory. *Journal of Neuroscience, 38*, 7020–7028.

Conway Morris, S. (2003). *Life's solution: Inevitable humans in a lonely universe.* Cambridge University Press.

Cossart, R., Dinocourt, C., Hirsch, J.C., Merchan-Perez, A., De Felipe, J., Ben-Ari, Y., Esclapez, M., & Bernard, C. (2001). Dendritic but not somatic GABAergic inhibition is decreased in experimental epilepsy. *Nature Neuroscience, 4*, 52–62.

Courchesne, E., & Pierce, K. (2005). Why the frontal cortex in autism might be talking only to itself: Local over-connectivity but long-distance disconnection. *Current Opinion in Neurobiology, 15*, 225–230.

Crick, F. (1994). *The astonishing hypothesis: The scientific search for the soul.* Scribners.

Crick, F., & Koch, C. (1998). Constraints on cortical and thalamic projections: The no-strong-loops hypothesis. *Nature, 391*, 245–250.

Crutchfield, J. P. (2012). Between order and chaos. *Nature Physics, 8*, 17–24. https://doi.org/10.1038/NPHYS2190

Curry, O. S., Mullins, D. A., & Whitehouse, H. (2019). Is it good to cooperate? Testing the theory of morality-as-cooperation in 60 societies. *Current Anthropology, 60*(1), 47–69.

Curtin, J. J., & Fairchild, B. A. (2003). Alcohol and cognitive control: Implications for regulation of behavior during response conflict. *Journal of Abnormal Psychology, 112*(3), 424–436. https://doi.org/10.1037/0021-843X.112.3.424

Dakin, S., & Frith, U. (2005). Vagaries of visual perception in autism. *Neuron, 48*, 497–507.

Dalmau, J., Lancaster, E., Martinez-Hernandez, E., Rosenfeld, M. R., & Balice-Gordon, R. (2011). Clinical experience and laboratory investigations in patients with anti-NMDAR encephalitis. *Lancet Neurology, 10*, 63–74.

Dawkins, R. (2016). *The selfish gene.* 40th anniversary edition. Oxford University Press.

DeFelipe, J. (2010). *Cajal's butterflies of the soul: Science and art.* Oxford University Press.

DeFelipe, J. (2011). The evolution of the brain, the human nature of cortical circuits, and intellectual creativity. *Frontiers in Neuroanatomy, 5*, 29. https://doi.org/10.3389/fnana.2011.00029

DeFelipe, J. (2015). The anatomical problem posed by brain complexity and size: A potential solution. *Frontiers in Neuroanatomy, 9*, 104. https://doi.org/10.3389/fnana.2015.00104

de Fockert, J., Davidoff, J., Fagot, J., Parron, C., & Goldstein, J. (2007). More accurate size contrast judgements in the Ebbinghaus illusion by a remote culture. *Journal of Experimental Psychology: Human Perception and Performance, 33*, 738–742.

De Giorgio, A., & Granato, A. (2015). Reduced density of dendritic spines in pyramidal neurons of rats exposed to alcohol during early postnatal life. *International Journal of Developmental Neuroscience, 41*, 74–79. https://doi.org/10.1016/j.ijdevneu.2015.01.005

De Meyer, K., & Spratling, M. W. (2009) A model of non-linear interactions between cortical top-down and horizontal connections explains the attentional gating of collinear facilitation. *Vision Research, 49*(5), 553–568.

Dennett, D. C. (2004). *Freedom evolves.* Penguin.

Delle Fave, A., Brdar, I., Wissing, M.P., Araujo, U., Castro Solano, A., Freire, T., Hernández-Pozo, M.D.R., Jose, P., Martos, T., Nafstad, H.E., Nakamura, J., Singh, K., & Soosai-Nathan, L. (2016). Lay definitions of happiness across nations: The primacy of inner harmony and relational connectedness. *Frontiers in Psychology*, *7*, 30. https://doi.org/10.3389/fpsyg.2016.00030

Dembrow, N., & Johnston, D. (2014). Subcircuit-specific neuromodulation in the prefrontal cortex. *Frontiers in Neural Circuits*, *8*, 54. https://doi.org/10.3389/fncir.2014.00054

Deneux, T., Harrell, E. R., Kempf, A., Ceballo, S., Filipchuk, A., & Bathellier, B. (2019). Context-dependent signaling of coincident auditory and visual events in primary visual cortex. *eLife*, *8*, e44006. https://doi.org/10.7554/eLife.44006

Doherty, M. J., Campbell, N. M., Tsuji, H., & Phillips, W. A. (2010). The Ebbinghaus illusion deceives adults but not young children. *Developmental science*, *13*(5), 714–721.

Doherty, M. J., Tsuji, H., & Phillips, W. A. (2008). The context sensitivity of visual size perception varies across cultures. *Perception*, *37*, 1426–1433.

Doron, G, Shin, J. N., Takahashi, N., Drüke, M., Bocklisch, C., Skenderi, S., de Mont, L., Toumazou, M., Ledderose, J., Brecht, M., Naud, R., & Larkum, M. E. (2020). Perirhinal input to neocortical layer 1 controls learning. *Science*, *370*(6523), eaaz3136.

Douglas, R. J., & Martin, K. A. C. (2008). Recurrent neuronal circuits in the neocortex. *Current Biology*, *17*(13), R496.

Edelman, S. (2008). *Computing the mind*. Oxford University Press.

Egner, T., & Hirsch, J. (2005). Cognitive control mechanisms resolve conflict through cortical amplification of task-relevant information. *Nature Neuroscience*, *8*, 1784–1790. https://doi.org/10.1038/nn1594

Eichenbaum, H. (2000). A cortical-hippocampal system for declarative memory. *Nature Reviews Neuroscience*, *1*, 41–50. https://doi.org/10.1038/35036213

Eichenbaum, H. (2017). Prefrontal–hippocampal interactions in episodic memory. *Nature Reviews Neuroscience*, *18*, 547–558. https://doi.org/10.1038/nrn.2017.74

Elliott, M. C., Tanaka, P. M., Schwark, R. W., & Andrade, R. (2018). Serotonin differentially regulates L5 pyramidal cell classes of the medial prefrontal cortex in rats and mice. *eNeuro*, *5*, ENEURO.0305-17.2018.

Elmore, L. C., Ma, W. J., Magnotti, J. F., Leising, K. J., Passaro, A. D., Katz, J. S., & Wright, A. A. (2011). Visual short-term memory compared in rhesus monkeys and humans. *Current Biology*, *21*(11), 975–979. https://doi.org/10.1016/j.cub.2011.04.031

Eyal, G., Verhoog, M. B., Testa-Silva, G., Deitcher, Y., Benavides-Piccione, R., DeFelipe, J., de Kock, C. P. J., Mansvelder, H. D., & Segev, I. (2018). Human cortical pyramidal neurons: From spines to spikes via models. *Frontiers in Cellular Neuroscience*, *12*, 181. https://doi.org/10.3389/fncel.2018.00181

Favorov, O. V., & Ryder, D. (2004). Sinbad: A neocortical mechanism for discovering environmental variables and regularities hidden in sensory input. *Biological Cybernetics*, *90*(3), 191–202.

Feldman, R. S., Meyer, J. S., & Quenzer, L. F. (1997). *Principles of neuropsychopharmacology*. Sinauer Associates.

Finlay, B. L., & Uchiyama R. (2014). Developmental mechanisms channeling cortical evolution. *Trends in Neuroscience*, *38*, 69–76. https://doi.org/10.1016/j.tins.2014.11.004

Firestone, C., & Scholl, B. J. (2016). Cognition does not affect perception: Evaluating the evidence for 'top-down' effects. *Behavioral and Brain Sciences*, *39*, e229. https://doi.org/10.1017/S0140525X15000965

Fletcher, L. N., & Williams, S. R. (2019). Neocortical topology governs the dendritic integrative capacity of layer 5 pyramidal neurons. *Neuron*, *101*, 76–90. doi.org/10.1016/j.neuron.2018.10.048

Fodor, J. A. (1983). *The modularity of mind*. MIT Press.

Fodor, J. A., & Pylyshyn, Z. W. (1988). Connectionism and cognitive architecture: A critical analysis. *Cognition, 28*, 3–72.

Freese, J. L., & Amaral, D. G. (2005). The organization of projections from the amygdala to visual cortical areas TE and V1 in the macaque monkey. *Journal of Comparative Neurology, 486*, 295–317.

Friston, K. J. (2010). The free-energy principle: A unified brain theory? *Nature Reviews Neuroscience, 11*, 127–128.

Frith, C., & Johnstone, E. (2003). *Schizophrenia: A very short introduction*. Oxford University Press.

Frith, U. (2003). *Autism: Explaining the enigma*. Blackwell.

Gazzaley, A., & Nobre, A. C. (2011). Top-down modulation: Bridging selective attention and working memory. *Trends in Cognitive Sciences, 16*, 129–135. doi.org/10.1016/j.tics.2011.11.014

Gelbard-Sagiv, H., Magidov, E., Sharon, H., Hendler, T., & Nir, Y. (2018). Noradrenaline modulates visual perception and late visually evoked activity. *Current Biology, 28*(14), 2239–2249. doi.org/10.1016/j.cub.2018.05.051

Gennari, S. P., MacDonald, M. C., Postle, B. R., & Seidenberg, M. S. (2007). Context-dependent interpretation of words: Evidence for interactive neural processes. *Neuroimage, 35*, 1278–1286.

Gervasoni, D., Lin, S. C., Ribeiro, S., Soares, E. S., Pantoja, J., & Nicolelis, M. A. (2004). Global forebrain dynamics predict rat behavioral states and their transitions. *Journal of Neuroscience, 24*(49), 11137–11147. https://doi.org/10.1523/JNEUROSCI.3524-04.2004

Gidon, A., Zolnik, T. A., Fidzinski, P., Bolduan, F., Papoutsi, A., Poirazi, P., Holtkamp, M., Vida, I., & Larkum, M. E. (2020). Dendritic action potentials and computation in human layer 2/3 cortical neurons. *Science, 367*(6473), 83–87. https://doi.org/10.1126/science.aax6239

Gilbert, C. D., & Sigman, M. (2007). Brain states: Top-down influences in sensory processing. *Neuron, 54*, 677–696.

Godenzini, L., Shai, A. S., & Palmer, L. M. (2022). Dendritic compartmentalization of learning-related plasticity. *eNeuro, 9*(3), ENEURO.0060-22.2022.

Granato, A. (2006). Altered organization of cortical interneurons in rats exposed to ethanol during neonatal life. *Brain Research, 1069*(1), 23–30. https://doi.org/10.1016/j.brainres.2005.11.024

Granato, A., & De Giorgio, A. (2014). Alterations of neocortical pyramidal neurons: Turning points in the genesis of mental retardation. *Frontiers in Pediatrics, 2*, 86. https://doi.org/10.3389/fped.2014.00086

Granato, A., Di Rocco, F., Zumbo, A., Toesca, A., & Giannetti, S. (2003). Organization of cortico-cortical associative projections in rats exposed to ethanol during early postnatal life. *Brain Research Bulletin, 60*(4), 339–344. https://doi.org/10.1016/S0361-9230(03)00052-2

Granato, A., & Merighi, A. (2021). Dendrites of neocortical pyramidal neurons: The key to understand intellectual disability. *Cellular and Molecular Neurobiology, 42*(1), 147–153. https://doi.org/10.1007/s10571-021-01123-1

Granato, A., Palmer, L. M., De Giorgio, A., Tavian, D., & Larkum, M. E. (2012). Early exposure to alcohol leads to permanent impairment of dendritic excitability in neocortical pyramidal neurons. *Journal of Neuroscience, 32*(4), 1377–1382. https://doi.org/10.1523/JNEUROSCI.5520-11

Grewal, K., Forest, J., Cohen, B. P., & Ahmad, S. (2021). Going beyond the point neuron: Active dendrites and sparse representations for continual learning. *bioRxiv* [preprint]. https://doi.org/10.1101/2021.10.25.465651

Grice, H. P. (1975). Logic and conversation. *Syntax and Semantics, 3*, 41–58.

Grice, H. P. (1989). *Studies in the way of words*. Harvard University Press.

Gruber, H. E. (1974). *Darwin on man: A psychological study of scientific creativity*. Wildwood House.

Guerri, C., Bazinet, A., & Riley, E. P. (2009). Foetal alcohol spectrum disorders and alterations in brain and behaviour. *Alcohol and Alcoholism*, *44*, 108–114.

Guo, K., Yamawaki, N., Svoboda, K., & Shepherd, G. M. G. (2018). Anterolateral motor cortex connects with a medial subdivision of ventromedial thalamus through cell type specific circuits, forming an excitatory thalamocortico- thalamic loop via layer 1 apical tuft dendrites of layer 5B pyramidal tract type neurons. *Journal of Neuroscience*, *38*, 8787–8797.

Guo, K., Yamawaki, N., Barrett, J. M., Tapies, M., & Shepherd, G. M. (2020). Cortico-thalamo-cortical circuits of mouse forelimb S1 are organized primarily as recurrent loops. *Journal of Neuroscience*, *40*(14), 2849–2858.

Haas, H. L. (2008). Histamine in the nervous system. *Physiological Reviews*, *88*, 1183–1241. https://doi.org/10.1152/physrev.00043.2007

Haberl, M. G., Zerbi, V., Veltien, A., Ginger, M., Heerschap, A., & Frick, A. (2015). Structural-functional connectivity deficits of neocortical circuits in the Fmr1 (−/y) mouse model of autism. *Science Advances*, *1*(10), e1500775.

Haga, T., & Fukai, T. (2018). Dendritic processing of spontaneous neuronal sequences for single-trial learning. *Scientific Reports*, *8*, 15166. https://doi.org/10.1038/s41598-018-33513-9

Hahn, N., Snedeker, J., & Rabagliati, H. (2015). Rapid linguistic ambiguity resolution in young children with autism spectrum disorder: Eye tracking evidence for the limits of weak central coherence. *Autism Research*, *8*, 717–726. https://doi.org/10.1002/aur.1487

Halford, G. S., Cowan, N., & Andrews, G. (2007). Separating cognitive capacity from knowledge: A new hypothesis. *Trends in Cognitive Sciences*, *11*, 236–242.

Halassa, M. M., & Kastner, S. (2017) Thalamic functions in distributed cognitive control. *Nature Neuroscience*, *20*, 1669–1679.

Halassa, M. M., & Sherman, S. M. (2019). Thalamocortical circuit motifs: A general framework. *Neuron*, *103*, 762–770.

Hancock, P. J. B., Walton, L., Mitchell, G., Plenderleith, Y., & Phillips, W. A. (2008). Segregation by onset asynchrony. *Journal of Vision*, *8*(7), 1–21. https://doi.org/10.1167/8.7.21

Happé, F. (1999). Autism: Cognitive deficit or cognitive style? *Trends in Cognitive Sciences*, *3*, 216–222.

Harari, Y. N. (2011). *Sapiens: A brief history of humankind*. Penguin.

Harder, M. Salge, C., & Polani, D. (2013). Bivariate measure of redundant information. *Physical Review E*, *87*, 012130.

Harley, T. A. (2021). *The science of consciousness*. Cambridge University Press.

Harnett, M. T., Magee, J. C., & Williams, S. R. (2015). Distribution and function of HCN channels in the apical dendritic tuft of neocortical pyramidal neurons. *Journal of Neuroscience*, *35*(3), 1024–103.

Harnett, M. T., Xu, N.-L., Magee, J. C., & Williams, S. R. (2013). Potassium channels control the interaction between active dendritic integration compartments in layer 5 cortical pyramidal neurons. *Neuron*, *79*, 516–529.

Harris, K. D., & Shepherd, G. M. (2015). The neocortical circuit: Themes and variations. *Nature Neuroscience*, *18*, 170–181.

Hebb, D. O. (1949). *The organization of behavior*. Wiley.

Heeger, D. J., & Mackey, W. E. (2019). Oscillatory recurrent gated neural integrator circuits (ORGaNICs), a unifying theoretical framework for neural dynamics. *Proceedings of the National Academy of Sciences of the United States of America*, *116*(45), 22783–22794.

Heeger, D. J., & Zemlianova, K. O. (2020). A recurrent circuit implements normalization, simu-lating the dynamics of V1 activity. *Proceedings of the National Academy of Sciences of the United States of America*, *117*(36), 22494–22505.

Helmsley, D. R. (1998). The disruption of the 'sense of self' in schizophrenia: Potential links with disturbances of information processing. *British Journal of Medical Psychology*, *71*, 115–124.

Herculano-Houzel, S. (2017). Numbers of neurons as biological correlates of cognitive cap-ability. *Current Opinion in Behavioral Science*, *16*, 1–7. https://doi.org/10.1016/j.cob eha.2017.02.004

Hertag, L., & Sprekeler, H. (2019). Amplifying the redistribution of somato-dendritic inhibition by the interplay of three interneuron types. *PLoS Computational Biology*, *15*(5), e1006999. https://doi.org/10.1371/journal.pcbi.1006999

Hobson, J. A. (2009). REM sleep and dreaming: Toward a theory of protoconsciousness. *Nature Reviews Neuroscience*, *10*, 803–813. https://doi.org/10.1038/nrn2716

Hobson, J. A., Hong, C. C-H., & Friston, K. J. (2014). Virtual reality and consciousness infer-ence in dreaming. *Frontiers in Psychology*, *5*, 1133. https://doi.org/10.3389/fpsyg.2014.01133

Hyde, T. M., & Weinberger, D. R. (1997). Seizures and schizophrenia. *Schizophrenia Bulletin*, *23*(4), 611–622. https://doi.org/10.1093/schbul/23.4.611

Ibrahim, L. A., Mesik, L., Ji, X. Y., Fang, Q., Li, H. F., Li, Y. T., Zingg, B., Zhang, L. I., & Tao, H. W. (2016). Cross-modality sharpening of visual cortical processing through layer-1-mediated inhibition and disinhibition. *Neuron*, *89*(5), pp.1031–1045.

Ibrahim, L. A., Schuman, B., Bandler, R., Rudy, B., & Fishell, G. (2020). Mining the jewels of the cortex's crowning mystery. *Current Opinion in Neurobiology*, *63*, 154–161. doi.org/10.1016/j.conb.2020.04.005

Inoue, S., & Matsuzawa, T. (2007). Working memory of numerals in chimpanzees. *Current Biology*, *17*(23), R1004.

Intrator, N., & Cooper, L. N. (1995). BCM theory of visual cortical plasticity. In M. A. Arbib (Ed.), *The handbook of brain theory and neural networks* (pp. 153–157). MIT Press.

Iurilli, G., Ghezzi, D., Olcese, U., Lassi, G., Nazzaro, C., Tonini, R., Tucci, V., Benfenati, F., & Medini, P. (2012). Sound-driven synaptic inhibition in primary visual cortex. *Neuron*, *73*(4), 814–828. https://doi.org/10.1016/j.neuron.2011.12.026

Jachim, S., Warren, P. A., McLoughlin, N., & Gowen, E. (2015). Collinear facilitation and con-tour integration in autism: Evidence for atypical visual integration. *Frontiers in Human Neuroscience*, *9*, 115. https://doi.org/10.3389/fnhum.2015.00115

Jadi, J. P., Behabadi, B. F., Poleg-Polsky, A., Schiller, J., & Mel, B. W. (2014). An augmented two-layer model captures nonlinear analog spatial integration effects in pyramidal neuron den-drites. *Proceedings of the IEEE*, *102*, 782–798.

James, W. (1890). *The principles of psychology*. Dover

James, W. (1902). *The varieties of religious experience*. The Modern Library.

James, W. (1904) Does 'consciousness' exist? The Journal of Philosophy, Psychology and Scientific Methods, *1*(18), 477–491.

Jarsky, T., Roxin, A., Kath, W. L., & Spruston, N. (2005). Conditional dendritic spike propaga-tion following distal synaptic activation of hippocampal CA1 pyramidal neurons. *Nature Neuroscience*, *8*, 1667–76.

Javitt, D.C., & Coyle, J.T. (2004) Decoding schizophrenia. *Scientific American*, *290*, 48–55.

Jaynes, E. T. (2003). *Probability theory: The logic of science* (G. L. Bretthorst, Ed.). Cambridge University Press.

Jiang, X., Wang, G., Lee, A. J., Stornetta, R. L., & Zhu, J. J. (2013). The organization of two new cortical interneuronal circuits. *Nature Neuroscience*, *16*(2), 210–218.

Johansson, P., & Hall, L. (2008). From change blindness to choice blindness. *Psychologia, 51,* 142–155.

Jones, E. G. (2001). The thalamic matrix and thalamocortical synchrony. *Trends in Neuroscience, 24*(10), 595–601. https://doi.org/10.1016/s0166-2236(00)01922-6

Kaaronen, R. O. (2018). A theory of predictive dissonance: Predictive processing presents a new take on cognitive dissonance. *Frontiers in Psychology, 9,* 2218. https://doi.org/10.3389/fpsyg.2018.02218

Khan, A. G., & Hofer, S. B. (2018). Contextual signals in visual cortex. *Current Opinion in Neurobiology, 52,* 131–138.

Kahneman, D. (2011). *Thinking, fast and slow.* Farrar, Straus and Giroux.

Kaldy, Z., & Kovacs, I. (2003). Visual context integration is not fully developed in 4-year-old children. *Perception, 32,* 657–666.

Kalmbach, B. E., Buchin, A., Long, B., Close, J., Nandi, A., Miller, J. A., Bakken, T. E., Hodge, R. D., Chong, P., de Frates, R., & Dai, K. (2018). h-Channels contribute to divergent intrinsic membrane properties of supragranular pyramidal neurons in human versus mouse cerebral cortex. *Neuron, 100*(5), 1194–1208. doi.org/10.1016/j.neuron.2018.10.012

Kalmbach, B. E., Johnston, D., & Brager, D. H. (2015). Cell type-specific channelopathies in the prefrontal cortex of the fmr1-/y mouse model of Fragile X syndrome. *eNeuro, 2*(6), ENEURO.0114-15.2015.

Kampa, B., Letzkus, J. J., & Stuart, G. (2006). Requirement of dendritic calcium spikes for induction of spike-timing dependent synaptic plasticity. *Journal of Physiology, 574,* 283–290. https://doi.org/10.1113/jphysiol.2006.111062

Kapadia, M. K., Ito, M., Gilbert, C. D., & Westheimer, G. (1995). Improvement in visual sensitivity by changes in local context: Parallel studies in human observers and in V1 of alert monkeys. *Neuron, 15,* 843–856.

Karimi, A., Odenthal, J., Drawitsch, F., Boergens, K. M., & Helmstaedter, M. (2020). Cell-type specific innervation of cortical pyramidal cells at their apical dendrites. *Elife, 9,* e46876. doi.org/10.7554/eLife.46876

Karmiloff-Smith, A. (1998). Development itself is the key to understanding developmental disorders. *Trends in Cognitive Sciences, 2,* 389–398.

Karmiloff-Smith, A. (2009). Nativism vs neuroconstructivism: Rethinking developmental disorders. *Developmental Psychology, 45*(1), 56–63.

Karnani, M. M., Agetsuma, M., & Yuste, R. (2014). A blanket of inhibition: Functional inferences from dense inhibitory connectivity. *Current Opinion in Neurobiology, 26,* 96–102.

Kay, J. (1999). Neural networks for unsupervised learning based on information theory. In J. W. Kay & D. M. Titterington (Eds.), *Statistics and neural networks* (pp. 25–63). Oxford University Press.

Kay, J., Floreano, D., & Phillips, W. A. (1998). Contextually guided unsupervised learning using local multivariate binary processors. *Neural Networks, 11*(1), 117–140.

Kay, J. W., Ince, R. A. A., Dering, B., & Phillips, W. A. (2017). Partial and entropic information decompositions of a neuronal modulatory interaction. *Entropy, 19*(11), 560. https://doi.org/10.3390/e19110560

Kay, J. W., & Phillips, W. A. (2011). Coherent infomax as a computational goal for neural systems. *Bulletin of Mathematical Biology, 73,* 344–372. https://doi.org/10.1007/s11583-010-9564

Kay, J. W., & Phillips, W. A. (2020). Contextual modulation in mammalian neocortex is asymmetric. *Symmetry, 12,* 815. https://doi.org/10.3390/sym12050815

Kay, J. W., Schulz, J. M., & Phillips, W. A. (2022). A comparison of partial information decompositions using data from real and simulated layer 5b pyramidal cells. *Entropy, 24,* 1021. https://doi.org/10.3390/e24081021

Keane, B. P. (2018). Contour interpolation: A case study in modularity of mind. *Cognition, 174*, 1–18. https://doi.org/10.1016/j.cognition.2018.01.008

Keane, B. P., Silverstein, S. M., Wang, Y., & Papathomas, T. V. (2013). Reduced depth inversion illusions in schizophrenia are state-specific and occur for multiple object types and viewing conditions. *Journal of Abnormal Psychology, 122*, 506–512. https://doi.org/10.1037/a0032110

Keller, A. J., Roth, M. M., & Scanziani, M. (2020a). Feedback generates a second receptive field in neurons of the visual cortex. *Nature, 582*, 545–549.

Keller, A. J., Dipoppa, M., Roth, M. M., Caudill, M. S., Ingrosso, A., Miller, K. D., & Scanziani, M. (2020b). A disinhibitory circuit for contextual modulation in primary visual cortex. *Neuron, 108*(6), 1181–1193.

Kerlin, A., Mohar, B., Flickinger, D., MacLennan, B. J., Dean, M. B., Davis, C., Spruston, N., & Svoboda, K. (2019). Functional clustering of dendritic activity during decision-making. *eLife, 8*, e46966.

Khan, A. G., & Hofer, S. B. (2018). Contextual signals in visual cortex. *Current Opinion in Neurobiology, 52*(October), 131–138.

Kim, Y., Yang, G. R., Pradhan, K., Venkataraju, K. U., Bota, M., García Del Molino, L. C., Fitzgerald, G., Ram, K., He, M., Levine, J. M., Mitra, P., Huang, Z. J., Wang, X. J., & Osten, P. (2017). Brain-wide maps reveal stereotyped cell-type-based cortical architecture and subcortical sexual dimorphism. *Cell, 171*(2), 456–469.

The Kingsway Shakespeare. (1927). Introduction by F. D Losey. George G. Harrap.

Kirchgessner. M. A., Franklin A. D., & Callaway, E. M. (2021). Distinct 'driving' versus 'modulatory' influences of different visual cortico-thalamic pathways. *bioRxiv* [preprint]. doi.org/10.1101/2021.03.30.437715

Klink, P. C. R. (2017). Distinct feedforward and feedback effects of microstimulation in visual cortex reveal neural mechanisms of texture segregation. *Neuron, 95*, 209–220. http://dx.doi.org/10.1016/j.neuron.2017.05

Klink, P. C. R., van Wezel, R. J. A., & van Ee, R. (2012). United we sense, divided we fail: Context-driven perception of ambiguous visual stimuli. *Philosophical Transactions of the Royal Society B: Biological Sciences, 367*, 932–941. https://doi.org/10.1098/rstb.2011.0358

Koch, C. and Crick, F. (1994). Some further ideas regarding the neuronal basis of awareness. In C. Koch & J. L. Davis (Eds.), *Large-scale neuronal theories of the brain* (pp. 93–109). MIT Press.

Koch, C., Massimini, M., Boly, M., & Tononi, G. (2016). Neural correlates of consciousness: Progress and problems. *Nature Reviews Neuroscience, 17*(5), 307–321.

Kok, P., Rahnev, D., Jehee, J. F., Lau, H. C., & de Lange, F. P. (2012) Attention reverses the effect of prediction in silencing sensory signals. *Cerebral Cortex, 22*(9), 2197–2206

Kok, P., Jehee, J. F., & de Lange, F. P. (2012). Less is more: Expectation sharpens representations in the primary visual cortex. *Neuron, 75*(2), 265–270.

Kole, M. H., Bräuer, A. U., & Stuart, G. J. (2007). Inherited cortical HCN1 channel loss amplifies dendritic calcium electrogenesis and burst firing in a rat absence epilepsy model. *Journal of Physiology, 578*, 507–525.

Kolla, N. J., & Bortolato, M. (2020). The role of monoamine oxidase A in the neurobiology of aggressive, antisocial, and violent behavior: A tale of mice and men. *Progress in Neurobiology, 194*, 101875.

Komura, Y., Nikkuni, A., Hirashima, N., Uetake, T., & Miyamoto, A. (2013). Responses of pulvinar neurons reflect a subject's confidence in visual categorization. *Nature Neuroscience, 16*, 749–755.

Körding, K. P., & König, P. (2000). Learning with two sites of synaptic integration. *Network: Computation in Neural Systems, 11*, 1–15.

Kourtzi, Z., Tolias, A. S., Altmann, C. F., Augath, M., & Logothetis, N. K. (2003). Integration of local features into global shapes: Monkey and human fMRI studies. *Neuron*, *37*(2), 333–346. https://doi.org/10.1016/s0896-6273(02)01174-1

Kovacs, I., & Julesz, B. (1993). A closed curve is much more than an incomplete one: Effect of closure in figure-ground segmentation. *Proceedings of the National Academy of Sciences of the United States of America*, *90*, 7495–7497.

Kruth, K. A., Grisolano, T. M., Ahern, C. A., & Williams, A. J. (2020). *SCN2A* channelopathies in the autism spectrum of neuropsychiatric disorders: A role for pluripotent stem cells? *Molecular Autism*, *11*(1), 23. https://doi.org/10.1186/s13229-020-00330-9

Kubota, Y., Karube, F., Nomura, M., & Kawaguchi, Y. (2016). The diversity of cortical inhibitory synapses. *Frontiers in Neural Circuits*, *10*, 27. https://doi.org/10.3389/fncir.2016.00027

Kuchibhotla, K. V., Gill, J. V., Lindsay, G. W., Papadoyannis, E. S., Field, R. E., Sten, T. A., Miller, K. D., & Froemke, R. C. (2017). Parallel processing by cortical inhibition enables context-dependent behavior. *Nature Neuroscience*, *20*, 62–71.

Kuhn, T. S. (1962). *The structure of scientific revolutions*. University of Chicago Press.

Kursun, O., Dinc, S., & Favorov, O. V. (2021). Contextually guided convolutional neural networks for learning most transferable representations. *arXiv* [preprint], *2103*, 01566v2

Kusmierz, T., Isomura, T., & Toyoizumi, T. (2017). Learning with three factors: Modulating Hebbian plasticity with errors. *Current Opinion in Neurobiology*, *46*, 170–177.

Kveraga, K., Ghuman, A. S., & Bar, M. (2007). Top-down predictions in the cognitive brain. *Brain and Cognition*, *65*, 145–168.

Labarrera, C., Deitcher, Y., Dudai, A., Weiner, B., Kaduri Amichai, A., Zylbermann, N., & London, M. (2018). Adrenergic modulation regulates the dendritic excitability of layer 5 pyramidal neurons in vivo. *Cell Reports*, *23*, 1034–1044.

LaBerge, D. (2006). Apical dendrite activity in cognition and consciousness. *Consciousness and Cognition*, *15*, 235–257.

Limanowski, J. (2021). Precision control for a flexible body representation. *Neuroscience and Biobehavioral Reviews*, *134*, 104401. https://doi.org/10.1016/j.neubiorev.2021.10.023

Lamme, V. A. F. (2004a). Beyond the classical receptive field: Contextual modulation of V1 responses. In J. S. Werner & L. M. Chalupa (Eds.), *The visual neurosciences* (pp. 720–732). MIT Press.

Lamme, V. A. (2004b). Local versus global recurrency. Commentary on: Cortex, countercurrent context, and dimensional integration of lifetime memory by Bjorn Merker. *Cortex*, *40*, 580–581.

Lamme, V. A. F. (2020). Visual functions generating conscious seeing. *Frontiers in Psychology*, *11*, 83. https://doi.org/10.3389/fpsyg.2020.00083

Larkum, M. E. (2013). A cellular mechanism for cortical associations: An organizing principle for the cerebral cortex. *Trends in Neuroscience*, *36*, 141–151.

Larkum, M. E. (2022). Are dendrites conceptually useful? *Neuroscience*, *325*, 4–14.

Larkum, M. E., Nevian, T., Sandler, M., Polsky, A., & Schiller J. (2009) Synaptic integration in tuft dendrites of layer 5 pyramidal neurons: A new unifying principle. *Science*, *325*, 756–760.

Larkum, M. E., Petro, L. S., Sachdev, R. N. S., & Muckli, L. (2018). A perspective on cortical layering and layer-spanning neuronal elements. *Frontiers in Neuroanatomy*, *12*, 56. https://doi.org/10.3389/fnana.2018.00056

Larkum, M. E., & Phillips, W. A. (2016). Does arousal enhance apical amplification and disamplification? *Behavioral and Brain Sciences*, *39*, e215. https://doi.org/10.1017/S0140525X15001867

Larkum, M. E., Senn, W., & Lüscher, H.-R. (2004). Top-down dendritic input increases the gain of layer 5 pyramidal neurons. *Cerebral Cortex*, *14*, 1059–1070.

Larkum, M. E., Watanabe, S., Nakamura, T., Lasser-Ross, N., & Ross, W. N. (2003). Synaptically activated Ca2+ waves in layer 2/3 and layer 5 rat neocortical pyramidal neurons. *Journal of Physiology*, *549*, 471–488.

Larkum, M. E., Waters, J., Sakmann, B., & Helmchen, F. (2007). Dendritic spikes in apical dendrites of neocortical layer 2/3 pyramidal neurons. *Journal of Neuroscience*, *27*, 8999–9008.

Larkum, M. E., Zhu, J. J., & Sakmann, B. (1999). A new cellular mechanism for coupling inputs arriving at different cortical layers. *Nature*, *98*(6725), 338–341.

Larkum, M. E., Zhu, J. J., & Sakmann, B. (2001). Dendritic mechanisms underlying the coupling of the dendritic with the axonal action potential initiation zone of adult rat layer 5 pyramidal neurons. *Journal of Physiology*, *533*, 447–466.

LeCun, Y., Bengio, Y., & Hinton, G. (2015). Deep learning. *Nature*, *521*, 436–444. https://doi.org/10.1038/nature14539

Ledergerber, D., & Larkum, M. E. (2012). The time window for generation of dendritic pikes by coincidence of action potentials and EPSPs is layer specific in somatosensory cortex. *PLoS One*, *7*(3), e33146. doi.org/10.1371/journal.pone.0033146

LeDoux, J. (2002). *Synaptic self*. Viking Penguin Publishers.

Lee, M., Mueller, A., & Moore, T. (2020). Differences in noradrenaline receptor expression across different neuronal subtypes in macaque frontal eye field. *Frontiers in Neuroanatomy*, *14*, 574130. https://doi.org/10.3389/fnana.2020.574130

Lee, S., Kruglikov, I., Huang, Z. J., Fishell, G., & Rudy, B. (2013). A disinhibitory circuit mediates motor integration in the somatosensory cortex. *Nature Neuroscience*, *16*(11), 1662–1670.

Letzkus, J. J., Wolff, S. B., & Lüthi, A. (2015). Disinhibition, a circuit mechanism for associative learning and memory. *Neuron*, *88*:264–276.

Li, B., Chen, F., Ye, J., Chen, X., Yan, J., Li, Y., Xiong, Y., Zhou, Z., Xia, J., & Hu, Z. (2010). The modulation of orexin A on HCN currents of pyramidal neurons in mouse prelimbic cortex. *Cerebral Cortex*, *20*(7), 1756–1767. doi.org/10.1093/cercor/bhp241

Li, W., Piech, V., & Gilbert, C. D. (2006). Contour saliency in primary visual cortex. *Neuron*, *50*, 951–962.

Linsker, R. (1992). Local synaptic learning rules suffice to maximize mutual information in a linear network. *Neural Computation*, *4*, 691–702.

Liu, R-J., & Aghajanian, G. K. (2008). Stress blunts serotonin- and hypocretin-evoked EPSCs in prefrontal cortex: Role of corticosterone-mediated apical dendritic atrophy. *Proceedings of the National Academy of Sciences of the United States of America*, *105*, 359–364. www.pnas.org_cgi_doi_10.1073_pnas.0706679105

Lizier, J. T, Bertschinger, N., Jost, J., & Wibral, M. (2018). Information decomposition of target effects from multi-source interactions: Perspectives on previous, current and future work. *Entropy*, *20*(4), 307. https://doi.org/10.3390/e20040307

Llinás, R., Ribary, U., Contreras, D., & Pedroarena, C. (1998). The neuronal basis for consciousness. *Philosophical Transactions of the Royal Society of London. Series B: Biological Sciences*, *353*(1377), 1841–1849.

Luebke, J. I. (2017). Pyramidal neurons are not generalizable building blocks of cortical networks. *Frontiers in Neuroanatomy*, *11*, 11. https://doi.org/10.3389/fnana.2017.00011

Lundqvist, M., Herman, P., & Miller, E. K. (2018). Working memory: Delay activity, yes! Persistent activity? Maybe not. *Journal of Neuroscience*, *38*, 7013–7019. https://doi.org/10.1523/JNEUROSCI.2485-17.2018

Ma, W. J., Husain, M., & Bays, P. M. (2014). Changing concepts of working memory. *Nature Neuroscience*, *17*, 347–356.

MacIver, M. A., & Finlay, B. L. (2022). The neuroecology of the water-to-land transition and the evolution of the vertebrate brain. *Philosophical Transactions of the Royal Society B: Biological Sciences*, *377*(1844), 20200523.

Magee, J. C., & Cook, E. P. (2000). Somatic EPSP amplitude is independent of synapse location in hippocampal pyramidal neurons. *Nature Neuroscience, 3,* 895–903.

Mahler, S. V., Moorman, D. E., Smith, R. J., James, M. H., & Aston-Jones, G. (2014). Motivational activation: A unifying hypothesis of orexin/hypocretin function. *Nature Neuroscience, 17,* 1298–1303.

Major, G., Larkum, M. E., & Schiller, J. (2013). Active properties of neocortical pyramidal neuron dendrites. *Annual Review of Neuroscience, 36,* 1–24.

Mäki-Marttunen, T., Devor, A., Phillips, W. A., Dale, A. M., Andreassen, O. A., & Einevoll, G. T. (2019). Computational modelling of genetic contributions to excitability and neural coding in layer V pyramidal cells: Applications to schizophrenia pathology. *Frontiers in Computational Neuroscience, 13,* 66. https://doi.org/10.3389/fncom.2019.00066

Mäki-Marttunen, T., & Mäki-Marttunen, V. (2022). Excitatory and inhibitory effects of HCN channel modulation on excitability of layer V pyramidal cells. *bioRxiv* [preprint]. https://doi.org/10.1101/2022.03.30.486368

Mandon, S., & Kreiter, A. K. (2005). Rapid contour integration in macaque monkeys. *Vision Research, 45*(2005), 291–300.

Markov, N. T., & Kennedy, H. (2013). The importance of being hierarchical. *Current Opinion in Neurobiology, 23,* 187–194. dx.doi.org/10.1016/j.conb.2012.12.008

Markov, N.T., Vezoli, J., Chameau, P., Falchier, A., Quilodran, R., Huissoud, C., Lamy, C., Misery, P., Giroud, P., Ullman, S., Barone, P., Dehay, C., Knoblauch, K., & Kennedy, H. (2014). Anatomy of hierarchy: Feedforward and feedback pathways in macaque visual cortex. *Journal of Comparative Neurology, 522,* 225–259.

Marvan, T., Polák, M., Bachmann, T., & Phillips, W. A. (2021). Apical amplification—a cellular mechanism of conscious perception? *Neuroscience of Consciousness, 7*(2), 1–17. doi.org/10.1093/nc/niab036

Masse, N. Y., Rosen, M. C., & Freedman, D. J. (2020). Reevaluating the role of persistent neural activity in short-term memory. *Trends in Cognitive Sciences, 24,* 242–258

Mather, M., Clewett, D., Sakaki, M., & Harley, C. W. (2016). Norepinephrine ignites local hotspots of neuronal excitation: How arousal amplifies selectivity in perception and memory. *Behavioral and Brain Sciences, 1,* 1–100. https://doi.org/10.1017/S0140525X07000891

McCulloch, W. S., & Pitts, W. (1943). A logical calculus of the ideas immanent in nervous activity. *Bulletin of Mathematical Biophysics, 5,* 115–133.

McGinley, M. J., Vinck, M., Reimer, J., Batista-Brito, R., Zagha, E., Cadwell, C. R., Tolias, A.S., Cardin, J. A., & McCormick, D. A. (2015). Waking state: Rapid variations modulate neural and behavioral responses. *Neuron, 87,* 1143–1161.

McGinn, C. (2006). *Shakespeare's philosophy: Discovering the meaning behind the plays.* Harper Collins.

Meijer, G. T., Mertens, P. E., Pennartz, C. M., Olcese, U., & Lansink, C. S. (2019). The circuit architecture of cortical multisensory processing: Distinct functions jointly operating within a common anatomical network. *Progress in Neurobiology, 174,* 1–15.

Meredith, R. M., & Mansvelder, H. D. (2007). Increased threshold for spike-timing-dependent plasticity is caused by unreliable calcium signaling in mice lacking fragile X gene Fmr1. *Neuron, 54,* 627–638. https://doi.org/10.1016/j.neuron.2007.04.028

Merker, B. (2007). Consciousness without a cerebral cortex: A challenge for neuroscience and medicine. *Behavioral and Brain Sciences, 30,* 63–134.

Merker, B., Williford, K., & Rudrauf, D. (2022). The integrated information theory of consciousness: A case of mistaken identity. *Behavioral and Brain Sciences, 45,* e41. https://doi.org/10.1017/S0140525X21000881

Merrikhi, Y., Clark, K., Albarran, E., Parsa, M., Zirnsak, M., Moore, T., & Noudoost, B. (2017). Spatial working memory alters the efficacy of input to visual cortex. *Nature Communications*, 8(1), 1–10. https://doi.org/10.1038/ncomms15041

Meyer, K. (2015). The role of dendritic signaling in the anesthetic suppression of consciousness. *Anesthesiology*, 122, 1415–1431.

Migliore, M., & Shepherd, G. M. (2002). Emerging rules for the distributions of active dendritic conductances. *Nature Reviews Neuroscience*, 3, 362–370.

Mohamed, S., & Rezende, D. J. (2015). Variational information maximisation for intrinsically motivated reinforcement learning. *arXiv* [preprint], 1509, 08731.

Mongillo, G., Barak, O., & Tsodyks, M. (2008). Synaptic theory of working memory. *Science*, 319, 1543–1546.

Morey, C. C. (2018). The case against specialized visual–spatial short-term memory. *Psychological Bulletin*, 144(8), 849–883. https://doi.org/10.1037/bul0000155

Morgan, A. T., Petro, L. S., & Muckli, L. (2019). Scene representations conveyed by cortical feedback to early visual cortex can be described by line drawings. *Journal of Neuroscience*, 39(47), 9410–9423.

Mottron, L., Dawson, M., Soulières, I., Hubert, B., & Burack, J. A. (2006). Enhanced perceptual functioning in autism: An updated model, and eight principle of autistic perception. *Journal of Autism and Developmental Disorders*, 6, 1–17.

Muckli, L., De Martino, F., Vizioli, L., Petro, L. S., Smith, F. W., Ugurbil, K., Goebel, R., & Yacoub, E. (2015). Contextual feedback to superficial layers of V1. *Current Biology*, 25(20), 2690–2695. https://doi.org/10.1016/j.cub.2015.08.057

Munn, B. R., Müller, E. J., Wainstein, G., & Shine, J. M. (2021). The ascending arousal system shapes neural dynamics to mediate awareness of cognitive states. *Nature Communications*, 12(1), 1–9. doi.org/10.1038/s41467-021-26268-x

Murayama, M., & Larkum, M. E. (2009). Enhanced dendritic activity in awake rats. *Proceedings of the National Academy of Sciences of the United States of America*, 106, 20482–20486. http://dx.doi.org/10.1073/pnas.0910379106.

Murphy, S. C., Palmer, L. M., Nyffeler, T., Müri, R. M., & Larkum, M. E. (2016). Transcranial magnetic stimulation (TMS) inhibits cortical dendrites. *Elife*, 5, e13598. https://doi.org/10.7554/eLife.13598

Nagano, M., Zane, E., & Grossman, R. B. (2021). Structural and contextual cues in third-person pronoun interpretation by children with autism spectrum disorder and their neurotypical peers. *Journal of Autism and Developmental Disorders*, 51, 1562–1583. https://doi.org/10.1007/s10803-020-04645-7

Nakajima, M., & Halassa, M. M. (2017). Thalamic control of functional cortical connectivity. *Current Opinion in Neurobiology*, 44, 127–131.

Naud, R., & Sprekeler, H. (2018). Sparse bursts optimize information transmission in a multiplexed neural code. *Proceedings of the National Academy of Sciences of the United States of America*, 115, E6329–E6338. https://doi.org/10.1073/pnas.172099511

Nelson, A. D., & Bender, K. J. (2021). Dendritic integration dysfunction in neurodevelopmental disorders. *Developmental Neuroscience*, 43(3–4), 201–221. https://doi.org/10.1159/000516657

Newell, B. R., & Shanks, D. R. (2014). Unconscious influences on decision making: A critical review. *Behavioral and Brain Sciences*, 37, 1–19.

Nisbett, R. E., & Miyamoto, Y. (2005). The influence of culture: Holistic versus analytic perception. *Trends in Cognitive Sciences*, 9, 467–473.

Nikolić, D. (2022). Where is the mind within the brain? Transient selection of subnetworks by metabotropic receptors and G protein-gated ion channels. *arXiv* [preprint], 2207, 11249.

Nikolić, D. (2015). Practopoiesis: Or how life fosters a mind. *Journal of Theoretical Biology*, *373*, 40–61.

Noam, Y., Bernard, C., & Baram, T. Z. (2011). Towards an integrated view of HCN channel role in epilepsy. *Current Opinion in Neurobiology*, *21*, 873–879. https://doi.org/10.1016/j.conb.2011.06.013

Norris, D. (2017). Short-term memory and long-term memory are still different. *Psychological Bulletin*, *143*(9), 992–1009. http://dx.doi.org/10.1037/bul0000108

Oberauer, K., Lewandowsky, S., Awh, E., Brown, G. D. A., Conway, A., Cowan, N., Donkin, C., Farrell, S., Hitch, G. J., Hurlstone, M. J., Ma, W. J., Morey, C. C., Nee, D. E., Schweppe, J., Vergauwe, E., & Ward, G. (2018). Benchmarks for models of short-term and working memory. *Psychological Bulletin*, *144*(9), 885–958. https://doi.org/10.1037/bul0000153

Ochsner, K. N., & Gross, J. J. (2005). The cognitive control of emotion. *Trends in Cognitive Sciences*, *9*, 242–249.

Osiurak, F., & Reynaud, E. (2020). The elephant in the room: What matters cognitively in cumulative technological culture. *Behavioral and Brain Sciences*, *43*, e156. https://doi.org/10.1017/S0140525X19003236

Pal, D., Dean, J. G., Liu, T., Li, D., Watson, C. J., Hudetz, A. G., & Mashour, G. A. (2018). Differential role of prefrontal and parietal cortices in controlling level of consciousness. *Current Biology*, *28*(13), 2145–2152. doi.org/10.1016/j.cub.2018.05.025

Pally, R. (2005). Non-conscious prediction and a role for consciousness in correcting prediction errors. *Cortex*, *41*, 643–662.

Palmer, L. M. (2014). Dendritic integration in pyramidal neurons during network activity and disease. *Brain Research Bulletin*, *103*, 2–10.

Palmer, L. M., Shai, A. S., Reeve, J. E., Andersen, H. L., Paulsen, O., & Larkum, M. E. (2014). NMDA spikes enhance action potential generation during sensory input. *Nature Neuroscience*, *17*, 383–390.

Palmer, L. M., Schulz, J. M., & Larkum, M. E. (2013). Layer-specific regulation of cortical neurons by interhemispheric inhibition. *Communicative and Integrative Biology*, *6*, e23545.

Parr, T., Benrimoh, D. A., Vinent, P., & Friston, K. J. (2018). Precision and false perceptual inference. *Frontiers in Integrative Neuroscience*, *12*, 39.

Parr, T., & Friston, K. J. (2017). Working memory, attention, and salience in active inference. *Scientific Reports*, *7*(1), 14678.

Parr, T., & Friston, K. J. (2019). Attention or salience? *Current Opinion in Psychology*, *29*, 1–5.

Parrish, A. E., & Beran, M. J. (2014). When less is more: Like humans, chimpanzees (*Pan troglodytes*) misperceive food amounts based on plate size. *Animal Cognition*, *17*, 427–434. https://doi.org/10.1007/s10071-013-0674-3

Parron, C., & Fagot, J. (2007). Comparison of grouping abilities in humans (*Homo sapiens*) and baboons (*Papio papio*) with Ebbinghaus illusion. *Journal of Comparative Psychology*, *121*, 405–411. https://doi.org/10.1037/0735-7036.121.4.405

Paspalas, C. D., Wang, M., & Arnsten, A. F. T. (2013). Constellation of HCN channels and cAMP regulating proteins in dendritic spines of the primate prefrontal cortex: Potential substrate for working memory deficits in schizophrenia. *Cerebral Cortex*, *23*(7), 1643–1654. http://dx.doi.org/10.1093/cercor/bhs152

Patel, G. H., Yang, D., Jamerson, E. C., Snyder, L. H., Corbetta, M., & Ferrera, V. P. (2015). Functional evolution of new and expanded attention networks in humans. *Proceedings of the National Academy of Sciences of the United States of America*, *112*(30), 9454e9459. https://doi.org/10.1073/pnas.1420395112

Pedarzani, P., & Storm, J. F. (1995). Protein kinase A-independent modulation of ion channels in the brain by cyclic AMP. *Proceedings of the National Academy of Sciences of the United States of America*, *92*, 11716–11720.

Pessoa, L. (2017). A network model of the emotional brain. *Trends in Cognitive Sciences, 21*, 357–371.

Phillips, W. A. (1974). On the distinction between sensory storage and short-term visual memory. *Perception and Psychophysics, 16*, 283–290.

Phillips, W. A. (1983). Short-term visual memory. *Philosophical Transactions of the Royal Society of London B: Biological Sciences, 302*, 295–309.

Phillips, W. A. (2012). Self-organized complexity and coherent infomax from the viewpoint of Jaynes's probability theory. *Information, 3*(1), 1–15.

Phillips, W. A. (2015). Prenatal exposure to alcohol causes enduring brain damage. *Adoption and Fostering, 39*(3), 201–211.

Phillips, W. A. (2017). Cognitive functions of intracellular mechanisms for contextual amplification. *Brain and Cognition, 112*, 39–53. https://doi.org/10.1016/j.bandc.2015.09.005

Phillips, W. A., Bachmann, T., & Storm, J. F. (2018). Apical function in neocortical pyramidal cells: A common pathway by which general anesthetics can affect mental state. *Frontiers in Neural Circuits, 12*, 50.

Phillips, W. A., Chapman, K. L. S., and Berry, P. D. (2004). Size perception is less context-sensitive in males. *Perception, 33*, 79–86.

Phillips, W. A., & Christie, D. F. M. (1977). Interference with visualization. *Quarterly Journal of Experimental Psychology, 29*, 637–650.

Phillips, W. A., Clark, A., & Silverstein, S. M. (2015) On the functions, mechanisms, and malfunctions of intracortical contextual modulation. *Neuroscience and Biobehavioral Reviews, 52*, 1–20, https://doi.org/10.1016/j.neubiorev.2015.02.01027

Phillips, W. A., Hobbs, S. B., & Pratt, F. R. (1978). Intellectual realism in children's drawings of cubes. *Cognition, 6*, 15–33.

Phillips, W. A., Larkum, M. E., Harley, C. W., & Silverstein, S. M. (2016). The effects of arousal on apical amplification and conscious state. *Neuroscience of Consciousness, 2016*(1), niw015. https://doi.org/10.1093/nc/niw015

Phillips, W., Kay, J., & Smyth, D. (1995). The discovery of structure by multi-stream networks of local processors with contextual guidance. *Network: Computation in Neural Systems, 6*, 225–246.

Phillips, W. A., & Silverstein, S. M. (2003). Convergence of biological and psychological perspectives on cognitive coordination in schizophrenia. *Behavioral and Brain Sciences, 26*(1), 65–82; discussion 82–137.

Phillips, W. A., & Silverstein, S. M. (2013). The coherent organization of mental life depends on mechanisms for context-sensitive gain-control that are impaired in schizophrenia. *Frontiers in Psychology, 4*, 307. https://doi.org/10.3389/fpsyg.2013.00307

Phillips, W. A., & Singer, W. (1974). Function and interaction of on and off transients in vision: 1. Psychophysics. *Experimental Brain Research, 19*, 493–506.

Phillips, W. A., & Singer, W. (1997). In search of common foundations for cortical computation. *Behavioral and Brain Sciences, 20*(4), 657–683; discussion 683–722.

Phillips, W. A., von der Malsburg, C., & Singer, W. (2010). Dynamic coordination in brain and mind. In C. von der Malsburg, W. A. Phillips, & W. Singer (Eds.), *Dynamic coordination in the brain: From neurons to mind* (pp. 1–24). MIT Press.

Pica, G., Piasini, E., Chicharro, D., & Panzeri, S. (2017). Invariant components of synergy, redundancy, and unique information among three variables. *Entropy, 19*, 451. https://doi.org/10.3390/e19090451

Poirazi, P., & Papoutsi, A. (2020). Illuminating dendritic function with computational models. *Nature Reviews Neuroscience, 21*, 303–321. doi.org/10.1038/s41583-020-0301-7

Polák, M., & Marvan, T. (2019). How to mitigate the hard problem by adopting the dual theory of phenomenal consciousness. *Frontiers in Psychology*, *10*, 2837. https://doi.org/10.3389/fpsyg.2019.02837

Poolos, N. P., & Johnston, D. (2012). Dendritic ion channelopathy in acquired epilepsy. *Epilepsia*, *53*(Suppl 9), 32–40.

Postle, B. R. (2015). The cognitive neuroscience of visual short-term memory. *Current Opinion in Behavioral Sciences*, *1*, 40–46.

Pouille, F., Marin-Burgin, A., Adesnik, H., Atallah, B. V., & Scanziani, M. (2009). Input normalization by global feedforward inhibition expands cortical dynamic range *Nature Neuroscience*, *12*, 1577–1585.

Purushothaman, G., Marion, R., Li, K., & Casagrande, V. A. (2012). Gating and control of primary visual cortex by pulvinar. *Nature Neuroscience*, *15*(6), 905–912. https://doi.org/10.1038/nn.3106

Quartz, S. R., & Sejnowski, T. J. (1997). The neural basis of cognitive development: A constructivist manifesto. *Behavioral and Brain Sciences*, *26*(1), 537–556.

Radnikow, G., & Feldmeyer, D. (2018). Layer- and cell type-specific modulation of excitatory neuronal activity in the neocortex. *Frontiers in Neuroanatomy*, *12*, 1. doi https://doi.org/10.3389/fnana.2018.00001

Ramaswamy, S., & Markram, H. (2015). Anatomy and physiology of the thick-tufted layer 5 pyramidal neuron. *Frontiers in Cellular Neuroscience* [online], 26 June. doi.org/10.3389/fncel.2015.00233

Ramezanpour, H., & Fallah, M. (2022). The role of temporal cortex in the control of attention. *Current Research in Neurobiology*, *3*, 100038.

Ranson, A., Broom, E., Powell, A., Chen, F., Major, G., & Hall, J. (2019). Top-down suppression of sensory cortex in an NMDAR hypofunction model of psychosis. *Schizophrenia Bulletin*, *45*(6), 1349–1357. https://doi.org/10.1093/schbul/sby190

Rasch, B., & Born, J. (2013). About sleep's role in memory. *Physiological Reviews*, *93*, 681–766.

Ray, P. G., Meador, K. J., Smith, J. R., Wheless, J. W., Sittenfeld, M., & Clifton, G. L. (1999). Physiology of perception: Cortical stimulation and recording in humans. *Neurology*, *52*(5), 1044–1049.

Read, D. W., Manrique, H. M., & Walker, M. J. (2022). On the working memory of humans and great apes: Strikingly similar or remarkably different? *Neuroscience & Biobehavioral Reviews*, *134*, 104496.

Reimer, J., McGinley, M. J., Liu, Y., Rodenkirch, C., Wang, Q., McCormick, D. A., & Tolias, A. S. (2016). Pupil fluctuations track rapid changes in adrenergic and cholinergic activity in cortex. *Nature Communications*, *7*, 13289.

Reinhart, R. M. G., Heitz, R. P., Purcell, B. A., Weigand, P. K., Schall, J. D., & Woodman, G. F. (2012). Homologous mechanisms of visuospatial working memory maintenance in macaque and human: Properties and sources. *Journal of Neuroscience*, *32*(22), 7711–7722. https://doi.org/10.1523/jneurosci.0215-12.2012

Revina, Y., Petro, L. S., & Muckli, L. (2018). Cortical feedback signals generalise across different spatial frequencies of feedforward inputs. *NeuroImage*, *180*, 280–290.

Revina, Y., Petro, L. S., Denk-Florea, C. B., Rao, I. S., & Muckli, L. (2021). Increased region of surround stimulation enhances contextual feedback and feedforward processing in human V1. *bioRxiv* [preprint]. https://doi.org/10.1101/2021.02.27.433018

Reynolds, J. H., & Heeger, D. J. (2009). The normalization model of attention. *Neuron*, *61*(2), 168–185.

Richerson, P. J., Gavrilets, S., & de Waal, F. B. (2021). Modern theories of human evolution foreshadowed by Darwin's Descent of Man. *Science*, *372*(6544), eaba3776.

Ridley, M. (1996). *The origins of virtue*. Penguin.

Rilling, J. K., Gutman, D. A., Zeh, T. R., Pagnoni, G., Gregory S. Berns, G. S., & Kilts, C. D. (2002). A neural basis for social cooperation. *Neuron, 35*, 395–405.

Rinaldi, L., & Karmiloff-Smith, A. (2017). Intelligence as a developing function: A neuroconstructivist approach. *Journal of Intelligence, 5*, 18. https://doi.org/10.3390/jintellig ence5020018

Robbins, T. W., & Arnsten, A. F. (2009). The neuropsychopharmacology of frontoexecutive function: Monoaminergic modulation. *Annual Review of Neuroscience, 32*, 267–287.

Robbins, T. W., & Everitt, B. J. (1995). Arousal systems and attention. In M. S. Gazzaniga (Ed.), *The cognitive neurosciences* (pp. 703–720). MIT Press.

Roelfsema, P. R., & Holtmaat, A. (2019). Control of synaptic plasticity in deep cortical networks. *Nature Reviews Neuroscience, 19*(3), 166–180.

Roelfsema, P. R., & Super, H. (2003). Why do schizophrenic patients hallucinate? *Behavioral and Brain Sciences, 26*(1), 101–103.

Roldan, C. E., & Phillips, W. A. (1980). Functional differences between upright and rotated images. *Quarterly Journal of Experimental Psychology, 32*, 397–112.

Rolls, E. T. (2016). *Cerebral cortex: Principles of operation.* Oxford University Press.

Rollwage, M., Loosen, A., Hauser, T. U., Moran, R., Dolan, R. J., & Fleming, S. M. (2020). Confidence drives a neural confirmation bias. *Nature Communications, 11*(1), 1–11. https://doi.org/10.1038/s41467-020-16278-6

Rose, N. S., LaRocque, J. J., Riggall, A. C., Gosseries, O., Starrett, M. J., Meyering, E. E., & Postle, B. R. (2016). Reactivation of latent working memories with transcranial magnetic stimulation. *Science, 354*, 1136–1139.

Roth, M. M., Dahmen, J. C., Muir, D. R., Imhof, F., Martini, F. J., & Hofer, S. B. (2016). Thalamic nuclei convey diverse contextual information to layer 1 of visual cortex. *Nature Neuroscience, 19*(2), 299–307.

Rubio-Garrido, P., Perez-de-Manzo, F., Porrero, C., Galazo, M. J., & Clasca, F. (2009). Thalamic input to apical dendrites in neocortical layer 1 is massive and highly convergent. *Cerebral Cortex, 19*, 2380–2395.

Ryan, T. J., & Grant, S. G. N. (2009). The origin and evolution of synapses. *Nature Reviews Neuroscience, 10*, 701–712.

Sachs, J. L., Mueller, U. G., Wilcox, T. P., & Bull, J. J. (2004). The evolution of cooperation. *The Quarterly Review of Biology, 79*(2), 135–160.

Sadeh, S., & Clopath, C. (2021). Inhibitory stabilization and cortical computation. *Nature Reviews Neuroscience, 22*, 21–37.

Sakurai, T. (2007). The neural circuit of orexin (hypocretin): Maintaining sleep and wakefulness. *Nature Reviews Neuroscience, 8*, 171–181. https://doi.org/10.1038/nrn2092

Salinas, E., & Sejnowski, T. J. (2001). Gain modulation in the central nervous system: Where behavior, neurophysiology, and computation meet. *Neuroscientist, 7*, 430–440.

Sarter, M., Hasselmo, M. E., Bruno, J. P., & Givens, B. (2005). Unraveling the attentional functions of cortical cholinergic inputs: Interactions between signal-driven and cognitive modulation of signal detection. *Brain Research Reviews, 48*(1), 98–111. https://doi.org/10.1016/j.brainresrev.2004.08.006

Scerra, V. E., Costello, M. G., Salinas, E., & Stanford, T. R. (2019). All-or-none context dependence delineates limits of FEF visual target selection. *Current Biology, 29*(2), 294–305.

Schmitz, T. W., & Duncan, J. (2018). Normalization and the cholinergic microcircuit: A unified basis for attention. *Trends in Cognitive Sciences, 22*, 422–437. doi.org/10.1016/j.tics.2018.02.011

Schulz, J. M., Kay, J. W., Bischofberger, J., & Larkum, M. E. (2021). GABA$_B$ receptor-mediated regulation of dendro-somatic synergy in layer 5 pyramidal neurons. *Frontiers in Cellular Neuroscience, 15*, 718413. https://doi.org/10.3389/fncel.2021.718413

Schulz, J. M., Knoflach, F., Hernandez, M.-C., & Bischofberger, J. (2018). Dendrite-targeting interneurons control synaptic NMDA-receptor activation via nonlinear α5-GABA A receptors. *Nature Communications, 9*, 1–16.

Schuman, B., Dellal, S., Prönneke, A., Machold, R., & Rudy, B. (2021). Neocortical layer 1: An elegant solution to top-down and bottom-up integration. *Annual Review of Neuroscience, 44*, 221–252. doi.org/10.1146/annurev-neuro-100520-012117

Segev, I., Rinzel, J., & Shepherd, G. M. (Eds.). (1995). *The theoretical foundation of dendritic function: Selected papers of Wilfrid Rall.* MIT Press.

Self, M. W., Kooijmansa, R. N., Supèr, H., Lamme, V. A., & Roelfsema, P. R. (2012). Different glutamate receptors convey feedforward and recurrent processing in macaque V1. *Proceedings of the National Academy of Sciences of the United States of America, 109*, 11031–11036. http://dx.doi.org/10.1073/pnas.1119527109

Self, M. W., Peters, J. C., Possel, J. K., Reithler, J., Goebel, R., Ris, P., Jeurissen, D., Reddy, L., Claus, S., Baayen, J. C., & Roelfsema, P. R. (2016). The effects of context and attention on spiking activity in human early visual cortex. *PLoS Biology, 14*(3), e1002420

Self, M. W., van Kerkoerle, T., Supèr, H., & Roelfsema, P. R. (2013). Distinct roles of the cortical layers of area V1 in figure-ground segregation. *Current Biology, 23*(21), 2121–2129.

Shai, A. S., Anastassiou, C. A., Larkum, M. E., & Koch, C. (2015). Physiology of layer 5 pyramidal neurons in mouse primary visual cortex: Coincidence detection through bursting. *PLoS Computational Biology, 11*(3), e1004090. https://doi.org/10.1371/journal. pcbi.1004090

Shapson-Coe, A., Januszewski, M., Berger, D. R., Pope, A., Wu, Y., Blakely, T., Schalek, R. L., Li, P. H., Wang, S., Maitin-Shepard, J., Karlupia, N., Dorkenwald, S., Sjostedt, E., Leavitt, L., Lee, D., Bailey, L., Fitzmaurice, A., Kar, R., Field, B., … Lichtman, J. W. (2021). A connectomic study of a petascale fragment of human cerebral cortex. *bioRxiv* [preprint]. https://doi.org/ 10.1101/2021.05.29.446289

Shepherd, G. M. (2011). The microcircuit concept applied to cortical evolution: From three-layer to six-layer cortex. *Frontiers in Neuroanatomy, 5*, 30. https://doi.org/10.3389/ fnana.2011.00030

Shepherd, G. M. G., & Yamawaki, N. (2021). Untangling the cortico-thalamo-cortical loop: Cellular pieces of a knotty circuit puzzle. *Nature Reviews Neuroscience, 22*, 389–406. doi.org/10.1038/s41583-021-00459-3

Shine, J. M., Müller, E. J., Munn, B., Cabral, J., Moran, R. J., & Breakspear, M. (2021). Computational models link cellular mechanisms of neuromodulation to large-scale neural dynamics. *Nature Neuroscience, 24*(6), 765–776. doi.org/10.1038/s41593-021-00824-6

Shipp, S., Adams, D. L., Moutoussis, K., & Zeki, S. (2009). Feature binding in the feedback layers of area V2. *Cerebral Cortex, 19*, 2230–2239. http://dx.doi.org/10.1093/cercor/bhn243.

Shwartz-Ziv, R., & Tishby, N. (2017). Opening the black box of deep neural networks via information. *arXiv* [preprint], arXiv:1703.00810v3.

Siegel, M., Körding, K. P., & König, P. (2000). Integrating top-down and bottom-up sensory processing by somato-dendritic interactions. *Journal of Computational Neuroscience, 8*, 161–173.

Silverstein, S. M. (2016). Visual perception disturbances in schizophrenia: A unified model. *Nebraska Symposium on Motivation, 63*, 77–132. https://doi.org/10.1007/978-3-319-30596-7_4

Silverstein, S. M, Berten, S., Essex, B, Kovács, I., Susmaras, T., & Little, D. M. (2009). An fMRI examination of visual integration in schizophrenia. *Journal of Integrative Neuroscience, 8*(2), 175–202. https://doi.org/10.1142/s0219635209002113

Silverstein, S. M., Keane, B. P., Wang, Y., Mikkilineni, D., Paterno, D., Papathomas, T. V., & Feigenson, K. (2013). Effects of short-term inpatient treatment on sensitivity to a size contrast illusion in first-episode psychosis and multiple-episode schizophrenia. *Frontiers in Psychology, 24*(4), 466. https://doi.org/10.3389/fpsyg.2013.00466

Silverstein, S. M., Knight, R. A., Schwarzkopf, S. B., West, L. L., Osborn, L. M., & Kamin, D. (1996). Stimulus configuration and context effects in perceptual organization in schizophrenia. *Journal of Abnormal Psychology, 105*(3), 410–420. https://doi.org/10.1037//0021-843x.105.3.410

Silverstein, S. M., & Lai, A. (2021). The phenomenology and neurobiology of visual distortions and hallucinations in schizophrenia: An update. *Frontiers in Psychiatry, 12*, 684720. https://doi.org/10.3389/fpsyt.2021.684720

Simons, D. J., & Rensink, R. A. (2005). Change blindness: Past, present, and future. *Trends in Cognitive Sciences, 9*(1), 16–20.

Singer, W., & Phillips, W. A. (1974). Function and interaction of on and off transients in vision: 2. Neurophysiology. *Experimental Brain Research, 19*, 507–521.

Sirois, S., Spratling, M., Thomas, M. S. C., Westermann, G., Mareschal, D., & Johnson, M. H. (2008). Précis of neuroconstructivism: How the brain constructs cognition. *Behavioral and Brain Sciences, 31*, 321–356.

Sjöström, P. J., & Häusser, M. (2006). A cooperative switch determines the sign of synaptic plasticity in distal dendrites of neocortical pyramidal neurons. *Neuron, 51*, 227–238.

Sjöström, P. J., Rancz, E. A., Roth, A., & Häusser, M. (2008). Dendritic excitability and synaptic plasticity. *Physiological Reviews, 88*(2), 769–840.

Smith, R., & Lane R. D. (2015). The neural basis of one's own conscious and unconscious emotional states. *Neuroscience and Biobehavioral Reviews, 57*, 1–29. doi.org/10.1016/j.neubiorev.2015.08.003

Smyth, D., Phillips, W. A., & Kay, J. (1996). Measures for investigating the contextual modulation of information transmission. *Network: Computation in Neural Systems, 7*, 307–316.

Snyder, A. (2009). Explaining and inducing savant skills: Privileged access to lower level, less-processed information. *Philosophical Transactions of the Royal Society B: Biological Sciences, 364*, 1399–1405 https://doi.org/10.1098/rstb.2008.0290

Spagna, A., Hajhajate, D., Liu, J., & Bartolomeo, P. (2021). Visual mental imagery engages the left fusiform gyrus, but not the early visual cortex: A meta-analysis of neuroimaging evidence. *Neuroscience and Biobehavioral Reviews 122*, 201–217.

Sparing, R., Mottaghy, F. M., Ganis, G., Thompson, W. L., Topper, R., Kosslyn, S. M., & Pascual-Leone, A. (2002). Visual cortex excitability increases during visual mental imagery—a TMS study in healthy human subjects. *Brain Research, 938*, 92–97.

Sperber, D., & Wilson, D. (1986). *Relevance communication and cognition.* Blackwell.

Spratling, M. W. (2008) Predictive coding as a model of biased competition in visual attention. *Vision Research, 48*(12), 1391–1408.

Spratling, M. W., & Johnson, M. H. (2004). A feedback model of visual attention. *Journal of Cognitive Neuroscience, 16*, 219–237.

Spratling, M. W., & Johnson, M. H. (2006). A feedback model of perceptual learning and categorization. *Visual Cognition, 13*, 129–165.

Spratt, P. W. E, Ben-Shalom, R., Keeshen, C. M., Burke, K. J., Jr., Clarkson, R. L., Sanders, S. J., & Bender, K. J. (2019). The autism-associated gene *Scn2a* contributes to dendritic excitability and synaptic function in the prefrontal cortex. *Neuron, 103*(4), 673–685. https://doi.org/10.1016/j.neuron.2019.05.037

Stein, B. E., & Stanford, T. R. (2008). Multisensory integration: Current issues from the perspective of the single neuron. *Nature Reviews Neuroscience, 9*, 255–266. https://doi.org/10.1038/nrn2331

Stokes, M. G. (2015). 'Activity-silent' working memory in prefrontal cortex: A dynamic coding framework. *Trends in Cognitive Sciences, 19*, 394–405.

Storm, J. F., Pedarzani, P., Haug, T. M., & Winther, T. (2000). Modulation of K+ channels in hippocampal neurons: Transmitters acting via cyclic AMP enhance the excitability through kinase-dependent and -independent modulation of AHP- and h-channels. In K. Kuba, H. Higashida, D. A. Brown, & T. Yoshioka (Eds.), *Slow synaptic responses and modulation* (pp. 78–92). Springer-Verlag.

Sussman, R. W., & Cloninger, C. R. (Eds.). (2011). *Origins of altruism and cooperation* (Vol. 2, No. 12, pp. 395–399). Springer.

Suzuki, M., & Larkum, M.E. (2020). General anesthesia decouples cortical pyramidal neurons. *Cell, 180*, 666–676.

Sydnor, V. J., Larsen, B., Bassett, D. S., Alexander-Bloch, A., Fair, D. A., Liston, C., Mackey, A. P., Milham, M. P., Pines, A., Roalf, D. R., Seidlitz, J., Xu, T., Raznahan, A., & Satterthwaite, T. D. (2021). Neurodevelopment of the association cortices: Patterns, mechanisms, and implications for psychopathology. *Neuron, 109*(18), 2820–2846.

Symmonds, M., Moran, C. H., Leite, M. I., Buckley, C., Irani, S. R., Stephan, K. E., Friston, K. J., & Moran, R. J. (2018). Ion channels in EEG: Isolating channel dysfunction in NMDA receptor antibody encephalitis. *Brain, 141*, 1691–702.

Szalay, G., Judák, L., Katona, G., Ócsai, K., Juhász, G., Veress, M., Szadai, Z., Fehér, A., Tompa, T., Chiovini, B., & Maák, P. (2016). Fast 3D imaging of spine, dendritic, and neuronal assemblies in behaving animals. *Neuron, 92*, 723–738.

Takahashi, N., Ebner, C., Sigl-Glöckner, J., Moberg, S., Nierwetberg, S., & Larkum, M. E. (2020). Active dendritic currents gate descending cortical outputs in perception. *Nature Neuroscience, 23*(10), 1277–1285. https://doi.org/10.1038/s41593-020-0677-8

Takahashi, N., Oertner, T. G., Hegemann, P., & Larkum, M. E. (2016). Active cortical dendrites modulate perception. *Science, 354*(6319), 1587–1590. https://doi.org/10.1126/science.aah6066

Tantirigama, M. L. S., Zolnik, T., Judkewitz, B., Larkum, M. E., & Sachdev, R. N. S. (2020). Perspective on the multiple pathways to changing brain states. *Frontiers in Systems Neuroscience, 14*, 23. https://doi.org/10.3389/fnsys.2020.00023

Thomson, A. M. (2021) Circuits and synapses: Hypothesis, observation, controversy and serendipity – an opinion piece. *Frontiers in Neural Circuits, 15*, 732315. https://doi.org/10.3389/fncir.2021.732315

Tononi, G., & Koch, C. (2015) Consciousness: Here, there and everywhere? *Philosophical Transactions of the Royal Society B: Biological Sciences, 370*, 20140167. doi.org/10.1098/rstb.2014.0167

Tremblay, R., Lee, S., & Rudy, B. (2016). GABAergic interneurons in the neocortex: From cellular properties to circuits. *Neuron, 91*, 260–292. https://doi.org/10.1016/j.neuron.2016.06.033

Tsuno, Y., Schultheiss, N. W., & Hasselmo, M. E. (2013). In vivo cholinergic modulation of the cellular properties of medial entorhinal cortex neurons. *Journal of Physiology, 591*(10), 2611–2627. https://doi.org/10.1113/jphysiol.2012.250431

Tzilivaki, A., Kastellakis, G., & Poirazi, P. (2019). Challenging the point neuron dogma: FS basket cells as 2-stage nonlinear integrators. *Nature Communications, 10*, 3664.

Uhlhaas, P. J., Phillips, W. A., & Silverstein, S. M. (2005). The course and clinical correlates of dysfunctions in visual perceptual organization in schizophrenia during the remission of psychotic symptoms. *Schizophrenia Research, 75*(2–3), 183–192. https://doi.org/10.1016/j.schres.2004.11.005

Uhlhaas, P. J., & Singer, W. (2010). Abnormal neural oscillations and synchrony in schizophrenia. *Nature Reviews Neuroscience, 11*, 100–113. https://doi.org/10.1038/nrn2774

Uhlhaas, P. J., & Singer, W. (2006). Neural synchrony in brain disorders: Relevance for cognitive dysfunctions and pathophysiology. *Neuron, 52*(1), 155–168. https://doi.org/10.1016/j.neuron.2006.09.020

Uhlhaas, P. J., & Singer, W. (2012). Neuronal dynamics and neuropsychiatric disorders: Toward a translational paradigm for dysfunctional large-scale networks. *Neuron*, *75*(6), 963–980. doi.org/10.1016/j.neuron.2012.09.004

Unsworth, N., & Robison, M. K. (2017). A locus coeruleus-norepinephrine account of individual differences in working memory capacity and attention control. *Psychonomic Bulletin and Review*, *24*, 1282–1311. https://doi.org/10.3758/s13423-016-1220-5

Valenzuela, C. F., Morton, R. A., Diaz, M. R., & Topper, L. (2012). Does moderate drinking harm the fetal brain? Insights from animal models. *Trends in Neuroscience*, *35*(5), 284–292. https://doi.org/10.1016/j.tins.2012.01.006

Van der Hallen, R., Evers, K., Brewaeys, K., Van den Noortgate, W., & Wagemans, J. (2015). Global processing takes time: A meta-analysis on local–global visual processing in ASD. *Psychological Bulletin*, *141*(3), 549–573. https://doi.org/10.1037/bul0000004

van Kerkoerle, T., Self, M. W., & Roelfsema, P. R. (2017). Layer-specificity in the effects of attention and working memory on activity in primary visual cortex. *Nature Communications*, *8*, 13804.

van Versendaal, D., & Levelt, C. N. (2016). Inhibitory interneurons in visual cortical plasticity. *Cellular and Molecular Life Sciences*, *73*, 3677–3691.

Varela, F., Lachaux, J. P., Rodriguez, E., & Martinerie, J. (2001). The brainweb: Phase synchronization and large-scale integration. *Nature Reviews Neuroscience*, *2*(4), 229–239.

Vaswani, A., Shazeer, N., Parmar, N., Uszkoreit, J., Jones, L., Gomez, A. N., Kaiser, L., & Polosukhin, I. (2017). Attention is all you need. In I. Guyon, U. Von Luxburg, S. Bengio, H. Wallach, R. Fergus, S. Vishwanathan, & R. Garnett (Eds.), *NIPS'17: Proceedings of the 31st International Conference on Neural Information Processing Systems* (pp. 6000–6010). ACM.

Veissière, S. P. L., Constant, A., Ramstead, M. J. D., Friston, K. J., & Kirmayer, L. J. (2020). Thinking through other minds: A variational approach to cognition and culture. *Behavioral and Brain Sciences*, *43*, e90. https://doi.org/10.1017/S0140525X19001213

Velisavljević, L., & Elder, J. H. (2008). Visual short-term memory of local information in briefly viewed natural scenes: Configural and non-configural factors. *Journal of Vision*, *8*(16), 1–17, http://journalofvision.org/8/16/8/

Vetter, P., Bola, L., Reich, L., Bennett, M., Muckli, L., & Amedi, A. (2020). Decoding natural sounds in early 'visual' cortex of congenitally blind individuals. *Current Biology*, *30*, 3039–3044. doi.org/10.1016/j.cub.2020.05.071

Vetter, P., Smith, F. W., & Muckli, L. (2014). Decoding sound and imagery content in early visual cortex. *Current Biology*, *24*, 1256–1262. https://doi.org/10.1016/j.cub.2014.04.020.

Vieira, M. M., Jeong, J., & Roche, K. W. (2021). The role of NMDA receptor and neuroligin rare variants in synaptic dysfunction underlying neurodevelopmental disorders. *Current Opinion in Neurobiology*, *69*, 93–104. doi.org/10.1016/j.conb.2021.03.001

Vlaev, I. (2018). Local choices: Rationality and the contextuality of decision-making. *Brain Science*, *8*(1), 8. https://doi.org/10.3390/brainsci8010008

Völter, C. J., Reindl, E., Felsche, E., Civelek, Z., Whalen, A., Lugosi, Z., Duncan, L., Herrmann, E., Call, J., & Seed, A. M. (2022). The structure of executive functions in preschool children and chimpanzees. *Scientific Reports*, *12*(1), 1–16.

Wainstein, G., Rojas-Líbano, D., Medel, V., Alnæs, D., Kolskår, K. K., Endestad, T., Laeng, B., Ossandon, T., Crossley, N., Matar, E., & Shine, J. M. (2021). The ascending arousal system promotes optimal performance through mesoscale network integration in a visuospatial attentional task. *Network Neuroscience*, *5*(4), 890–910. https://doi.org/10.1162/netn_a_00205

Walker, M. (2017). *Why we sleep*. Penguin Books.

Walker, S. (1983). *Animal thought*. Routledge & K. Paul.

Wall, N. R., De La Parra, M., Sorokin, J. M., Taniguchi, H., Huang, Z. J., & Callaway, E. M. (2016). Brain-wide maps of synaptic input to cortical interneurons. *Journal of Neuroscience*, 36(14), 4000–4009.

Wang, L. and Krauzlis, R. J. (2018). Visual selective attention in mice. *Current Biology*, 28, 676–685. doi.org/10.1016/j.cub.2018.01.038

Wang, M., Ramos, B. P., Paspalas, C. D., Shu, Y., Simen, A., Duque, A. Vijayraghavan, S., Brennan, A., Dudley, A., Nou, E., Mazer, J. A., McCormick, D. A., & Arnsten, A. F. T. (2007). Alpha2A-adrenoceptors strengthen working memory networks b inhibiting cAMP-HCN channel signaling in prefrontal cortex. *Cell*, 129(2), 397–410. https://doi.org/10.1016/j.cell.2007.03.015

Wang, R., Martin, C. D., Lei, A. L., Hausknecht, K. A., Ishiwari, K., Richards, J. B., Haj-Dahmane, S., & Shen, R.-Y. (2020). Prenatal ethanol exposure leads to attention deficits in both male and female rats. *Frontiers in Neuroscience*, 14, 12. https://doi.org/10.3389/fnins.2020.00012

Wang, X.-J., Tegnér, J., Constantinidis, C., & Goldman-Rakic, P. S. (2004). Division of labor among distinct subtypes of inhibitory neurons in a cortical microcircuit of working memory. *Proceedings of the National Academy of Sciences of the United States of America*, 101, 1368–1373. www.pnas.org_cgi_doi_10.1073_pnas.0305337101

Wang, X.-J., & Yang, G. R. (2018). A disinhibitory circuit motif and flexible information routing in the brain. *Current Opinion in Neurobiology*, 49, 75–83.

Weintraub, D. J. (1979). Ebbinghaus illusion: Context, contour, and age influence the judged size of a circle amidst circles. *Journal of Experimental Psychology: Human Perception and Performance*, 5, 353–364.

Wibral, M., Finn, C., Wollstadt, P., Lizier, J. T., & Priesemann, V. (2017). Quantifying information modification in developing neural networks via partial information decomposition. *Entropy*, 19, 494.

Wibral, M., Lizier, J. T., & Priesemann, V. (2015a). Bits from brains for biologically inspired computing. *Frontiers in Robotics and AI*, 2, 1–25.

Wibral, M., Priesemann, V., Kay, J. W., Lizier, J. T., & Phillips, W. A. (2015b). Partial information decomposition as a unified approach to the specification of neural goal functions. *Brain and Cognition*, 112, 25–38. http://dx.doi.org/10.1016/j.bandc.2015.004

Williams, R. (1961). *Culture and society 1780–1050*. Penguin Books Ltd.

Williams L. E., & Holtmaat A. (2019). Higher-order thalamocortical inputs gate synaptic long-term potentiation via disinhibition. *Neuron*, 101, 91–102. https://doi.org/10.1016/j.neuron.2018.10.049

Williams, S. R., & Fletcher, L. N. (2019). A dendritic substrate for the cholinergic control of neocortical output neurons. *Neuron*, 101, 1–14. https://doi.org/10.1016/j. neuron.2018.11.035

Williams S. R., & Stuart G. J. (2002). Dependence of EPSP efficacy on synapse location in neocortical pyramidal neurons. *Science*, 295, 1907–1910.

Wills, C., & Bada, J. (2000). *The spark of life. Darwin and the primeval soup*. Oxford University Press.

Wilson, J. T. (1981). Visual persistence at both onset and offset of stimulation. *Perception & Psychophysics*, 30, 353–356.

Wilting, J., & Priesemann, V. (2019). Between perfectly critical and fully irregular: A reverberating model captures and predicts cortical spike propagation. *Cerebral Cortex*, 29(6), 2759–2770. https://doi.org/10.1093/cercor/bhz049

Wingfield, T., McHugh, C., Vas, A., Richardson, A., Wilkins, E., Bonington, A., & Varma, A. (2011). Autoimmune encephalitis: A case series and comprehensive review of the literature. *QJM*, 104(11), 921–931.

Wolff, M. J., Jochim, J., Akyürek, E. G., & Stokes, M. G. (2017). Dynamic hidden states underlying working-memory-guided behavior. *Nature Neuroscience*, 20(6), 864–871.

Xu, N.-L., Harnett, M. T., Williams, S. R., Huber, D., O'Connor, D. H., Svobda, K., & Magee, J. C. (2012). Nonlinear dendritic integration of sensory and motor input during an active sensing task. *Nature*, *492*(7428), 247–251.

Xu, Y. (2017) Reevaluating the sensory account of visual working memory storage. *Trends in Cognitive Science*, *21*, 794–81.

Yang, Y., Liu, D. Q., Huang, W., Deng, J., Sun, Y., Zuo, Y., & Poo, M. M. (2016). Selective synaptic remodeling of amygdalocortical connections associated with fear memory. *Nature Neuroscience*, *19*(10), 1348–1355.

Yizhar, O., Fenno, L. E., Prigge, M., Schneider, F., Davidson, T. J., O'Shea, D. J., Sohal, V. S., Goshen, I., Finkelstein, J., Paz, J. T., & Stehfest, K. (2011). Neocortical excitation/inhibition balance in information processing and social dysfunction. *Nature*, *477*(7363), 171–178.

You, W-K., & Mysore, S. P. (2020). Dynamics of visual perceptual processing in freely behaving mice. *bioRxiv* [preprint]. doi.org/10.1101/2020.02.20.958652

Záborszky, L., Gombkoto, P., Varsanyi, P., Gielow, M. R., Poe, G., Role, L. W., Ananth, M., Rajebhosale, P., Talmage, D. A., Hasselmo, M. E., & Dannenberg, H. (2018). Specific basal forebrain–cortical cholinergic circuits coordinate cognitive operations. *Journal of Neuroscience*, *38*(44), 9446–9458. https://doi.org/10.1523/JNEUROSCI.1676-18.2018

Zagha, E., & McCormick, D. A. (2014). Neural control of brain state. *Current Opinion in Neurobiology*, *29*, 178–186. doi.org/10.1016/j.conb.2014.09.010

Zhang, S., Xu, M., Kamigaki, T., Hoang Do, J. P., Chang, W. C., Jenvay, S., Miyamichi, K., Luo, L., & Dan, Y. (2014a). Long-range and local circuits for top-down modulation of visual cortex processing. *Science*, *345*(6197), 660–665. https://doi.org/10.1126/science.1254126

Zhang, Y., Bonnan, A., Bony, G., Ferezou, I., Pietropaolo, S., Ginger, M., Sans, N., Rossier, J., Oostra, B., LeMasson, G., & Frick, A. (2014b). Dendritic channelopathies contribute to neocortical and sensory hyperexcitability in Fmr1–/y mice. *Nature Neuroscience*, *17*(12), 1701–1709. https://doi.org/10.1038/nn.3864

Zhou, H., Shafer, R. J., & Desimone, R. (2016). Pulvinar-cortex interactions in vision and attention *Neuron*, *89*, 209–220. doi.org/10.1016/j.neuron.2015.11.034

Zhu, J. J. (2000). Maturation of layer 5 neocortical pyramidal neurons: Amplifying salient layer 1 and layer 4 inputs by Ca2+ action potentials in adult rat tuft dendrites. *Journal of Physiology*, *526*(3), 571–587.

Zikopoulos, B., & Barbas, H. (2013). Altered neural connectivity in excitatory and inhibitory cortical circuits in autism. *Frontiers in Human Neuroscience*, *7*, 609. https://doi.org/10.3389/fnhum.2013.00609

Zipser, K., Lamme, V. A. F., & Schiller, P. H. (1996). Contextual modulation in primary visual cortex. *Journal of Neuroscience*, *15*, 7376–7389.

neurobiology
autism spectrum disorders, 244–46
foetal alcohol spectrum disorders, 253
interdisciplinary interactions, 21–22
neurocomputational studies, context
sensitivity, 261–62
neuroconstructivism, 220f, 220–21
neuroimaging studies
autism spectrum disorders, 249–50
cortical activity, 160
foetal alcohol spectrum disorders, 253
functional neuroimaging, 146–47
prefrontal cortex, 157
see also functional magnetic resonance imaging
(fMRI); magnetic resonance imaging (MRI);
transcranial magnetic stimulation (TMS)
neuromodulators
apical dendrites and neocortical
dynamics, 89–93
conscious experience, 137–40
cooperative neuron regulation, 294–99
neocortical activity, 75
prefrontal cortex, 163–64
temporal maitenance information, 162–64
neuronal motor outflow, information, 276
neurons
neocortex, 28
numbers and cognition, 303
signals amplification, 13
neurophysiology, context-sensitivity evidence, 71
neurotransmitters, 50
mental state transitions, 80–83, 81f
NGF (neuralgiform) interneurons, 62–64
Nietzsche, Friedreich, 168–69
N-methyl-D-aspartate (NMDA) receptors, 57
autism spectrum disorders, 250
context amplification, 119–20
schizophrenia spectrum disorders, 237–39
nonconsciousness, consciousness *vs.*, 103
non-cortical sites, output to, 204–5
nonsynaptic voltage-dependent ion
channels, 50–51
noradrenaline (NA), 75–76
adrenergic arousal and, 297–98
conscious experience, 137–38
consciousness, 103
locus coeruleus, 297
neocortical arousal, 81–83
neocortical effects, 80
norepinephrine *see* noradrenaline (NA)
normalization, inhibitory interneurons, 129
Nutt, David, 8

object recognition, 125
objectivity, modification, 312

openness, 99–100
orbitofrontal cortex (OFC), 125
orexin, 88
apical dendrites, 87–89
clinical utility and, 296–97
conscious experience, 137–38
neocortex, 80, 295, 296
prefrontal cortex, 146–47
wakefulness, 88–89
organized complexity, 9
Orwell, George, 114
oscillatory dynamics, autism spectrum
disorders, 241–42
output amplification, pyramidal cells, 16–17
output information decomposition, 273–74
oxytocin, 93

pain perception, oxytocin, 93
parallel distributed processing (PDP), 274
parietal regions
frontal eye field and, 148
neglect disorders, 143
visual input, 156–57
visuospatial short-term memory, 156–58
partial information decomposition (PID), 262–
63, 275
partial seizures, 233
parvalbumin (PV), 304–5
basket cells, 127
evolution, 206–7
interneurons, 62–64
patch-clamp recordings
apical dendrite–soma communication, 51–52
context sensitive computation, 269–70
multi-site patch clamping, 286
pathologies, 229–56
PDP (parallel distributed processing), 274
Penrose triangle, 33–34
perception
context, 316
context-sensitivity *see* context-sensitive
perception
emotional tone, 174
experiences, 213f, 221–22
frontal region, 157–58
multimodal regions, 121–22, 122f
objectivity, 304
sensory input, 316–17
veracity of, 101–2
perceptual abstraction
development of, 223
neocortex, 33
perceptual systems
external world information, 62
outputs *vs.* amplification, 57–58